Nursing Practice: Advanced Concepts and Clinical Perspectives

Nursing Practice: Advanced Concepts and Clinical Perspectives

Edited by Helen Hayden

hayle medical

New York

Hayle Medical,
750 Third Avenue, 9th Floor,
New York, NY 10017, USA

Visit us on the World Wide Web at:
www.haylemedical.com

ISBN: 978-1-63241-810-4

Cataloging-in-Publication Data

Nursing practice : advanced concepts and clinical perspectives / edited by Helen Hayden.
    p. cm.
Includes bibliographical references and index.
ISBN 978-1-63241-810-4
1. Nursing--Practice. 2. Nursing. 3. Care of the sick. 4. Clinical medicine. I. Hayden, Helen.
RT86.7 .N87 2019
610.73--dc23

Table of Contents

Preface..**VII**

Chapter 1 **Patient satisfaction with prehospital emergency care following a hip
fracture: a prospective questionnaire-based study** 1
Glenn Larsson, Ulf Strömberg, Cecilia Rogmark and Anna Nilsdotter

Chapter 2 **Patient safety culture in nursing homes – a cross-sectional study among nurses
and nursing aides caring for residents with diabetes**..................**10**
Irit Titlestad, Anne Haugstvedt, Jannicke Igland and Marit Graue

Chapter 3 **Student evaluation of the impact of changes in teaching style on their
learning: a mixed method longitudinal study** **18**
Susan Jones, Somasundari Gopalakrishnan, Charles A. Ameh, Brian Faragher,
Betty Sam, Roderick R. Labicane, Hossinatu Kanu, Fatmata Dabo,
Makally Mansary, Rugiatu Kanu and Nynke van den Broek

Chapter 4 **Knowledge, attitude, and practice of breast Cancer among nurses
in hospitals**..**27**
Amanuel Kidane Andegiorgish, Eyob Azeria Kidane and Merhawi Teklezgi Gebrezgi

Chapter 5 **Medium-fidelity simulation in clinical readiness: a phenomenological study
of student midwives concerning teamwork** **34**
Zukiswa Brenda Ntlokonkulu, Ntombana Mc'deline Rala and Daniel Ter Goon

Chapter 6 **Birth preparedness and complication readiness among pregnant women in
Tehulederie district**..**42**
Demlie Belete Endeshaw, Lema Derseh Gezie and Hedija Yenus Yeshita

Chapter 7 **"I see myself as part of the team" – family caregivers' contribution to safety
in advanced home care**...**51**
Christiane Schaepe and Michael Ewers

Chapter 8 **Exploring the perceived factors that affect self-medication among nursing
students**...**61**
Ali Soroush, Alireza Abdi, Bahare Andayeshgar, Afsoon Vahdat and
Alireza Khatony

Chapter 9 **Voluntary stopping of eating and drinking (VSED) as an unknown challenge
in a long-term care institution**.......................................**68**
Nadine Saladin, Wilfried Schnepp and André Fringer

Chapter 10 **Predictors of organizational commitment among university
nursing Faculty**...**82**
Rekha Timalsina, Sarala K. C., Nilam Rai and Anita Chhantyal

Chapter 11   **From apprehension to advocacy: a qualitative study of undergraduate
nursing student experience in clinical placement in residential aged care** 90
Heather Moquin, Cydnee Seneviratne and Lorraine Venturato

Chapter 12   **Design and evaluation of the StartingTogether App for home visits in
preventive child health care** 101
Olivier Anne Blanson Henkemans, Marjolein Keij, Marc Grootjen,
Mascha Kamphuis and Anna Dijkshoorn

Chapter 13   **Surgical patients' perspectives on nurses' education on post-operative care
and follow up** 117
Bernard Atinyagrika Adugbire and Lydia Aziato

Chapter 14   **Caring for late preterm infants: public health nurses' experiences** 126
Genevieve Currie, Aliyah Dosani, Shahirose S. Premji, Sandra M. Reilly,
Abhay K. Lodha and Marilyn Young

Chapter 15   **What relatives of older medical patients want us to know - a mixed-methods
study** 134
Ditte Maria Sivertsen, Louise Lawson-Smith and Tove Lindhardt

Chapter 16   *Heart health whispering*: **A randomized, controlled pilot study to promote
nursing student perspective-taking on carers' health risk behaviors** 143
Michelle Lobchuk, Lisa Hoplock, Gayle Halas, Christina West, Cheryl Dika,
Wilma Schroeder, Terri Ashcroft, Kathleen Chambers Clouston and
Jocelyne Lemoine

Chapter 17   **A hermeneutic study of integrating psychotherapist competence in postnatal
child health care: nurses' perspectives** 154
Katarina Kornaros, Sofia Zwedberg, Eva Nissen and Björn Salomonsson

Chapter 18   **Non-application of the nursing process at a hospital in Accra, Ghana** 164
Joana Agyeman-Yeboah and Kwadwo Ameyaw Korsah

Chapter 19   **Quality of nursing work life and turnover intention among nurses of tertiary
care hospitals** 171
Bayan Kaddourah, Amani K. Abu-Shaheen and Mohamad Al-Tannir

Chapter 20   **Advancing mobile learning in Australian healthcare environments: nursing
profession organisation perspectives and leadership challenges** 178
Carey Ann Mather, Elizabeth Anne Cummings and Fred Gale

Chapter 21   **Neonatal nasogastric tube feeding in a low-resource African setting – using
ergonomics methods to explore quality and safety issues in task sharing** 191
Gregory B. Omondi, George Serem, Nancy Abuya, David Gathara,
Neville A. Stanton, Dorothy Agedo, Mike English and Georgina A. V. Murphy

Permissions

List of Contributors

Index

Preface

Every book is a source of knowledge and this one is no exception. The idea that led to the conceptualization of this book was the fact that the world is advancing rapidly; which makes it crucial to document the progress in every field. I am aware that a lot of data is already available, yet, there is a lot more to learn. Hence, I accepted the responsibility of editing this book and contributing my knowledge to the community.

Nursing is a diverse healthcare profession. It has applications in the areas of pediatrics, gynecology and obstetrics, women's health and mental health, among others. It is concerned with the promotion and optimization of health, disease prevention and alleviation of pain. It also includes the maintenance of a quality of life for patients and their family. Nursing can be further divided into focused branches such as cardiac nursing, perioperative nursing, palliative nursing, obstetrical nursing, telenursing, etc. From theories to research to practical applications, case studies related to all contemporary topics of relevance to nursing have been included in this book. Some of the diverse topics covered herein address the varied branches that fall under this discipline. As this field is emerging at a rapid pace, the contents of this book will help the readers understand the modern concepts and applications of the subject.

While editing this book, I had multiple visions for it. Then I finally narrowed down to make every chapter a sole standing text explaining a particular topic, so that they can be used independently. However, the umbrella subject sinews them into a common theme. This makes the book a unique platform of knowledge.

I would like to give the major credit of this book to the experts from every corner of the world, who took the time to share their expertise with us. Also, I owe the completion of this book to the never-ending support of my family, who supported me throughout the project.

Editor

Patient satisfaction with prehospital emergency care following a hip fracture: a prospective questionnaire-based study

Glenn Larsson[1,2*], Ulf Strömberg[4], Cecilia Rogmark[2,3] and Anna Nilsdotter[2,4]

Abstract

Background: Older patients with a hip fracture require specialized emergency care and their first healthcare encounter before arriving at the hospital is often with the ambulance service. Since 2005 there has been a registered nurse on the crew of every ambulance in Sweden in order to provide prehospital emergency care and to prepare the patients for hospitalization. It is important to investigate patient satisfaction with prehospital emergency care following a hip fracture to ensure that their expectations of good care are met.
The aim of this study was to investigate patient satisfaction with prehospital emergency care following a hip fracture by comparing two similar emergency care contexts.

Methods: The study was conducted using the Consumer Emergency Care Satisfaction Scale (CECSS) on patients treated for hip fracture in prehospital emergency care. The data were collected within a randomized controlled study for the purpose of comparing prehospital fast track care (PFTC) and the traditional type of transport to an accident and emergency department (A&E).

Results: Questionnaire data from 287 patients, 188 women (66%) and 99 men (34%) with a mean age of 80.9 years, were analysed. More than 80% of the patients selected the most positive response alternatives, but 16% were dissatisfied with the nursing information provided. Patients in PFTC responded more positively on specific caring behaviour than those transported to the A&E department in the traditional way.

Conclusion: Patient satisfaction with prehospital emergency care following a hip fracture is an important outcome and this study highlights the fact that patients expressed a high level of satisfaction with the prehospital emergency care provided by ambulance nurses in both care contexts under study. However, some areas need to be improved in terms of nursing information.

Keywords: Prehospital emergency care, Patient satisfaction, Hip fracture, Ambulance nurse

Background

Prehospital emergency care is an essential part of the healthcare system. Measuring patient satisfaction is of great importance for ensuring that ambulance service care meets expectations and provides the best possible experience. To improve prehospital emergency care and prepare patients for hospitalization, all ambulance organizations in Sweden have upgraded their level of competence by the inclusion of registered nurses since 2015 [1].

Patient dissatisfaction is multidimensional and includes management, quality of health care and the relationship between patients and health care professionals. Moreover, complaints often concern treatment and communication [2].

A study found that patients were dissatisfied with the information provided, organization/rules and perceived that healthcare providers defend themselves when patients complain [3]. Patients also expressed dissatisfaction about waiting times at the A&E for admission to a hospital ward, ineffective communication and lack of environmental control [4].

Dissatisfaction with care is often linked to staff insensitivity and communication failure and healthcare professionals find

* Correspondence: Glenn.larsson@regionhalland.se
[1]Department of Ambulance and Prehospital Care, Region Halland, Health Centre Nyhem, 302 49 Halmstad, Sweden
[2]Department of Orthopaedics, Lund University, Lund, Sweden
Full list of author information is available at the end of the article

it challenging to meet patients' expectations of receiving an explanation and an apology [5]. Other causes of dissatisfaction are lack of knowledge or competence on the part of staff members [6].

Patient satisfaction is a multidimensional concept that measures patients' experiences of medical competence, including not only clinical and technical skills but also healthcare professionals' interpersonal skills, attitudes and provision of information [7, 8]. Another dimension of patient satisfaction is associated with patients' expectations. Patient satisfaction is widely used as a basis for evaluating waiting times and nursing skills in emergency care [9, 10].

Ambulance nurses are qualified to perform assessment, nursing care, medical treatment and information in addition to collaborating with other professionals. Moreover, the National Board of Health and Welfare states that the same standards of diagnosis, treatment and safety should apply in prehospital emergency care as in hospital care [11, 12].

It is well known that older patients suffering from hip fracture require comprehensive care and in Sweden the annual number of cases is predicted to increase from 18,000 today to 30,000 in 2050 [13]. The ambulance service is often the patients' first care encounter before arriving at the hospital. Progress has been made in prehospital nursing care and many interventions have been transferred from the hospital to the ambulance service [14]. As hip injuries are painful and in most cases the patients are frail, they require specialized emergency care [15]. Registered nurses in ambulance organizations provide care at the scene and during transportation, which includes various forms of assessment, pain treatment, stabilization of the patient's condition, sending the electrocardiogram (ECG) results to the hospital and providing information to the patient and subsequent caregivers [12]. The prehospital guidelines [16] for patients with suspected hip fracture recommend either the standard procedure with transport to the accident and emergency department (A&E) or prehospital fast track care (PFTC). PFTC means that the ambulance nurse provides a greater number of interventions and prepares the patient for immediate transport to the radiology department and admission to the orthopaedic ward, instead of first transporting her/him to the A&E department.

Several studies describe a lack of satisfaction with ambulance care from the patient perspective. In Finland, dissatisfaction was reported when patients considered that their needs were not met, staff members did not introduce themselves and they did not transport the patients to the hospital they wished to go to [17].

Two studies from the U.S. describe the lack of a professional attitude, rude behaviour, inadequate medical assessment and patient dissatisfaction with the choice of destination [18, 19]. On the other hand, one study from England found that patients experienced ambulance care as very positive [20]. However, the results of studies carried out in Sweden differ and although patients are generally satisfied [21], hip fracture care needs to be improved [22]. Nevertheless, Hommel et al. presented positive statements from patients, which described short waiting times for an ambulance and a fast process on arrival at the hospital and upon admission to an orthopaedic ward [23].

Little is known about patient satisfaction with prehospital emergency care following a hip fracture and whether the ambulance service has succeeded in its mission to strengthen clinical and technical skills as well as sensitive, two-way interpersonal communication with patients.

Greater knowledge in this area will enhance ambulance nurses' understanding of patients' expectations, thus providing a valuable basis for guiding knowledge acquisition and competence development in the prehospital area.

The aim of this study was to investigate patients' satisfaction with prehospital emergency care following a hip fracture by comparing two similar emergency care contexts.

Methods
Study design, sample and setting
The patients in this study were recruited from participants in a randomized, controlled trial [24]. The purpose of the original study was to compare two pathways: PFTC and traditional transport to the A&E department, focusing on outcomes in terms of time to radiographic examination and surgery, postoperative complications, length of hospital stay and mortality.

During the study period all patients who were assessed as having a suspected hip fracture by an ambulance nurse were eligible for inclusion. The ambulance nurses informed the patient about the research project and explained the differences in the nursing interventions between the two pathways (PFTC and A&E). If a patient agreed to participate in the study, the randomization took place at the scene by the ambulance nurses using a closed, opaque envelope. In cases where patients were unable to give their consent because of dementia or cognitive deficit, a relative could do so on their behalf. The patients were allocated either to the PFTC (intervention) or to traditional transport to the A&E department (control group).

The inclusion procedure consisted of the ambulance nurse using a study folder marked with the ambulance journal number for each patient who agreed to participate in the study.

The present study was designed as a sub-study of the original study, for the purpose of examining patient satisfaction with prehospital emergency care following a hip fracture.

Prehospital fast track care (PFTC)

The ambulance nurse administered and assessed a 12-Lead ECG and sent it to the hospital database. Blood samples were taken to analyse plasma glucose level. The ambulance nurse provided the patient with an ID-bracelet and called the receptionist or the triage nurse at the A&E department and asked for an x-ray referral to be sent to the radiology department. A phone call was made to the orthopaedic surgeon on duty for confirmation or advice when the ambulance nurse was unsure about the patient's condition. The orthopaedic ward nurse received information by phone from the ambulance nurse about the patient's current condition. The patient was transported straight to the radiology department instead of to the A&E department. If the x-ray verified a hip fracture, the patient was transported directly to the orthopaedic ward for preoperative care. If the x-ray did not verify a hip fracture, the patient was transported to the A&E department for further assessment and a decision about treatment.

Accident and emergency (A&E) department

Patients randomized to A&E were transported to the A&E department and the ambulance nurse reported the patient to the admissions nurse. An A&E nurse gave the patient an ID-bracelet and administered blood tests and an ECG. The patient was placed in an examination room or a corridor along with other orthopaedic patients to await the orthopaedic surgeon. Following examination by the surgeon, the patient was moved to the radiology department for radiographic examination and then back to the A&E department to await the treatment decision. Thereafter the patient was admitted to an orthopaedic department. The A&E nurse then reported the patient to the orthopaedic department and the patient was transported there.

The study was carried out between July 2012 and May 2014 at the ambulance organization in the Region of Halland, Sweden. The organization consists of eight ambulance stations and provides a population of 305,000 people with prehospital emergency care and transport to two emergency hospitals.

Patients in the study

All patients in the study were assessed by the Rapid Emergency Triage and Treatment System (RETTS) [25] and cared for in accordance with the ambulance organization's guidelines on pain treatment, oxygen therapy and intravenous liquid substitution.

The inclusion criteria were verified hip fracture, awake, adequate vision and hearing as well as sufficiently lucid to answer the questionnaire. Patients were excluded if they had other injuries or were affected by dementia (judged by clinical appearance or a known diagnosis) or other conditions that made participation impossible.

Instrument

The study was conducted using the Consumer Emergency Care Satisfaction Scale (CECSS), which consists of a patient questionnaire that was developed to measure patient satisfaction with A&E nursing care [26]. The instrument was developed in Australia and has been evaluated for validity and reliability when measuring the quality of A&E care from the patient perspective. It contains 19 statements and a 5-point Likert scale is used to measure the patient's response from *completely agree* = 5 to *completely disagree* = 1.

The CECSS measures patient satisfaction with A&E nursing care in the areas of care and discharge teaching. There are 12 items for care, 3 for discharge teaching and 4 for reducing response bias. The total score ranges from 15 to 75 [27].

A modified version of the instrument was used [21] in which all of the 16 questions measured patient satisfaction, 12 with care (information, clinical and technical skills) as well as 4 negative items (attitude and behaviour) that were summarized separately.

Three items concerning patient teaching were excluded because they measure patient satisfaction before leaving the A&E department and were thus not relevant for this study. The total score was 12–60 for the care subscale and 4–20 for the negative items. A total score of ≥36 on the care subscale indicates patient satisfaction, while < 36 indicates dissatisfaction. For the negative items, ≤12 indicates patient satisfaction and > 12 dissatisfaction.

Data collection

Patients with a verified hip fracture were admitted to an orthopaedic ward either by means of PFTC or from the A&E department. During the patient's stay at the orthopaedic ward, a designated nurse from the ambulance service administration, who was not a member of the research team, distributed a modified version of the questionnaire coded with the patient's ambulance journal number (specific case number, no patient identity). The nurse explained the instructions for filling in the questionnaire pertaining to satisfaction with prehospital emergency care. The patients completed the questionnaire during their hospital stay and returned it to an orthopaedic nurse who stored the questionnaires in the orthopaedic nurses' office. The designated nurse returned to the orthopaedic ward at a later date and collected the completed questionnaires.

For those patients who did not meet the inclusion criteria and were therefore excluded, the nurse documented the reason for exclusion in the study protocol. Such patients were not provided with information about the questionnaire and their data were not analysed.

Information about age, gender and allocation to either PFTC or A&E was retrieved from the ambulance data.

Data for comparison with other studies

In order to compare patient satisfaction, the mean score on the care subscale and the number of most positive response alternatives in the present study were compared with the corresponding data from six previous studies conducted between 2002 and 2016 in five different countries [21, 28–32]. The number of patients included varied from 40 to 573. The studies used for comparison were conducted in different emergency care contexts with mixed patient groups and variation in age, gender, ethnicity, priority and nursing interventions.

Analyses

The outcome data were summarized using descriptive statistics. For comparison between the PFTC and A&E groups, the Mann-Whitney U-Test (with corrections for ties) was employed for ordinal outcomes on individual items and the Chi-square test for the categorized subscale scores. The patients' sum scores were categorized into 60–48, 47–36 and 35–12 for the care subscale and 4–8, 9–12 and 13–20 for the negative-item subscale.

The analyses were carried out using IBM Statistics for Windows version 20.0.2 [IBM Corp. Armonk, NY, USA].

Results

Inclusion and patient characteristics

During the study period, the ambulance organization cared for 571 patients with a suspected hip fracture. Of these patients, 284 were excluded (no fracture, $n = 171$; dementia, $n = 73$; other reasons such as declining participation, not remembering being transported or having died during the hospital stay, $n = 26$; failure to complete the questionnaire, $n = 13$; and inadequate knowledge of the Swedish language, $n = 1$). Hence, 287 patient questionnaires were included and analysed (Fig. 1).

Of the included patients, 188 were women (66%) and 99 were men (34%) with a mean age of 80.9 years. The patient characteristics are presented in Table 1.

Comparison of the CECSS in PFTC and A&E

There were no significant differences between the PFTC ($n = 137$) and the A&E ($n = 150$) groups in the care subscale; 98% of the patients in both groups indicated satisfaction ($p = 0.98$), with only two from each group reporting dissatisfaction. Considering the negative items, 14% of the patients in the A&E group indicated less satisfaction compared with 6% in the PFTC group ($p = 0.07$) (Table 2). The responses to the two individual negative

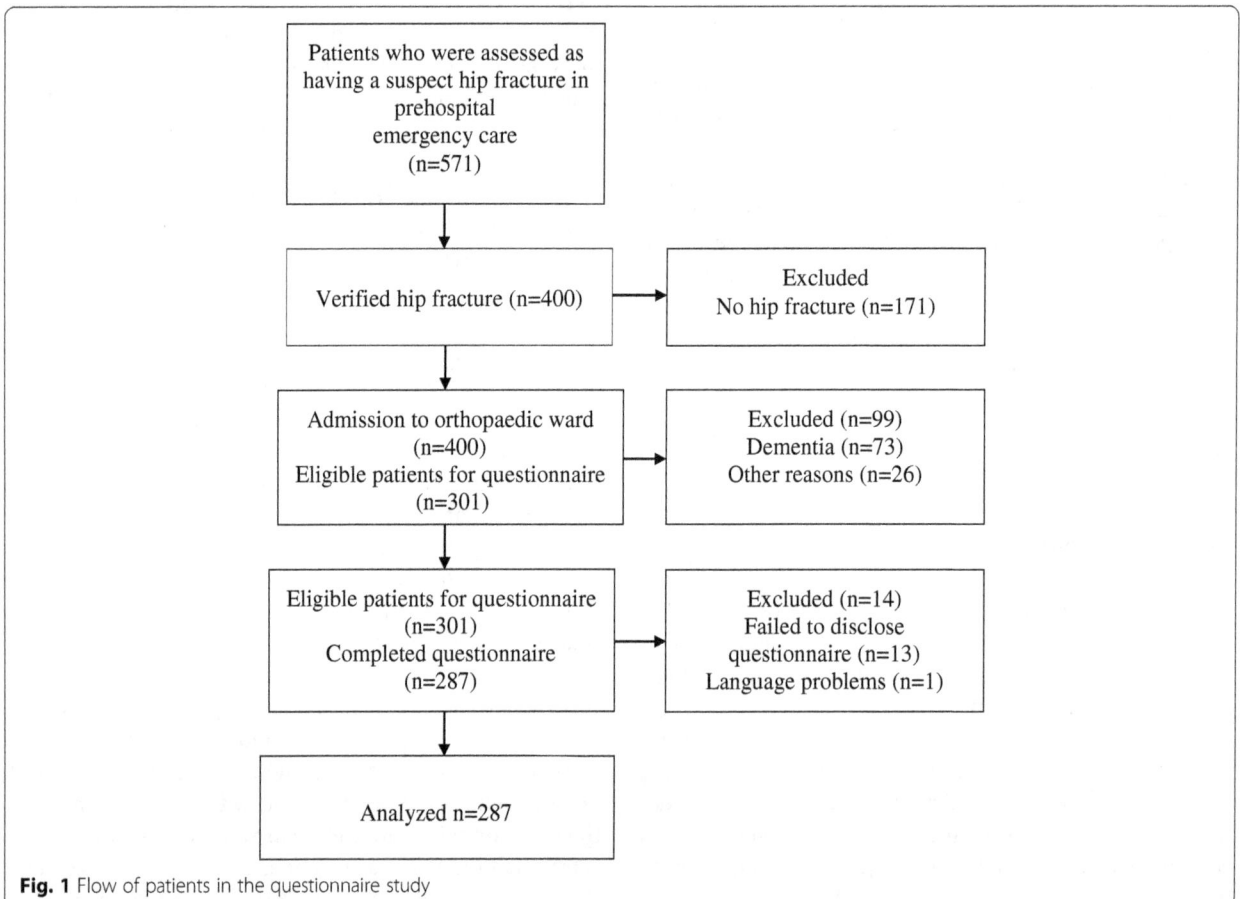

Fig. 1 Flow of patients in the questionnaire study

Table 1 Characteristics of hip fracture patients in prehospital emergency care (n = 287) based on the CECSS

Variables of prehospital care	N (%)
PFTC	137 (48)
A&E	150 (52)
Men	99 (34)
Women	188 (66)
Age, mean (years) ± SD[a]	80.9 ± 9.4
Median	83
Min-Max	51–100
ECG	152 (53)
P-glucose	157 (55)
Pain treatment	273 (95)
Oxygen	162 (56)
Infusion	162 (56)
Sedative	81 (28)
Antiemetic	22 (8)

[a]SD Standard deviation

items, *"The nurse treated me as a 'case' instead of as a person"* and *"The nurse was not very friendly"*, differed noticeably between the groups, with a higher proportion of the most favourable response alternatives in the PFTC group (85.4% vs. 80.7%, $p = 0.21$, and 97.1% vs. 85.3%, $p < 0.01$, respectively).

Patient satisfaction – Distribution of responses
The distribution of responses on patient satisfaction for each item on the care subscale and negative item scale is presented in Table 3 with the number and percentage for each response. More than 80% of the patients selected the most positive response alternative on both the care subscale and the negative questions. However, two items on the care subscale concerning nursing information, namely *"The nurse gave me a chance to ask questions"* and *"The nurse made sure that all my questions were answered"*, revealed that 16.4 and 16.7% respectively of the patients were dissatisfied. Mean scores

Table 2 Comparison of patient satisfaction scores for the care subscale and the negative items

	Score	PFTC (n = 137)	A&E (n = 150)	P value
[a]Care subscale (12 items)	60–48	124	135	0.98[c]
	47–36	11	13	
	35–12	2	2	
[b]Negative items (4 items)	4–8	129	129	0.07[c]
	9–12	6	14	
	13–20	2	7	

[a] ≥36 indicates patient satisfaction in care items
[b] ≤ 12 indicates patient satisfaction in negative items
[c] Chi-2 test was used for comparison of the category scores

for the care subscale and the negative items were 55.47 (SD 5.7) and 5.52 (SD 2.8) respectively.

Comparison with other studies using the CECSS
Four out of six studies reported a high level of patient satisfaction. In five of the studies, the mean scores on the care subscale ranged from 43.46 to 57.60. One study reported the results as percentages of the most positive response alternatives. Two studies reported a higher level of patient satisfaction compared with the present study, one with a mean score on the care subscale and the other with the most positive response alternatives (Table 4).

Discussion
This study demonstrates that patients with a hip fracture were satisfied with the care provided by registered nurses during ambulance assignments. A majority of the patients selected the most positive response alternative on the care subscale and also in response to the negative questions. Some responses, especially on the care subscale regarding "skills, knowledge and concern", indicate a very high level of patient satisfaction with prehospital emergency care.

No significant difference was observed between the PFTC and the A&E groups on the care subscale. A streamlined process with faster admission to a hospital had no effect on patient satisfaction in our study, although there was a difference in terms of satisfaction with the greater number of nursing interventions associated with PFTC. The waiting time and competence associated with fast track care at A&E have previously been reported to be a predictor of patient satisfaction [33]. However, there was a tendency towards less patient satisfaction in the A&E group compared with the PFTC group on the negative items. Patients in the PFTC group responded more positively on specific aspects of nurses' caring behaviour. The importance for patient satisfaction might be on negative items, possibly highlighting the importance that the patient attributes to the fact that the ambulance nurse facilitated faster admission on arrival at the hospital. Accordingly, this study suggests a possible area in which patient satisfaction could be improved.

Patients with a hip fracture often suffer severe pain and anxiety. Ambulance nurses provide immediate care at the scene comprising pain relief, examination, removal and transport to hospital. It is reasonable to assume that the positive response largely depends on the rapid aid as well as the competence and carefulness of the ambulance nurses, which together result in patients feeling better, due to a reduction in their pain and anxiety. A recently published study describes positive experiences when ambulance personnel used different pain management strategies for patients with a suspected hip fracture [34].

Table 3 Number and percentage distribution of CECSS item responses (n = 287)

Item	N (%)				
	Total agreement		Total disagreement		
	5	4	3	2	1
1.The nurse performed her/his duties with skill	266(92.4)	16(5.6)	4 (1.4)	0 (0.0)	1 (0.3)
2.The nurse seemed to know something about my illness/problem	263 (91.6)	18 (6.3)	5 (1.7)	1 (0.3)	0 (0.0)
3.The nurse knew what treatment I needed	246 (85.7)	19 (6.6)	16(5.6)	3 (1.0)	3 (1.0)
4.The nurse should have been more attentive than he/she was	21 (7.3)	6 (2.1)	3 (1.0)	16(5.6)	241 (84.0)
5.The nurse explained all procedures before they were carried out	225 (78.4)	26 (9.1)	19 (6.6)	10 (3.5)	7 (2.4)
6.The nurse seemed too busy to spend time talking to me	16(5.6)	3 (1.0)	7 (2.4)	13 (4.5)	248 (86.4)
7.The nurse explained things in terms I could understand	246 (85.7)	17 (5.9)	14 (4.9)	7 (2.4)	3 (1.0)
8.The nurse was understanding when listening to my problem	230 (80.1)	20 (7.0)	19 (6.6)	12 (4.2)	6 (2.1)
9.The nurse seemed genuinely concerned about my pain, fear and anxiety	237 (82.6)	22 (7.7)	15 (5.2)	7 (2.4)	6 (2.1)
10.The nurse was as gentle as he/she could be when performing painful procedures	258 (89.9)	16(5.6)	9 (3.1)	2 (0.7)	2 (0.7)
11.The nurse treated me as a "case" instead of as a person	23 (8.0)	4 (1.4)	8 (2.8)	14 (4.9)	238 (82.9)
12.The nurse seemed to understand how I felt	239 (83.3)	26 (9.1)	15 (5.2)	5 (1.7)	2 (0.7)
13.The nurse gave me a chance to ask questions	172 (59.9)	25 (8.7)	43 (15.0)	24 (8.4)	23 (8.0)
14.The nurse was not very friendly	14 (4.9)	3 (1.0)	3 (1.0)	6 (2.1)	261 (90.9)
15.The nurse appeared to take time to meet my needs	239 (83.3)	27 (9.4)	11 (3.8)	7 (2.4)	3 (1.0)
16 The nurse made sure that all my questions were answered	174 (60.6)	24 (8.4)	41 (14.3)	27 (9.4)	21 (7.3)
Care subscale (12 items)	233 (81.2)	21 (7.3)	18 (6.2)	9 (3.1)	6 (2.0)
Negative item subscale (4 items)	19 (6.6)	4 (1.4)	5 (1.7)	12 (3.9)	247 (86)

"The nurse seemed genuinely concerned about my pain, fear and anxiety" is one example of a statement that received a high level of the most positive response alternatives, which definitely underlines the high quality of care provided by ambulance nurses. One previous study describes patients' positive experiences of prehospital emergency care, but also certain negative effects of medical treatment, such as confusion and the need to ask questions about what really happened in the ambulance [22].

Dissatisfaction with care is often related to lack of information and communication [6].

The present study reveals a positive response to questions dealing with these areas, which may be due to the development of prehospital guidelines and awareness of the importance of high-quality care for this vulnerable group of patients.

Despite the acute situation, the ambulance nurse has time to talk and listen to the patient. Informing a patient about what is going to happen and reporting the patient's condition to the next level of care ensure a continuum of care. However, 16% of patients were dissatisfied with the nursing information received. Despite the generally very positive responses from patients, this is an important finding and indicates areas that require improvement. Another prehospital study describes the patients' deep need for appropriate information to enhance their experience.

Table 4 Studies employing the CECSS for comparison with the present study

Author	Year	Number of patients	Country	Result	Score or most positive response alternatives
Cunado et al. [28]	2002	96	Spain	High satisfaction	50.50[a]
Chan JN, Chau J. [29]	2005	56	Hong Kong	Satisfaction	43.93[a]
Ekwall A, Davies BA. [30]	2010	157	Sweden	High satisfaction	45.9–52.6[a]
Johansson et al. [21]	2011	40	Sweden	High satisfaction	93% most positive response alternatives[b]
Wright et al. [31]	2013	573	USA	High satisfaction	55.9–57.6[a]
Messina et al. [32]	2014	259	Italy	Satisfaction	43.46[a]
Larsson et al.[c]	2018	287	Sweden	High satisfaction	55.47[a] 82.5% most positive response alternatives[b]

[a] Mean score on the care subscale
[b] Proportion of the most positive response alternatives
[c] The present study

Relational skills together with technical knowledge contributed to patients' perception of professionalism in the ambulance service [35]. Accordingly, an increased focus on physical, emotional and social needs might contribute to greater patient satisfaction.

In addition, communicational and behavioural skills have previously been described as important for ambulance nurses' competence [36].

Comparison with other studies

Despite the fact that The National Board of Health and Welfare has stated that prehospital emergency care standards should be identical to those in hospital emergency care, there is a gap in the literature concerning patient satisfaction with nursing care in the ambulance service. We therefore compared patient satisfaction from two similar emergency care contexts using the same questionnaire.

The CECSS has been used in several studies and different emergency care contexts. While we are aware that the modified version for ambulance care has not been tested for reliability and validity, we believe the two contexts to be comparable.

In comparison with other studies, our result indicates a high level of patient satisfaction.

Only one other study presents a higher mean score on the care subscale than the present study [31]. However, the score level of all the studies indicates satisfaction or a very high level of satisfaction [28–30, 32]. When compared with a previous study from Sweden on the ambulance service, the present study indicates a very high level of patient satisfaction [21]. In addition, comparable studies describe patient satisfaction in different and unspecified patient groups. Another aspect that should be considered is that the present study focused on a large and specific patient group requiring skilled nursing care, thus contributing reliable information about satisfaction with prehospital emergency care in patients with a hip fracture.

Strengths and limitations

The response rate was high, indicating a great willingness to participate in the study.

It is reasonable to assume that the result can be generalized to other ambulance organizations in which ambulance nurses provide care and use similar guidelines for this patient group.

Some considerations should be borne in mind. For example, patients with dementia were excluded. One solution might have been for relatives to answer the questionnaire. A previous study using the CECSS describes options for the participation of accompanying persons [37].

As one cannot rely on relatives being present at the scene, either in the ambulance or at the hospital, we decided not to use the option of proxy answers for individuals with dementia.

Investigating patient satisfaction and gaining knowledge of how to achieve quality improvements in healthcare are recognised as challenging [38]. Studies using questionnaires are relatively simple to implement and constitute an approved method for investigating quality of care. However, as several studies have concluded that all participants were more or less satisfied, it is possible that patient satisfaction is far too general a parameter to be examined by means of a questionnaire and that the instrument is not specific enough about what patients are satisfied or dissatisfied with. It is reasonable to assume that patients' expectations of ambulance care vary between individuals, depending on morbidity and other factors that may affect individual patient satisfaction. In order to increase knowledge about patient satisfaction with prehospital emergency care, it will be necessary to develop new methods, probably with a more individual approach, such as phone calls, e-mails or deep interviews, where patients themselves can decide and explain what they are satisfied or dissatisfied with.

Although the quality of ambulance care is often defined by waiting times for life-threatening conditions, some authors have addressed the need for quality indicators in prehospital emergency care [39]. Patients may have low expectations of prehospital emergency care, knowing little about it in its modern form. They assume they will just be given basic assistance at the scene and then transportation, not the more advanced types of care provided today [40]. This might explain the high level of satisfaction in the present study.

In other words, patients' expectations are met if they feel that they receive adequate physical care and encounter a friendly attitude [14]. Although it is challenging to investigate patient satisfaction, the results of the present study indicate certain areas that require further research. Firstly, patient expectations must be addressed individually and in detail to understand the background and reasons for individual patient satisfaction. No two patients are likely to be identical in this respect. Secondly, improving the nursing information given to patients is essential, as is the actual delivery of information in an effective and authoritative manner. Thirdly, evaluations of patient expectations and satisfaction should be undertaken on a regular, systematic basis in order to guide the development of competence in the ambulance service. Fourthly, more prehospital emergency care outcomes need to be documented from the patient perspective, leading to the establishment of a set of quality indicators. Other authors have also described the need for quality indicators in prehospital emergency care [41]. These four indications thus point conclusively to the need for further research on several aspects of the topic investigated in this study.

Conclusion

It is essential to examine patient satisfaction with prehospital emergency care following a hip fracture. This study highlights patients' high level of satisfaction with the prehospital emergency care provided by ambulance nurses. The ambulance service has succeeded in its mission to develop and strengthen prehospital emergency skills in the care of patients with a hip fracture. However, several areas can be improved in terms of nursing information, regular evaluations and the establishment of a set of quality indicators for prehospital emergency care.

Abbreviations

A&E: Accident and emergency department; CECSS: Consumer Emergency Care Satisfaction Scale; ECG: Electrocardiogram; PFTC: Prehospital fast track care; RETTS: Rapid Emergency Triage and Treatment System

Acknowledgements

A special thanks to Susanne Svensson, director of the Department of Prehospital Emergency Care who gave the ambulance nurses the opportunity to conduct research.

Funding

We thank the Department of Prehospital Emergency Care and the Scientific Council of Region Halland for generously funding this project.

Authors' contributions

GL: Study design, data collection, statistics, data analyses, interpretation and critical revision of the manuscript for important intellectual content and preparation of the manuscript.
US: Study design, statistics, data analyses, interpretation and critical revision of the manuscript for important intellectual content and preparation of the manuscript. CR: Study design, data analyses, interpretation and critical revision of the manuscript for important intellectual content. AN: Study design, data analyses, interpretation and critical revision of the manuscript for important intellectual content and preparation of the manuscript. All authors have read, edited and approved the final manuscript.

Competing interests

The authors declare that they have no competing interests.

Author details

[1]Department of Ambulance and Prehospital Care, Region Halland, Health Centre Nyhem, 302 49 Halmstad, Sweden. [2]Department of Orthopaedics, Lund University, Lund, Sweden. [3]Skane University Hospital, Malmö, Sweden. [4]Department of R&D, Sahlgrenska University Hospital, Göteborg, Sweden.

References

1. Sjolin H, Lindstrom V, Hult H, Ringsted C, Kurland L. What an ambulance nurse needs to know: a content analysis of curricula in the specialist nursing programme in prehospital emergency care. Int Emerg Nurs. 2015 Apr;23(2): 127–32.
2. Reader TW, Gillespie A, Roberts J. Patient complaints in healthcare systems: a systematic review and coding taxonomy. BMJ Qual Saf. 2014 Aug;23(8): 678–89.
3. Skalen C, Nordgren L, Annerback EM. Patient complaints about health care in a Swedish County: characteristics and satisfaction after handling. Nurs Open. 2016;3(4):203–11.
4. Lee AV, Moriarty JP, Borgstrom C, Horwitz LI. What can we learn from patient dissatisfaction? An analysis of dissatisfying events at an academic medical center. J Hosp Med. 2010;5(9):514–20.
5. Cave J, Dacre J. Dealing with complaints. BMJ. 2008;336(7639):326–8.
6. Sverige. Socialstyrelsen. Nationella indikatorer för god vård: hälso- och sjukvårdsövergripande indikatorer: indikatorer i Socialstyrelsens nationella riktlinjer. Stockholm: Socialstyrelsen; 2009. http://www.socialstyrelsen.se/ publikationer2009/2009-126-72
7. Dinh M, Walker A, Parameswaran A, Enright N. Evaluating the quality of care delivered by an emergency department fast track unit with both nurse practitioners and doctors. Australia Emerg Nurs J. 2012;15(4):188–94.
8. Taylor C, Benger JR. Patient satisfaction in emergency medicine. Emerg Med J. 2004;21:528–32.
9. Jennings N, Clifford S, Fox AR, O'Connell J, Gardner G. The impact of nurse practitioner services on cost, quality of care, satisfaction and waiting times in the emergency department: a systematic review. Int J Nurs Stud. 2015; 52(1):421–35.
10. Shital S, Anay K, Rumoro Dino P, Samuel HF. Managing patient expectations at emergency department triage. Patient Exp J. 2015;2(2):31–44.
11. Suserud B-O. A new profession in the pre-hospital care field - the ambulance nurse. Nurs Crit Care. 2005;10(6):269–71.
12. Socialstyrelsen. SOSFS 2009:10. Socialstyrelsens föreskrifter om ambulanssjukvård m.m; 2009. p. 1–12. http://www.socialstyrelsen.se/sosfs/ 2009-10
13. Rosengren BE, Karlsson MK. The annual number of hip fractures in Sweden will double from year 2002 to 2050: projections based on local and nationwide data. Acta Orthop. 2014;85(3):234–7.
14. Melby V, Ryan A. Caring for older people in prehospital emergency care: can nurses make a difference? J Clin Nurs. 2005;14(9):1141–50.
15. Hwang U, Richardson LD, Sonuyi TO, Morrison RS. The effect of emergency department crowding on the management of pain in older adults with hip fracture. J Am Geriatr Soc. 2006 Feb;54(2):270–5.
16. Suserud B, Lundberg L. Prehospital emergency care. 2, [revised and extended] ed. Liber: Stockholm; 2016.
17. Kuisma M, Maatta T, Hakala T, Sivula T, Nousila-Wiik M. Customer satisfaction measurement in emergency medical services. Acad Emerg Med. 2003;10(7): 812–5.
18. Colwell CB, Pons PT, Pi R. Complaints against an EMS system. J Emerg Med. 2003;25(4):403–8.
19. Doering GT. Customer care. Patient satisfaction in the prehospital setting. Emerg Med Serv. 1998;27(9):69. 71–4
20. Halter M, Marlow T, Tye C, Ellison GT. Patients' experiences of care provided by emergency care practitioners and traditional ambulance practitioners: a survey from the London ambulance service. Emerg Med J. 2006;23(11):865–6.
21. Johansson A, Ekwall A, Wihlborg J. Patient satisfaction with ambulance care services: survey from two districts in southern Sweden. Int Emerg Nurs. 2011;19(2):86–9.
22. Aronsson K, Bjorkdahl I, Wireklint SB. Prehospital emergency care for patients with suspected hip fractures after falling - older patients' experiences. J Clin Nurs. 2014;23(21–22):3115–23.
23. Hommel A, Kock ML, Persson J, Werntoft E. The Patient's view of nursing care after hip fracture. ISRN Nurs. 2012;2012:863291.
24. Larsson G, Stromberg RU, Rogmark C, Nilsdotter A. Prehospital fast track care for patients with hip fracture: impact on time to surgery, hospital stay, post-operative complications and mortality a randomised, controlled trial. Injury. 2016;47(4):881–6.

25. Widgren BR, Jourak M. Medical emergency triage and treatment system (METTS): a new protocol in primary triage and secondary priority decision in emergency medicine. J Emerg Med. 2011;40(6):623–8.

26. Davis BA, Bush HA. Developing effective measurement tools: a case study of the consumer emergency care satisfaction scale. J Nurs Care Qual. 1995;9(2): 26–35.

27. Davis BA, Kiesel CK, McFarland J, Collard A, Coston K, Keeton A. Evaluating instruments for quality: testing convergent validity of the consumer emergency care satisfaction scale. J Nurs Care Qual. 2005;20(4):364–8.

28. Cunado BA, Garcia CB, Rial CC, Garcia LF. Spanish validation of an instrument to measure the quality of nursing care in hospital emergency units. J Nurs Care Qual. 2002;16(3):13–23.

29. Chan JN, Chau J. Patient satisfaction with triage nursing care in Hong Kong. J Adv Nurs. 2005;50(5):498–507.

30. Ekwall A, Davis BA. Testing a Swedish version of the consumer emergency care satisfaction scale in an emergency department and 2 observation wards. J Nurs Care Qual. 2010;25(3):266–73.

31. Wright G, Causey S, Dienemann J, Guiton P, Coleman FS, Nussbaum M. Patient satisfaction with nursing care in an urban and suburban emergency department. J Nurs Adm. 2013;43(10):502–8.

32. Messina G, Vencia F, Mecheroni S, Dionisi S, Baragatti L, Nante N. Factors affecting patient satisfaction with emergency department care: an Italian rural hospital. Glob J Health Sci. 2014;7(4):30–9.

33. Dinh MM, Enright N, Walker A, Parameswaran A, Chu M. Determinants of patient satisfaction in an Australian emergency department fast-track setting. Emerg Med J. 2013;30(10):824–7.

34. Jakopovic D, Falk AC, Lindstrom V. Ambulance personnel's experience of pain management for patients with a suspected hip fracture: a qualitative study. Int Emerg Nurs. 2015;23(3):244–9.

35. Togher FJ, Davy Z, Siriwardena AN. Patients' and ambulance service clinicians' experiences of prehospital care for acute myocardial infarction and stroke: a qualitative study. Emerg Med J. 2013;30(11):942–8.

36. Wihlborg J, Edgren G, Johansson A, Sivberg B. Reflective and collaborative skills enhances ambulance nurses' competence - a study based on qualitative analysis of professional experiences. Int Emerg Nurs. 2017;32:20–7.

37. Kristensson J, Ekwall A. Psychometric properties of the consumer emergency care satisfaction scale: tested on persons accompanying patients in emergency department. J Nurs Care Qual. 2008;23(3):277–82.

38. Al-Abri R, Al-Balushi A. Patient satisfaction survey as a tool towards quality improvement. Oman Med J. 2014;29(1):3–7.

39. Price L. Treating the clock and not the patient: ambulance response times and risk. Qual Saf Health Care. 2006;15(2):127–30.

40. Ahl C, Nystrom M, Jansson L. Making up one's mind:--patients' experiences of calling an ambulance. Accid Emerg Nurs. 2006;14(1):11–9.

41. Pittet V, Burnand B, Yersin B, Carron PN. Trends of pre-hospital emergency medical services activity over 10 years: a population-based registry analysis. BMC Health Serv Res. 2014;14:380. 6963–14–380

Patient safety culture in nursing homes – a cross-sectional study among nurses and nursing aides caring for residents with diabetes

Irit Titlestad[1,2], Anne Haugstvedt[1], Jannicke Igland[1,3] and Marit Graue[1*]

Abstract

Background: Due to the high morbidity and disability level among diabetes patients in nursing homes, the conditions for caregivers are exceedingly complex and challenging. The patient safety culture in nursing homes should be evaluated in order to improve patient safety and the quality of care. Thus, the aim of this study was to examine the perceptions of patient safety culture of nursing personnel in nursing homes, and its associations with the participants' (i) profession, (ii) education, (iii) specific knowledge related to their own residents with diabetes, and (iv) familiarity with clinical diabetes guidelines for older people.

Methods: Cross-sectional survey design. The study included 89 nursing home personnel (38 registered nurses and 51 nurse aides), 25 (28%) with advanced education, at two nursing homes. We collected self-reported questionnaire data on age, profession, education and work experience, diabetes knowledge and familiarity with diabetes guidelines. In addition, we applied the Nursing Home Survey on Patient Safety Culture instrument, with 42 items and 12 dimensions.

Results: In general, those with advanced education scored higher in all patient safety culture dimensions than those without, however statistically significant only for the dimensions "teamwork" (mean score 81.7 and 67.7, $p = 0.042$) and "overall perceptions of resident safety" (mean score 90.0 and 74.3, $p = 0.016$). Nursing personnel who were familiar with diabetes guidelines for older people had more positive perceptions in key areas of patient safety culture, than those without familiarity with the guidelines.

Conclusions: The findings from this study show that advanced education and familiarity with current diabetes guidelines was related to adequate evaluations on essential areas of patient safety culture in nursing homes.

Keywords: Nursing home, Nursing personnel, Patient safety culture, Diabetes

Background

The increasing prevalence of diabetes worldwide as well as the increasing number of older individuals in many societies will lead to an expected rise in the number of older individuals with diabetes in nursing homes in the years to come [1–3]. A systematic review has shown a variation in the prevalence of diabetes in nursing homes from 8 to 53%, with a mean prevalence of 18.5% [4]. Studies in Norway have indicated the prevalence of diabetes in Norwegian nursing homes to be 15–17% [5, 6]. Nursing home residents with diabetes have a higher burden of comorbidity and are considered to be a vulnerable and neglected group of patients who suffer from a high level of both physical and cognitive impairment [3]. Thus, residents with diabetes are a complex and challenging care group in nursing homes [2]. Nursing personnel must handle an extensive list of medications, treatments and care deficiencies that are both complicated and time-consuming. National clinical diabetes guidelines are intended to support and give concrete recommendations in relation to

* Correspondence: marit.graue@hvl.no
[1]Faculty of Health and Social Sciences, Western Norway University of Applied Sciences, Postbox 7030, N-5020 Bergen, Norway
Full list of author information is available at the end of the article

diabetes care, to ensure patient safety and minimize adverse events and variations in clinical practice [7, 8]. In Norway, the municipalities are responsible for providing care for inhabitants in need, and almost all nursing homes are public. The main groups of nursing personnel in the nursing homes are registered nurses (with education on university/university college level), nursing aides (with education on upper secondary school level) and assistants without any formal education. Nurses and nursing aides authorized to administer medication, are primarily the nursing personnel who need the knowledge and expertise to secure high quality care for residents with diabetes.

Patient safety is a topic that internationally has received increased professional and political attention in recent years [9, 10]. It is recommended to evaluate the patient safety culture (PSC) in health care institutions to subsequently improve patient safety and quality of care [11–16]. Research has shown that there is a relationship between weak PSC and clinical outcomes, where a higher perception of PSC is associated with better patient outcomes [17, 18]. The health providers' knowledge and expertise, and familiarity with national clinical recommendations in relation to treatment and care within a specific clinical field, might influence PSC and thus partially explain the observed associations between PSC and clinical outcomes. Clinical guidelines intends to ensure the best possible patients safety by serving as a tool for health professionals and patients to take proper and responsible decisions, and also by contributing to less adverse variations in practice and improved quality of health care [7]. However, studies have shown that diabetes guidelines in nursing homes are not followed closely enough and that the quality of care could be improved by better use of the guidelines [4].

In a previous study, we have shown insufficient diabetes knowledge among nurses, nursing aides and nursing assistants in nursing homes in Norway [19]. Although the nurses reported better diabetes knowledge than the nursing aides and nursing assistants, all groups lacked knowledge on important topics related to diabetes treatment and care. In that study we did, however, not study the participants familiarity with clinical diabetes guidelines or if the lack of knowledge was related to PSC. Thus, in this study, we will explore possible associations between PSC and nursing personnel's knowledge and expertise, and familiarity with clinical diabetes guidelines in relation to diabetes treatment and care for older people.

Methods

Aim

We aimed to examine the perception of PSC among nursing home personnel, and its associations with the participants' (i) profession (registered nurses vs. nursing aides), (ii) education (with or without advanced education), (iii) specific knowledge related to their own residents with diabetes, and (iv) familiarity with clinical diabetes guidelines for older people.

Design and study population

We conducted the study from August to September 2015. We invited registered nurses and nursing aides at two nursing homes in Western Norway to participate in this cross-sectional study. The nursing homes had respectively 123 and 107 residents divided on long-term care units (for about 80% of the residents), short-term units and rehabilitation units. Of the respectively 89 and 93 registered nurses and nursing aides working in the two nursing homes, 31 (35%) and 36 (39%) was registered nurses. Thus, nursing aides constituted the largest personnel group in the nursing homes.

Measures

Demographic variables

We collected data on age ("18–29 years", "30–39 years", "40–49 years", "50–59 years" or "60 years or older"); profession ("registered nurse", "nursing aides" or "other"), continuing education (with advanced education or without) and time since completing education ("less than 5 years", "5–10 years", "11–15 years", "16–20 years" or "more than 20 years"). The nursing personnel was not asked specifically what their advanced education included, but for nurses advanced education typically included geriatric or palliative education while for nursing aides was geriatric or psychiatric courses. In addition, nursing home work experience ("1–5 years", "6–10 years", "11–15 years", "16–20 years" or "21 years or more"), status of employment ("permanent" or "temporary"), ("full" or "part-time") and work shift ("day, evening and night", "day and evening", "only night" or "others") were assessed.

Specific knowledge related to their own residents with diabetes

The questionnaire included questions about the participants' familiarity with clinical diabetes guidelines for older people ("yes", "no"), if they administered insulin ("yes", "no", "don't know") and whether they knew if any of their residents were on glucose lowering drugs which could cause hypoglycaemia ("yes", "no","don't know"). In addition, specific knowledge related to their own residents with diabetes included questions about glycaemic treatment goals, routines for blood glucose monitoring and risk assessment in relation to hypoglycaemia [20].

Nursing home survey on patient safety culture

We used the Nursing Home Survey on Patient Safety Culture (NHSPSC) to collect data on the participants' perceptions of PSC [21]. The NHSPSC was developed in 2008 by the Agency for Healthcare Research and Quality to measure PSC among nursing homes personnel [12, 22], and has been translated into Norwegian by Cappelen et al. [23]. The NHSPSC is composed of a total of 42 items divided into 12 dimensions with three to four items in each dimension, and items can be either positively and negatively worded [21]. The 12 dimensions are: the respondents' perception of "teamwork", "staffing", "compliance with procedures", "training and skills", "response to mistakes", "handoffs (information concerning patient transition)", "feedback and communication about incidents", "communication openness", "supervisor expectations and actions promoting resident safety", "overall resident safety", "management support for resident safety" and "organizational learning". The response alternatives on these items are either "strongly disagree", "disagree", "neither", "agree", "strongly agree", and "not applicable/do not know" or "never", "rarely", "sometimes", "most of the time" and "always". The answers "agree" and "strongly agree" were defined as a positive response on positively worded items, while "disagree" and "strongly disagree" were defined as positive responses on negatively worded items. In addition, the instrument contains two single questions about (i) the respondents' general opinion about the PSC in the nursing home and (ii) the number of reported adverse events during the past year [21]. A respondents' individual score for each NHSPSC dimension was estimated by calculating the number of positive responses for each dimension, divided by the number of items in the dimension, and multiplying by 100. In cases where a participant did not answer one or more items (missing), the dimension score was calculated according to the actual number of items each individual had responded to. Individual dimension scores are ranged from 0 to 100, where higher scores indicate a more positive response [21]. The method used in the present study to calculate individual scores have been used in previous studies [14] and results in mean scores which will be equal to the score for the total study population according to the instructions in the manual [21]. Mean scores in the present study can therefore be compared with the results from studies in which scores are calculated at the institutional level [24]. A validation study of the Norwegian version of the NHSPSC by Cappelen et al. [23], indicated satisfactory internal consistency with Cronbach's alpha for the different dimensions ranging from 0.55 to 0.90. However, results from confirmatory factor analyses gave improved model fit after merging of the three last dimensions ("organizational learning", "overall perceptions of patient safety" and "management support for patient safety"), resulting in 10 dimensions instead of 12 [23]. In our study, Cronbach's alpha ranged from 0.50 to 0.73 for the 12 dimensions. We also made a combination of the three last dimensions in accordance with Cappelen et al. [23] in order to explore if this changed any of our results for comparison of PSC between groups. Reliability analysis of the new combined dimension proved to have a good Cronbach's alpha value (0.77), while each dimension separately was found to have a Cronbach's alpha score lower than 0.60.

Data analysis

The study population was characterized using descriptive statistics (counts and percentages) (Table 1). Association between categorical variables were tested using chi-square tests. The associations between NHSPSC dimension scores and demographic- and diabetes-related questions were analysed by independent sample t-tests, and reported as mean, standard deviation and P-values. In addition to analyses for each of the 12 original dimensions, we also did analyses for the combination of the three last dimensions according to the dimension suggested by Cappelen et al. [23]. The SPSS statistical program package Version 21; SPSS Inc.Chicago, IL, USA was used, and statistical significance was defined as $P < 0.05$.

Ethics

The head nurses in the two participating nursing homes participated in the planning phase of the study. The Norwegian Centre for Research Data approved the study (Ref No: 2015/43349). All participants gave informed consent. Data collection took place at specially allotted rooms outside the participants' work unit in the nursing home.

Results

Of the 182 eligible nursing personnel from the two included nursing homes 89 individuals completed the study questionnaire. This gave response rates in the two nursing homes of 56 and 44%, respectively. Of the 89 responders, 38 (43%) were registered nurses and 51 (57%) were nursing aides (Table 1). Furthermore, 25 (28%) of the 89 participants had any kind of advanced education with a non-significant difference between professions (36.8% among nurses and 22.4% among nursing aides, $p = 0.14$). Totally 49 (55%) of the participants reported that they were familiar with the Norwegian diabetes guidelines for older people with diabetes in nursing homes, with a slightly higher proportion among nurses, but not significant (60.5% among nurses and 51.0% among nursing aides, $p = 0.37$). Advanced education in itself was not significantly associated with familiarity to the diabetes guidelines (44% among nursing personnel with advanced education and 58.1% among nursing personnel without advanced education reported familiarity to the diabetes guidelines, $p = 0.23$). In total 58 (65%) of the participants answered "yes" on the question whether they knew if any of their residents were on glucose lowering drugs which could cause hypoglycaemia, and 73 (82%) reported that they administered insulin with a significantly higher proportion among nurses compared to nursing aides (92.1% versus 74.5%, $p = 0.03$).

Table 1 Characteristics of the study population ($N = 89$)

	n (%)
Profession group	
Registered Nurses	38 (42.7)
Nurse Aides	51 (57.3)
Nursing home	
Nursing home 1	50 (56.2)
Nursing home 2	39 (43.8)
Age (years)	
18–29	5 (5.6)
30–39	14 (15.7)
40–49	29 (32.6)
50–59	28 (31.5)
≥ 60	12 (13.5)
Missing	1 (1.1)
Time since completing education (years)	
< 5	13 (14.6)
5–10	22 (24.7)
11–15	19 (21.4)
16–20	13 (14.6)
> 20	22 (24.7)
Advanced education	
Yes	25 (28.1)
No	62 (69.7)
Missing	2 (2.2)
Work experience from nursing home (years)	
1–5	5 (5.6)
6–10	24 (27.0)
11–15	17 (19.1)
16–20	18 (20.2)
≥ 21	25 (28.1)
Conditions of employment	
Permanent	88 (98.9)
Temporary	1 (1.1)
Job content	
Full	52 (58.4)
Part-time	36 (40.5)
Missing	1 (1.1)
Work shift	
Day, evening and night	7 (7.9)
Day and evening	76 (85.4)
Only night	1 (1.1)
Others	5 (5.6)

Nurses had significantly higher score on the PSC dimension "communication openness" compared to nursing aides (mean 71.0 versus 47.4, $p = 0.004$). For the other dimensions, including the new combined dimension, no significant differences between nurses and nursing aides were identified (results not shown in tables). We identified that nursing personnel with advanced education reported significantly more positive perceptions of the dimensions "teamwork" and "overall perceptions of resident safety" compared to those without advanced education, whereas the dimension "management support for resident safety" was borderline significant ($p = 0.051$) (Table 2). The difference was also significant for the new combined dimension. The ones with advanced education also responded more positively to all the other patient safety dimensions, but the differences were not statistically significant. We found a borderline significant difference on perception of "compliance with procedures" between the nursing personnel who did not know if their patients' blood glucose lowering drugs could cause hypoglycaemia and those who did have such knowledge, with highest score among those without knowledge (mean 67.9 versus 52.6, $P = 0.050$). For the other dimensions, including the new combined dimension, there were no significant differences between nursing personnel with and without knowledge of patients on glucose lowering drugs. However, the differences between the groups in four of the dimensions were higher than 5–10 points; "staffing" (mean 45.4, versus 38.4 $p = 0.183$), "training and skills" (mean 55.6 versus 46.8, $p = 0.303$), "nonpunitive response to mistakes" (mean 73.8 versus 67.1, $p = 0.387$) and "overall perceptions of resident safety" (mean 87.7 versus 75.7, $p = 0.079$).

Our study indicated significant associations between the participants' perceived familiarity with the Norwegian diabetes guidelines for older nursing homes residents and their perceptions of several NHSPSC dimensions (Table 3). Those who claimed to be familiar with the guidelines on average had more positive scores on a larger proportion of questions within the dimensions "handoffs" (60.9 versus 42.9, $P = 0.013$), "supervisor expectations and actions promoting resident safety" (85.4 versus 67.5, $P = 0.015$), "management support for resident safety" (54.3 versus 30.0, $P < 0.003$) and "organizational learning" (63.4 versus 44.9, $P = 0.014$). The total patient safety culture scores were 11% higher among those who were familiar with the guidelines compared to those who were not ($P = 0.021$). Those who were familiar with the guidelines also scored significantly higher for the new combined dimension ($p = 0.003$).

Discussion
To our knowledge, this is the first study examining PSC among nursing home personnel and its associations with the participants' familiarity with diabetes guidelines for older people. We found that personnel with advanced education and familiarity with guidelines had a more

Table 2 Nursing personnel's with and without advanced education mean patient safety culture score for the 12 dimensions in the NHSPSC[a] (N = 87)

	With advanced education Mean (SD) n = 25	Without advanced education Mean (SD) n = 62	P Value [b]
Positive responses to			
1. Teamwork	81.7 (25.7)	67.7 (33.8)	0.042[b]
2. Staffing	43.7 (16.4)	37.2 (25.7)	0.169
3. Compliance with procedures	62.5 (33.1)	54.3 (35.8)	0.319
4. Training and skills	54.0 (33.1)	44.6 (38.1)	0.258
5. Nonpunitive response to mistakes	69.0 (30.0)	68.5 (34.2)	0.952
6. Handoffs (information concerning patient transition)	54.3 (31.1)	50.7 (34.9)	0.634
7. Feedback and communication about incidents	86.0 (28.9)	82.3 (26.5)	0.579
8. Communication openness	63.3 (34.7)	55.6 (39.9)	0.375
9. Supervisor expectations and actions promoting resident safety	85.3 (32.0)	73.2 (34.9)	0.127
10. Overall perceptions of resident safety	90.0 (23.6)	74.3 (32.9)	0.016[b]
11. Management support for resident safety	54.3 (32.3)	37.4 (39.9)	0.051
12. Organizational learning	64.3 (30.7)	50.7 (36.1)	0.082
Combined dimension (10, 11 and 12)	69.6 (23.5)	54.1 (31.6)	0.016[b]

[a]Score for each person is calculates as percent positive responses within each dimension. Score for each dimension may vary between 0 and 100%. Higher scores indicate more positive responses
[b]Significantly different t-test at P < 0.05

positive perception in key areas of PSC. Moreover, safety culture perceptions differed significantly between registered nurses and nursing aides relative to the dimension, "communication openness" in the NHSPSC. It might be that registered nurses are more able to speak up about problems and at the same time, their suggestions might be more valued than those of nursing aides. Castle [25] also discusses this matter, related to differences in perception of PSC among professions. In that study, higher perception of PSC was associated with higher registered nurse staffing levels. As nursing aides represent a large part of the staffing in nursing homes in many countries, the low positive scoring on "communication openness" among nursing aides in our study (47.7%) may arouse some concerns. Communication between nursing personnel is a particularly important concern for quality of care and may therefore influence on patient safety. Other researchers have also suggested that failure of communication between personnel within the health system might be associated with individual and structural factors and lack of knowledge and skills [26] putting patient safety and patient outcomes in danger [11]. Sinclair [3] points out that there are a number of important barriers to improving diabetes care in nursing homes. One obstacle is inadequate training of nursing personnel in basic diabetes care, and lack of resources for such training. In our study, 35% of the participants' lack knowledge about which of the glucose lowering medications that can give hypoglycaemia. Another important barrier for improving care is miscommunication

between nursing personnel, which occur due to the lack of clear professional boundaries and responsibilities, as well as the lack of national standards for diabetes care in nursing homes [3]. According to Danielsson et al. [27], efforts for improving PSC have to take into account the profession groups' values, norms, and assumptions related to patient safety.

This study also showed that advanced education was associated with better perception of PSC. Even though there were statistically significant differences only in three dimensions, the difference between the groups in nine of the dimensions was higher than 5–10 points. For a variety of questionnaire-based scales, changes between 5 and 10% (or five to 10 points on a 100-point scale) might be considered large enough to be noticed by people and thus regarded as important [28]. We do therefore think that also the non-significant differences are noteworthy. In our sample, we did not have the power to elaborate this further; however, further research might examine more in detail whether advanced education, and the duration of training in itself, might play a role for patient safety. Nursing home patients with diabetes usually have several additional chronic conditions, and therefore treatment and care for this group of patients is more challenging [3, 29]. The higher the competence among nursing personnel are, the more knowledge, skills and abilities to handle different situations, both in terms of direct patient contact, cooperation between nursing personnel, and between different professions. Nursing personnel with higher competence may

Table 3 Nursing personnel's mean patient safety culture score for the 12 dimensions in the NHSPSC in relation to familiarity to the Norwegian clinical diabetes guidelines for elderly nursing home residents[a] (N = 89)

	Nursing personnel who reported familiarity to the Norwegian clinical diabetes guidelines Mean (SD) n = 49	Nursing personnel who reported no familiarity to the Norwegian clinical diabetes guidelines Mean (SD) n = 40	P Value [b]
Positive responses to:			
Teamwork	77.2 (26.2)	65.2 (36.8)	0.088
Staffing	39.8 (25.8)	38.8 (20.9)	0.833
Compliance with procedures	56.9 (35.0)	56.7 (34.8)	0.970
Training and skills	53.1 (39.6)	42.9 (33.7)	0.196
Nonpunitive response to mistakes	73.1 (34.1)	62.3 (32.1)	0.127
Handoffs (information concerning patient transition)	60.9 (33.2)	42.9 (33.0)	0.013[b]
Feedback and communication about incidents	87.6 (24.1)	78.1 (29.5)	0.107
Communication openness	58.5 (36.8)	56.7 (40.1)	0.824
Supervisor expectations and actions promoting resident safety	85.4 (29.9)	67.5 (36.6)	0.015[b]
Overall perceptions of resident safety	84.0 (29.0)	73.8 (32.7)	0.126
Management support for resident safety	54.3 (37.1)	30.0 (36.6)	0.003[b]
Organizational learning	63.4 (31.4)	44.9 (36.1)	0.014[b]
Combined dimension (10, 11 and 12)	67.7 (27.5)	49.0 (30.1)	0.003[b]

[a]Score for each person is calculates as percent positive responses within each dimension. Score for each dimension may vary between 0 and 100%. Higher scores indicate more positive responses
[b]Significantly different t-test at P < 0.05

take a more comprehensive approach to nursing and patient safety. Findings from a large survey that was carried out among nurses working in municipal health care in Norway showed that approximately 70% of the participants reported that the need for more nurses with advanced education or a master's degree is increasing [26]. This relates to the increasing number of older people with higher burden of comorbidity and a range of chronic conditions requiring demanding medical treatment and procedures [2]. Findings from the study of Agarwal et al. [30] showed that nursing personnel reported a need for more training and updating of knowledge on various topics related to diabetes.

Findings concerning whether nursing personnel had knowledge of which patients were using blood glucose lowering drugs that can cause hypoglycaemia show that those who claimed to lack this knowledge scored borderline significantly higher in one dimension ("compliance with procedures") than those who claimed to have the knowledge. They scored higher in six other dimensions as well, but without statistically significant differences. However, the differences between the groups in four of the dimensions were higher than 5–10 points and were therefore perceived as being important [28]. Knowledge of which patients are using these medications appears to be important for the perception of patient safety because hypoglycaemia among frail elderly may lead to worsening of chronic diseases, cognitive impairment, increased morbidity and mortality [31]. In a way, it makes sense to

assume that those with knowledge of which patients were using blood glucose lowering drugs that can cause hypoglycaemia also would report higher scores on perception of PSC. On the other hand, they might not have had the knowledge about how to handle side effects, such as hypoglycaemia. Thus, the knowledge of which patients who are on blood glucose lowering drugs might not necessarily play a role related to differences in perception of PSC. The somewhat unexpected result led us to consider that these findings were influenced by other variables that we did not examine in this study.

We found associations between some areas of PSC, and whether or not nursing personnel reported familiarity with diabetes guidelines for older people. Kuehn [32] points to studies suggesting that guidelines can help ensure quick application of new knowledge in practice, reducing undesirable variations and improving safety and quality. However, in routine practice not all patients may actually receive the most appropriate treatment based on research evidence [33]. The fact that only 55% of the participants in this study reported familiarity with the diabetes guidelines for older nursing home residents can raise questions about where in the system dissemination of new and relevant knowledge fails, and why. Promoting the implementation of clinical guidelines in Norwegian nursing homes and not at least appropriate use of guidelines can lead to awareness among nursing personnel of the need to take informed decisions [34], which can enhance patient safety [7].

Limitations

The sample was a nonprobability sample, which can be exposed to bias [35]. In addition, the sample was small, with a relatively low response rate, which made it difficult to identify significant differences between groups. Moreover, we did not have access to background information on those who chose not to participate (except for their profession) and whether they differed from those who participated, for example in relation to gender, age and their educational level. These variables may affect the variation in PSC scores and could therefore have an impact on the results. The study included only two nursing homes and was conducted in only one municipality. Thus, generalizing should be done with caution. In addition, the results should be interpreted with caution when comparing the findings from this study to studies from other countries, as also stated in previous studies on PSC [36]. Differences between countries may be related to differences in how reporting of adverse events is treated and to variation in composition of the work force [36]. Because of the high number of comparisons between groups, there is also an increased risk of type I error and thus a possibility that some of the significant findings were just chance findings. Another limitation is that the questions about knowledge used in the study only capture the nursing personnel's perceptions about knowledge and not the actual knowledge.

Conclusions

Advanced education and familiarity with diabetes guidelines among nursing home personnel were associated with positive perceptions in key areas of PSC and may therefore play an important role concerning patient safety and quality of care. Further research is warranted to explore whether training programs to increase diabetes knowledge and promote the implementation of clinical guidelines in nursing homes can be related to the perception of PSC level.

Abbreviations

NHSPSC: the Nursing Home Survey on Patient Safety Culture; PSC: Patient safety culture

Acknowledgements

We would like to thank all the nursing personnel for participating in the study.

Funding

The present study is part of a larger study funded by a grant from the Norwegian Research Council (project number 221065) and from Western Norway University of Applied Sciences.

Authors' contributions

MG, AH and IT designed the study. AH and IT collected the data. IT, JI and MG contributed to data analysis. IT, JI, AH and MG contributed to drafting the manuscript. All authors read and approved the final manuscript.

Competing interests

The authors declare that they have no competing interests

Author details

[1]Faculty of Health and Social Sciences, Western Norway University of Applied Sciences, Postbox 7030, N-5020 Bergen, Norway. [2]Kleppestø Nursing Home, Askøy Municipality, Bergen, Norway. [3]Department of Global Public Health and Primary Care, University of Bergen, Bergen, Norway.

References

1. International Diabetes Federation (IDF). IDF Diabetes Atlas. Seventh edition : International Diabetes Federation; 2015 [Accessed 17 November 2016]. Available from: http://www.idf.org/diabetesatlas.
2. Kirkman M, Briscoe V, Clark N, Florez H, Haas L, Halter J, et al. Diabetes in Older Adults. Consensus report Diabetes Care. 2012;35(12):2650–64. https://doi.org/10.2337/dc12-1801.
3. Sinclair AJ, Diabetes UK. Position Statements and Care Recommendations. Good clinical practice guidelines for care home residents with diabetes: an executive summary (report). Diabet Med. 2011;28(7):772–7. https://doi.org/10.1111/j.1464-5491.2011.03320.x.
4. Garcia TJ, Brown SA. Diabetes Management in the Nursing Home. A systematic review of the literature. The Diabetes Educator. 2011;37(2):167–87.
5. Andreassen LM, Sandberg S, Kristensen GBB, Sølvik UØ, Kjome RLS. Nursing home patients with diabetes: prevalence, drug treatment and glycemic control. Diabetes Res Clin Pract. 2014;105(1):102–9. https://doi.org/10.1016/j.diabres.2014.04.012.
6. Drageset J, Nygaard HA, Eide GE, Bondevik M, Nortvedt MW, Natvig GK. Sense of coherence as a resource in relation to health-related quality of life among mentally intact nursing home residents - a questionnaire study. Health Qual Life Outcomes. 2008;6:85. https://doi.org/10.1186/1477-7525-6-85.
7. Helsedirektoratet. Veileder for utvikling av kunnskapsbaserte retningslinjer. Oslo: Helsediretoratet; 2012. Available from: https://helsedirektoratet.no/retningslinjer/veileder-for-utvikling-av-kunnskapsbaserte-retningslinjer Accessed 11 Aug 2016.
8. Hølleland G, Sunnevåg K. Diabetes i sykehjem - Fagprosedyre fra et fagringarbeid høsten 2011. Bergen: Nasjonalt nettverk for fagprosedyrer; 2011. Available from: http://www.helsebiblioteket.no/microsite/fagprosedyrer/fagprosedyrer/diabetes-i-sykehjem-behandling [Accessed 11 Oct 2014].
9. Ot.prp. nr. 91 (2010-2011). Lov om kommunale helse- og omsorgstjenester m.m. (helse- og omsorgstjenesteloven). Oslo: Helse- og omsorgsdepartementet.
10. World Health Organization (WHO). Health topics: Patient safety. World Health Organization; 2016. Available from: http://www.who.int/topics/patient_safety/en/. Accessed 7 Sep 2016
11. Ammouri AA, Tailakh AK, Muliira JK, Geethakrishnan R, Al Kindi SN. Patient safety culture among nurses. Int Nurs Rev. 2015;62(1):102–10. https://doi.org/10.1111/inr.12159.
12. Castle GN, Wagner ML, Perera CS, Ferguson MJ, Handler MS. Assessing resident safety culture in nursing homes: using the nursing home survey on resident safety. Journal of Patient Safety. 2010;6(2):59–67. https://doi.org/10.1097/PTS.0b013e3181bc05fc.

13. Hughes CM, Lapane KL. Nurses' and nursing assistants' perceptions of patient safety culture in nursing homes. Int J Qual Health Care. 2006;18(4):281–6. https://doi.org/10.1093/intqhc/mzl020.

14. Handler SM, Castle NG, Studenski SA, Perera S, Fridsma DB, Nace DA, et al. Patient safety culture assessment in the nursing home. Quality and Safety in Health Care. 2006;15(6):400–4.

15. Castle GN, Sonon KE. A culture of patient safety in nursing homes. Quality and Safety in Health Care. 2006;15(6):405–8. https://doi.org/10.1136/qshc.2006.018424.

16. Castle GN, Wagner LM, Ferguson JC, Handler SM. Nursing home deficiency citations for safety. Journal of Aging & Social Policy. 2010;23(1):34–57. https://doi.org/10.1080/08959420.2011.532011.

17. Thomas KS, Hyer K, Castle NG, Branch LG, Andel R, Weech-Maldonado R. Patient safety culture and the association with safe resident Care in Nursing Homes. Gerontologist. 2012;52(6):802–11. https://doi.org/10.1093/geront/gns007.

18. Bonner AF, Castle NG, Men A, Handler SM. Certified nursing Assistants' perceptions of nursing home patient safety culture: is there a relationship to clinical outcomes? J Am Med Dir Assoc. 2009;10(1):11–20. https://doi.org/10.1016/j.jamda.2008.06.004.

19. Haugstvedt A, Aarflot M, Igland J, Landbakk T, Graue M. Diabetes knowledge in nursing homes and home-based care services: a validation study of the Michigan diabetes knowledge test adapted for use among nursing personnel. BMC nursing 2016; DOI: https://doi.org/10.1186/s12912-016-0159-1, URL: http://www.biomedcentral.com/1472-6955/15/40

20. Dunning T, Duggan N, Svage BA. The McKellar guidelines for managing older people with diabetes in residential and other care setting. Geelong, Australia: Deakin University and Barwon Health; 2014.

21. Sorra J, Franklin M, Streagle S. Survey User's guide. Nursing home survey on patient safety culture. Rockville: Agency for Healthcare Research and Quality; 2008. Available from: http://www.ahrq.gov/sites/default/files/publications/files/nhguide.pdf [Accessed 8 Oct 2015].

22. Sorra J, Famolaro T, Yount N, Burns W, Liu H, Shyy M. AHRQ Nursing Home Survey on Patient Safety Culture: 2014 User Comparative Database Report. Rockville, MD: 2014. Available from: http://www.ahrq.gov/sites/default/files/wysiwyg/professionals/quality-patient-safety/patientsafetyculture/nursing-home/2014/nhsurv14-ptl.pdf [Accessed 8 Oct 2016].

23. Cappelen K, Aase K, Storm M, Hetland J, Harris A. Psychometric properties of the nursing home survey on patient safety culture in Norwegian nursing homes. BMC Health Serv Res. 2016;16(1):446. https://doi.org/10.1186/s12913-016-1706-x.

24. Famolaro T, Yount ND, Greene K, Hare R, Thornton S, Sorra J. Nursing Home Survey on Patient Safety Culture 2016 User Comparative Database Report. Rockville, MD: 2016. Available from: http://www.ahrq.gov/sites/default/files/wysiwyg/professionals/quality-patient-safety/patientsafetyculture/nursing-home/2016/nhsurv16-pt1.pdf [Accessed 2 Nove 2016].

25. Castle GN. Nurse Aides' ratings of the resident safety culture in nursing homes. Int J Qual Health Care. 2006;18(5):370–6. https://doi.org/10.1093/intqhc/mzl038.

26. Øgar B. Kommunikasjon for bedre kvalitet i helsetjenesten. Anmeldelser. Tidsskrift for Den norske legeforening. 2011;131(20):2039–40.

27. Danielsson M, Nilsen P, Ohrn A, Rutberg H, Fock J, Carlfjord S. Patient safety subcultures among registered nurses and nurse assistants in Swedish hospital care: a qualitative study. BMC Nurs. 2014;13(1):39. https://doi.org/10.1186/s12912-014-0039-5.

28. Fayers PM, Machin D. Quality of life. The assessment, analysis and interpretation of patient-reported outcomes. 2nd. Chichester: John Wiley & Sons Ltd; 2007. p. 391–454.

29. Migdal A, Yarandi SS, Smiley D, Umpierrez GE. Update on diabetes in the elderly and in nursing home residents. J Am Med Dir Assoc. 2011;12(9):627–32. https://doi.org/10.1016/j.jamda.2011.02.010.

30. Agarwal G, Sherifali D, Kaasalainen S, Dolovich L, Akhtar-Danesh N. Nurses' perception and comfort level with diabetes management practices in long-term care. Can J Diabetes. 2014;38(5):314–9. https://doi.org/10.1016/j.jcjd.2013.12.003.

31. Singhal A, Segal A, Munshi M. Diabetes in long-term care facilities. Current Diabetes Reports. 2014;14(3):1–9. https://doi.org/10.1007/s11892-013-0464-y.

32. Kuehn BM. IOM sets out "gold standard" practices for creating guidelines, systematic reviews. The Journal of the American Medical Association. 2011;305(18):1846–8.

33. Flottorp S, Aakhus E. Implementeringsforskning: vitenskap for forbedring av praksis. Norsk Epidemiologi. 2013;23(2):187-96. DOI: https://doi.org/10.5324/nje.v23i2.1643

34. Heimro LS, Haugstvedt A. Dokumentasjon og oppfølging av bebuarar med diabetes i sjukeheim. Sykepleie forskning. 2015;10(3):216–26.

35. Polit DF, Beck CT. Nursing research: generating and assessing evidence for nursing practice. 9 ed. Philadelphia: Wolters Kluwer Health; 2012.

36. Buljac-Samardzic M, van Wijngaarden JDH, Dekker-van Doorn CM. Safety culture in long-term care: a cross-sectional analysis of the safety attitudes questionnaire in nursing and residential homes in the Netherlands. BMJ Quality & Safety. 2015;25(6):1–9. https://doi.org/10.1136/bmjqs-2014-003397.

Student evaluation of the impact of changes in teaching style on their learning: a mixed method longitudinal study

Susan Jones[1*], Somasundari Gopalakrishnan[2], Charles A. Ameh[2], Brian Faragher[2], Betty Sam[3], Roderick R. Labicane[4], Hossinatu Kanu[5], Fatmata Dabo[6], Makally Mansary[5], Rugiatu Kanu[5] and Nynke van den Broek[2]

Abstract

Background: Maternal and Child Health Aides are the largest nursing cadre in Sierra Leone providing maternal and child health care at primary level. Poor healthcare infrastructure and persistent shortage of suitably qualified health care workers have contributed to high maternal and newborn morbidity and mortality. In 2012, 50% of the MCHAides cohort failed their final examination and the Government of Sierra Leone expressed concerns about the quality of teaching within the programmes. Lack of teaching resources and poor standards of teaching led to high failure rates in final examinations reducing the number of newly qualified nurses available for deployment.

Methods: A mixed-methods approach using semi-structured observations of teaching sessions and completion of a questionnaire by students was used. Fourteen MCHAide Training Schools across all districts of Sierra Leone, 140 MCHAide tutors and 513 students were included in the study. In each school, teaching was observed by two researchers at baseline, 3 and 6 months after the tutor training programme. Students completed a questionnaire on the quality of teaching and learning in their school at the same time points.

Results: A total of 513 students completed the questionnaire, 120 tutors took part in the training and 66 lessons across all schools were observed. There was a statistically significant ($p < 0.05$) improvement in mean student evaluation of teaching and learning in 12/19 areas tested at follow-up compared to baseline. Observation of 66 teaching sessions demonstrated an increase in the number of student-focused, interactive teaching methods used.

Conclusion: Prior to the teaching and learning workshops there was little student-focused learning within the schools. Teaching was conducted predominantly using lectures even for practical sessions. Training tutors to move away from didactic teaching towards a more student-focused approach leads to increased student satisfaction with teaching and learning within the schools.

Keywords: Nurse education, Student satisfaction

Background

Sierra Leone is ranked 183rd among 187 nations in the Human Development Index and the country faces many challenges in providing maternal and newborn care. For a population of just over 6 million, there are 0.22 nurses-midwives and 1.66 medical doctors per 10,000 population. This demonstrates a lack of human resources when compared to the World Health Organization recommendation of 23 doctors, nurses and midwives per 10,000 population [1]. In 2000 Sierra Leone reported a maternal mortality ratio (MMR) of 1800 per 100,000 live births which improved steadily to 1495 in 2005 and 857 in 2008. However, in 2016, post the Ebola epidemic, there was again a rise in MMR to 1360, compared to the sub-Saharan African average of 546/100,000 [1].

Following the introduction in Sierra Leone of free health care for pregnant and lactating women in 2010, there has been a steady increase in the number of women attending for antenatal care, with 78% of women attending for 4 visits and nearly 97% attending at least

* Correspondence: S.jones@hud.ac.uk
[1]School of Human and Health Sciences, University of Huddersfield, Queensgate, Huddersfield HD1 3DH, UK
Full list of author information is available at the end of the article

one antenatal care (ANC) visit [1]. In working towards Millennium Development Goal 4 (to reduce child mortality by 2015) and 5 (to improve maternal health by 2015) Sierra Leone instituted measures to improve the number of deliveries attended by a skilled birth attendant (SBA). In 2000, 42% of births were attended by an SBA which rose to 97% in 2012 but dropped back to 60% in 2016 [2]. The causes of maternal death are well known with 80% being due to haemorrhage, infection, eclampsia, complications of unsafe abortion and obstructed labour [3]. |It is also well known that having healthcare workers who are skilled in providing the continuum of maternal and newborn care and are working in an enabling environment significantly reduces both newborn and maternal morbidity and mortality.

The shortage of healthcare workers in Sierra Leone has led to the introduction of new cadres of nurses. Maternal and Child Health Aide (MCHA) training was introduced in 1972 in four districts. Women who had at least 3 years of secondary education and were aged over 25 years of age were able to apply for training [4, 5]. A gradual roll-out of the programme meant that in 2012 all 14 districts of Sierra Leone had a MCHA training school. The most recent intake in 2012 saw a total enrolment of 750 students across all districts. In 2014 MCHAs constituted 46% of the total workforce for health, and provided the majority of maternal and newborn health care. Strengthening pre-service training to maximize the learning opportunities of MCHA is crucial if good quality maternal care is to be provided [6].

This study aimed to determine the impact of a tutor development programme on student satisfaction with teaching and learning. In 2012, a high failure rate (50%) of the MCHA student cohort led the Ministry of Health and Sanitation (MoHS) and partners to question how effective the teaching and learning was within the schools. With its funding partner, UNICEF, the MoHS requested the evaluation of the academic quality of the MCHA training programme including the involvement of the programme managers and staff responsible for the teaching and learning environment.

An observational study of the teaching styles employed within each MCHAide school in 2015 showed teaching was predominantly didactic, teaching aids were rarely used (less than 15%) and teaching was tutor focused rather than student focused [7]. Over-crowding in many of the schools, lack of appropriate classroom furniture and inconsistent electricity supply where findings contributing to a poor learning environment and academic output in these schools.

Studies have shown that there is a positive correlation between the quality of teaching and student satisfaction [8] and student satisfaction and grades [9]. Good teaching quality enhances student performance leading to higher scores and higher student satisfaction [10]. We therefore, looked at student satisfaction as an indicator for changes in the quality of teaching. This allowed us to determine quality of teaching without adding the additional burden of further assessments to the students and the school. Results from the student final examinations were also recorded as a measure of student performance.

The research team were asked to work with the MCHA schools to improve the quality of teaching and the learning environment in the Schools. The aims of this study were: 1) to examine the impact of a training programme to equip tutors with the skills to increase the number of student-focused lessons; and 2) to determine the impact of changes in teaching on student satisfaction.

Style of teaching, subject matter and student learning styles all combine to influence how well a student learns and how satisfied they will be with their education [11]. The high failure rate in the 2012 MCHA cohort of students indicates a breakdown in one or more of these areas. For nursing students to become competent and independent practitioners who can recall theory and practice in sometimes stressful situations, requires an education system that encourages student focused learning, reflective practice and takes account of the diversity of the teaching matter [12]. The global shift from traditional lectures to interactive and group based learning is based on the social constructivist theory that learners build on the experiences, previous knowledge, cultural backgrounds and social influences to become self-directed learners. In Sierra Leone students are used to being taught through a reductionist teacher focused approach; it is therefore important to understand how any changes in teaching practice influence student satisfaction and learning.

Concerns about the quality of pre-service education are not confined to Sierra Leone. Fullerton et al. [13] report on three sub Saharan African countries which continue to use didactic, lecture based training despite ongoing concerns about the quality of such training. As in the MCHA schools many of the teachers that Fullerton observed had no formal training in teaching and learning and were employed for their clinical rather than teaching expertise.

Methods

This longitudinal, mixed methods study used a phenomenographical approach which offers a more sophisticated and complex understanding of teaching and learning because it includes what is happening with both the tutors and the students [14–16]. Structured non-participant observation was used to observe the amount of student focused teaching in each school at baseline.

Participants

All students from all 14 MCHA schools were asked to participate in the study. Given the large number of students (750) self-administered questionnaires were used to determine student satisfaction with the learning and teaching environment. Each school takes approximately 40–60 students in each cohort with a total of 1258 h of taught theory from 10 teachers per school. At the request of the MoHS, all 14 schools were included in the programme to prevent any school being potentially disadvantaged. In addition to the tutor training, each school received skills room equipment and audio-visual aids to assist tutors in developing more interactive teaching methods.

Data collection

From 2013 to 2014 four education experts from the research team facilitated four district based, 2-day workshops for 10 core teaching staff (including the School coordinator) from each of the 14 MCHA schools (140 core staff in total). There were 35 tutors in each work shop. None of the MCHA tutors had a formal teaching qualification.

The workshop aimed to develop tutors understanding of teaching and learning theories and how to apply these in practice; to understand the concept of student focused learning; to understand how to apply different teaching methods within the classroom and to develop skills in reflective practice. The workshops covered active teaching and learning methods, lesson planning, writing learning outcomes, reflective practice, supportive supervision, mentorship and effective learning environments. During the final session of the 2-day workshop tutors developed an action plan for their own school to implement their learning from the workshop into practice. In addition, tutors also took part in formative teaching practice both in the classroom and simulation or skills room.

All workshops were completed within a two-week period and first follow up observations conducted 3 months afterwards. It was anticipated that this would allow tutors time to start implementing changes in some of their lessons. Observed classes included only those tutors who had been to the workshop.

A descriptive analysis of the age and entry qualification of MCHA students at the time of the study was conducted by reviewing admission records. This was to establish compliance with admission criteria as there is a high potential that less qualified students (on entry) may find it more difficult to cope with the curricula.

Prior to the tutors training programme a baseline visit was conducted for each of the 14 MCHA schools in August–September 2013. Three follow-up visits were planned to all 14 MCHA schools across Sierra Leone. The follow-up visits were timed to coincide with key dates during the MCHA training.

First follow-up was at the end of the students first year (3 months from baseline). Second follow-up occurred immediately prior to their second year examinations (6 months from baseline). Final follow-up was conducted at the end of the programme (12 months from baseline).

Due to the Ebola epidemic in Sierra Leone which occurred from May 2014 to December 2015 the MCHA schools were closed in August 2014. Only 10 of the 14 schools could be visited for the second follow-up and no schools could be visited for the third follow-up. Final results are based on the 10 schools seen at second follow-up only.

At each visit (baseline, 3 months and 6 months), both qualitative and quantitative methodology was used to gain as full a picture as possible of the teaching and learning within each school and allow for triangulation of data. Data collectors worked in pairs to administer the student questionnaire but conducted independent observation of the teaching using a standardised data collection tool.

The aim was to observe two one-hour teaching sessions at each visit in each MCHA school (2x14x3 visits = 84 observations) and ask 750 students to complete a questionnaire at each visit (3 × 750 = 2250 questionnaires). Outcome measures were student evaluation of teaching and learning an increase in student focused sessions, reduction in the use of didactic teaching methods and increase in student learning.

Both tutors and students were provided with written and verbal information about the study by the research team and asked to sign a consent form if they agreed to participate.

Observation of teaching

A structured non-participant observation method was used to observe teaching sessions in each school at each visit [17]. A full explanation was given to the MCHA tutors on the purpose of the planned visits to their schools by the research team and their consent for this sought. Event sampling was used to select the teaching sessions and keep disruption of the normal school timetable to a minimum [18]. There is an underlying assumption when using structured observation that the researchers are familiar with, and understand, the activity being observed [19]. Each member of the research team was involved with and experienced in teaching and learning at a pre and/or post registration level. A modified pre-designed structured observation form was used that assessed teaching methods, student learning and student involvement.

Researchers also took notes during the observations which were subsequently transcribed. Transcription was completed by the same members of the research team to aid with familiarisation of the data which is a key aspect of the framework approach [20]. One member of the research team independently coded the transcripts from four schools which gave an initial coding framework. Though a deductive approach was used to provide an initial structure for the observations an inductive open-coding approach was taken for the final coding [20]. Informal feedback was provided to tutors after the observations by the research team.

Student questionnaires

Students were asked to evaluate the teaching and learning within their own school through an anonymised self-administered questionnaire. Questionnaires were adapted for language and clarity in partnership with MoHS from those used at the Liverpool School of Tropical Medicine to obtain student feedback on teaching. Students rated the lessons in three areas, teaching methods, student learning and student involvement, as these are thought to be the key components which influence teaching and learning [Clark 11]. A 19 question, 5-point Likert scale was used. Basic demographics including the student's highest academic qualification on entry to the programme and their age were also obtained. Students completed the questionnaire immediately after the lesson being observed. MCHA tutors were asked to leave the classroom during the completion of the questionnaire.

Data analysis

Qualitative data analysis was completed using the Framework Analysis approach. This approach is useful where data covers similar topics or key issues and so can be categorised [20]. In this study the structured observation form used a deductive approach to pre-select key themes of teaching and learning which could be considered as the key issues [20]. It was expected that other sub themes may also occur at follow-up visits which would be incorporated into the Framework analysis.

All student questionnaires were electronically scanned and processed using Formic. SPSS version 22 was used for analysis. New random samples were selected on each occasion, so most students completed a questionnaire at just one of the three assessment times; these samples were considered to be statistically independent. One-way analyses of variance (ANOVA) were used to evaluate the changes in mean student satisfaction scores across the three assessment points; statistical significance was set at the conventional alpha level of 5% ($p \leq 0.05$). Each of the test items (questions) were analysed individually and then the total score across all 19 items was evaluated; Cronbach's alpha (coefficient of reliability) was calculated to ensure adequate internal reliability of this total score.

Results

Student evaluation of teaching and learning

Five hundred thirteen students completed the questionnaire at baseline; 518 at first follow-up and 466 at second follow-up. All students on the MCHA programme are female. Descriptive analysis of the age and qualification on entry showed that not all students met the admission criteria of; 1) being between the ages of 26–40 years; 2) have completed level-3 at senior secondary school, and; 3) at least attempted but not necessarily passed the West Africa Senior School Certificate Examination (WASSCE) or GCE O-level (Table 1). Sixty-three (12.5%) students had failed to attain the minimum academic entry criteria. In total, 44% (222) had a higher qualification than WASSCE on entry to the programme. Of the 504 students who completed the baseline questionnaire, 276 (55%) had not passed their final examination at the end of their secondary school education.

Positive evaluation of teaching and learning by the students increased from baseline to second follow up as the number of student focused lessons increased. Twelve (1) out of 19 areas assessed obtained a statistically significant higher mean score ($p < 0.05$). Only 4 areas did not show an increase in mean scores over time (Table 2). In particular students positively evaluated the usefulness of teaching methods ($p = 0,002$) as more student focused methods were used.

Variables which could be considered to be important in developing more student-focused learning and therefore to be influenced by the training workshop included; the teaching methods used, being encouraged to think and to ask questions, the availability of tutors outside of lessons and the breath of learning and student interest in the subject. There was a statistically significant increase in student scores at follow-up compared to

Table 1 Age and qualification of students on entry to Maternal and Child Health Aide training

Age at entry n (%)					
Student age in years	18–25	26–33	34–41	42–50	Meet criteria n (%)
	108 (21%)	230 (45%)	146 (28%)	20 (4%)	376 (75%)
Educational qualification at entry n (%)					
SSS3	Passed WASSC	Attempted WASSC	GCE O level	Other	Meet criteria n (%)
63 (12.5%)	6 (1%)	213 (42%)	133 (26%)	89 (18%)	441 (88%)

SSS3 3rd year of senior secondary school, *WASSCE* West Africa Senior School Certificate Examination

baseline. Students also reported that lessons were better organised and tutors more respectful to their students. A decrease in the number of students reporting that lessons were difficult from baseline to follow-up may indicate the positive impact of the new teaching styles on student learning as they moved into their second year.

There was a statistically significant increase in the positive evaluation by students of variables which could be considered to be indirectly influenced by what goes on in the classroom; these included students completing homework and the numbers attending all lessons. Students continued to report that it was difficult to find time for self-study which may be influenced by commitments outside of the school including family.

Cronbach's alpha for the total score using all 19 questions was 0.71; this increased to 0.72 when the question on 'Hours of self-study' was not included and to 0.79 when the questions on 'Content of lesson too hard', 'Hours of self-study' and 'Difficult to find time' were not included. This total score increased highly significantly between baseline and the first follow-up assessment but there was only a very modest and non-significant increase between the first and second follow-ups.

Observation of teaching

Across all 14 schools 120 85%) tutors took part in the teaching and learning workshop. A total of 26 lessons were observed at baseline, 21 at the first follow-up and 19 at the second follow-up (66 of 84 planned observations = 78.6%). Following transcription, qualitative data was coded using Framework analysis into a total of 10 key themes and 48 sub themes (Table 3).

Student participation, teacher preparation and style of teaching

Observed methods of teaching were classified into two groups based on the amount of student involvement (Table 4). Tutor-focused lessons had minimal student involvement, relied on didactic methods and centred on students answering questions as a group rather than as individuals. Student-focused lessons were those which encouraged individual questions and answers and employed interactive teaching methods such as role play, discussion groups or practical's. At baseline 58% out of the 26 lessons were described as using didactic (tutor-focused) methods, this decreased to 33% of lessons at first follow-up and to 31% of lessons at second follow-up. There was a corresponding increase in student-focused (interactive) lessons from 4% at baseline, to 29% at first follow-up and 21% at second follow-up. The number of lessons described as being well organised also increased from baseline to follow up.

The learning and teaching environment

The quality of the learning and teaching environment varied across the schools with some having well ventilated, well-lit classrooms with electricity and of an adequate size, to those that were too small for the number of students, poorly ventilated and without electricity. However, following the training workshops tutors did try and make better use of the limited space and facilities they had and included more student-focused teaching such as group work and discussions. Despite the many challenges that the schools face there were good relationships in each school between the students and their tutors, particularly with the co-ordinators for each school who also provided the majority of teaching.

Each training schools was provided with audio visual equipment (projectors, a desktop and laptop computer) and skills equipment including mannequins and anatomical models to develop a skills room.

Lesson content, depth of learning and student feedback

The depth of student learning was found to be an important issue, especially at baseline where the majority of teaching was didactic with rote learning, memorising and little synthesising of information. Tutors sometimes ran out of time to meet all of the lessons learning outcomes or were repeating previous lessons when timetabled tutors did not attend their sessions. A lack of individualized student feedback was noted, with peer feedback given only in the form of applause by the whole class in any particular session. No formative or summative assessments were observed during the study.

Discussion

Teaching and learning is a complex mix of many components which all contribute to the overall learning experience of the student. Studies suggest that students learn in different ways and that tutors should adopt a teaching methodology that takes into account these different learning styles [11]. Matching teaching styles with each student's individual learning style can be difficult if not impossible for large student groups. Using diverse teaching styles is therefore important in order to maximize learning [12]. In many countries teaching has moved away from didacticism to a more facilitative approach which sees the student rather than the tutor as the focus of the classroom. The aim of such a student-focusedapproach is to equip students with skills in critical thinking, problem-solving and independent learning [21]. This is particularly important in dynamic areas of work such as nursing. Discerning how students evaluate the impact of changes in teaching styles is important to fully understand their impact on learning. Changes in teaching style are not just challenging to faculty but also to students and this has to be

Table 2 Student assessment following programme to strengthen teaching at MCHAide schools across Sierra Leone

Name of variable in student questionnaire	Baseline			3-month follow-up			6-month follow-up			p value*
	Number of students n	Mean score (1–5)	95% CI	Number of students n	Mean score (1–5)	95% CI	Number of students n	Mean score (1–5)	95% CI	
1. Clarity of objectives	509	4.72	4.66–4.79	516	4.79	4.73–4.85	466	4.80	4.75–4.86	0.107
2. Easy explanations given	510	4.67	4.61–4.73	516	4.78	4.73–4.83	465	4.80	4.75–4.85	0.003
3. Useful teaching methods used	510	4.52	4.44–4.60	516	4.71	4.65–4.77	466	4.75	4.70–4.80	0.002
4. Tutor encourages questions	510	4.73	4.67–4.79	517	4.83	4.78–4.87	466	4.81	4.76–4.85	0.066
5. Lesson is well organised	506	4.33	4.23–4.43	518	4.72	4.67–4.78	464	4.68	4.62–4.73	<0.001
6. Tutor encourages thinking	508	4.28	4.19–4.37	515	4.55	4.48–4.62	465	4.55	4.49–4.61	<0.001
7. Tutor is available for extra support	512	3.65	3.52–3.78	515	3.93	3.82–4.05	464	4.00	3.88–4.11	0.001
8. Tutor treats students respectfully	512	4.38	4.27–4.48	515	4.28	4.18–4.38	465	4.56	4.49–4.63	0.005
9. Wide breadth of learning	513	4.64	4.58–4.71	518	4.81	4.76–4.85	464	4.83	4.79–4.87	<0.001
10. Level of student Interest in subject	511	4.63	4.56–4.69	518	4.73	4.68–4.79	463	4.75	4.69–4.80	0.011
11. Students think subject taught is important	513	4.89	4.85–4.93	518	4.90	4.87–4.93	463	4.88	4.85–4.92	0.402
12. Students attend all lessons	505	4.64	4.57–4.71	516	4.61	4.54–4.67	462	4.59	4.53–4.65	0.004
13. Students complete homework	496	3.85	3.73–3.97	510	4.24	4.16–4.33	459	4.33	4.26–4.40	<0.001
14. Students participate in class discussions	509	4.67	4.62–4.73	512	4.68	4.63–4.73	463	4.68	4.63–4.74	0.706
15. Students expectations of breadth of learning	510	4.56	4.48–4.64	513	4.81	4.76–4.85	463	4.81	4.77–4.86	<0.001
16. Students think lessons are difficult	501	2.98	2.85–3.11	509	2.62	2.49–2.74	457	2.86	2.73–3.00	<0.001
17. Students find time for Self-study	500	3.88	3.76–4.00	513	3.85	3.74–3.96	463	3.95	3.85–4.06	0.673
18. Students find it difficult to find time for self-study	507	3.02	2.88–3.16	514	2.74	2.61–2.87	463	3.11	2.98–3.24	<0.001
19. Hours of self-study by student	511	2.93	2.84–3.02	517	2.81	2.73–2.89	464	2.87	2.79–2.96	0.239
Total (out of 95)	460	71.3	70.61–72.03	471	73.6	73.10–74.12	445	73.8	73.24–74.36	<0.001

*p value for comparison of scores at follow up with those obtained at baseline

Table 3 Observation of teaching: key themes and sub themes identified using framework analysis

Key Theme	Sub themes
Student participation	• use of local language • role play • examples from students • answering questions • asking questions • student reflection • students summarise key points of lecture • note taking • student tasks
Lesson preparedness by tutor	• lesson notes/guide • learning outcomes • teaching plan • adherence to timetable • organization • pace of teaching • Interruption of session by tutor
Use of visual aids/teaching equipment	• blackboard • IT • diagrams • use of equipment/anatomical models
Depth of learning	• memorisation • rote learning • understanding • synthesising information • meeting learning outcomes/objectives
Style of teaching	• lectures • discussions • links to future lectures • links to previous lectures • practical demonstrations • links to practice • scenarios
Provides students with feedback	• individualized feedback given • lack of formative feedback • student peer feedback given
Content	• depth • appropriateness • repeated topic • did not complete content
Assessment	• formative • summative
Teaching environment	• ventilation • light • space • desks and chairs available • adapted teaching style to fit environment
Student/tutor relationship	• student commitment • tutor commitment • student/tutor rapport • control of class

Table 4 Classification and characteristics of observed teaching styles

Didactic/Tutor-focused	Interactive/Student group-focused
Lecture	Student practical
Group Q&A	Scenarios
Tutor demonstration	Role play
	Seminar discussion
	1:1 tutoring
	Individual Q&A
	Tutorial

being 'active teaching methods' have a more positive impact on students learning outcomes [22]. In nursing using a didactic, information-giving teaching approach does not equip students with the ability to question and synthesize multiple sources of information, skills which will be needed by nurses in their daily practice [23].

The introduction of task shifting and of new cadres of healthcare workers in Sierra Leone has meant that new training schools have been set up; bringing challenges in finding suitably qualified tutors to deliver a new and expanded curriculum in often shorter than conventional time frames. Task shifting generally involves shorter, more focused training programmes to equip healthcare workers for specific settings [24]. Sierra Leone is not unique within Africa in providing education from junior to higher education through a didactic teaching process [25]. There is a need to develop an education system that provides training for the tutors (often senior healthcare providers) whose capacity and enthusiasm to deliver the new curriculum using new teaching methodology is critical to the success of the programmes. In addition, in most settings, there is an identified urgent need to improve the quality of the learning environment [26, 27].

Main findings

Both tutors and students contribute to the success of teaching and learning. From a tutor's perspective how they engage and work with students can contribute to the overall effectiveness of their teaching. The workshop intervention was deemed successful in encouraging tutors to change their methods of teaching with a decrease in tutor-focused and an increase in student-focused methods of teaching. The aim of the training workshop was to train and encourage tutors to use a wider variety of teaching methods and move away from simple didactic teaching, and in this respect the workshop was successful. However, this change in teaching also needs to be recognised as being useful by the students for their learning.

acknowledged if they are to be effective. In this study students recognized the changes in teaching style and positively evaluated their usefulness to their learning.

Some argue that the most effective teaching style is the one that the tutor feels most comfortable using, despite the students learning style. However, teaching activities and styles that can generally be classified as

Data from the student questionnaires showed a positive evaluation of teaching and learning in the schools as the number of student focused lessons increased. Interactive teaching methods have increased in popularity in high resource areas but less so in low resource areas such as Sierra Leone. Where there is a lack of education and information technology resources then the teaching methods used take on an even higher importance as they are often the only information resource available to students. Encouraging students to be part of developments in teaching by asking them to evaluate new methods can further help to develop the learning and teaching environment.

Though there is an agreed minimum qualification for entry to the MCHA training programme in Sierra Leone, 12.5% of the students did not have this and this may have affected their ability to learn at the required level. At follow-up there was a decrease in students who reported finding the lessons difficult (mean 2.98 at baseline compared to 2.86 at second follow up follow-up). Despite the difficulty of lessons increasing as the students moved into their second and final year when more complex subjects were taught. This may be a reflection of the impact that the move from didactic to student focused teaching was having with students reporting an increase in being encouraged to think, ask questions and a greater breadth of learning.

Some areas of learning and teaching are less easy for tutors to influence (hours of self-study, finding time to study) and it is reasonable to expect that just changing the methods of teaching could not influence these. Nevertheless, it is important for the overall picture of teaching and learning within the MCHA schools to know if there are factors outside of the classroom that may hinder learning. All of the students are female who have family commitments outside of their studies and which could reasonably be expected to impact on their self-study time. The majority of students lived in homes without a regular electricity supply further hampering study at home. Further research is needed to understand which particular enablers of student learning can be strengthened and how in this context.

Researchers were surprised to find that tutors advised students not to take notes. There is contradictory evidence on the effectiveness of in-class note taking and if this benefits students understanding or is a distraction. Though it would seem appropriate, given the lack of other reference material available, that the MCH Aide students should be allowed to take notes or have these provided by their tutors [28, 29]. Where students have limited or no access to learning materials or libraries the information provided within the classroom may take on a higher importance. The provision of learning resources is particularly important for this group of students who additionally reported finding time for self-study outside of the MCHA School difficult.

This study has important findings which need to be considered by countries looking at task shifting health care and introducing new cadres of nursing. The increase in numbers of healthcare workers in formal education programmes is not necessarily enough to meet the health needs of a country. The quality of the education programme and standards of teaching need to be addressed if such programmes are to successfully bridge the human resource shortages.

Strengths and limitations

The study involved both tutors and students and therefore obtained a comprehensive view of teaching and learning within the schools. Observation of teaching was new to the MCHA tutors but appropriate within the context of the study to determine the styles of teaching used and was, in fact, welcomed by the tutors. The use of peer review of teaching (on which the observations were based) is well established in many academic institutions, the aim of which is to provide constructive feedback to tutors on their practice [30]. The presence of the observers may have altered the dynamics within the classroom [31].

A planned final follow-up visit at 12 months and focus groups with the tutors following tutor training could not be completed due to the Ebola epidemic which occurred from May 2014 to November 2015. This is unfortunate as it would have provided self-evaluation of the tutors and information on the sustainability of the observed changes within the schools. The researchers also planned to conduct student focus groups to explore their perceptions and experiences in more detail than can be done via a questionnaire, but again the Ebola epidemic prevented this.

Conclusion

Encouraging student evaluation of new teaching styles is important if they are to engage fully with the learning environment. Tutors provide feedback to students on their progress but it is also essential for students to provide feedback on how teaching methods are impacting on their learning if nurse education is to progress and meet the global shortage of qualified nurses.

The aim of the tutor training workshop was to increase the standard of teaching and learning within the schools and increase the number of students passing their examinations. In the State final examination for the 2012–2015 cohort 80% of students passed compared to a 50% pass rate in the previous 2010 cohort (MoHS verbal communication from the national MCHA Coordinator).

Abbreviations
ANC: Antenatal care; CMNH-LSTM: Centre for Maternal and Newborn Health at the Liverpool School of Tropical Medicine; MCHAides: Maternal and Child Health Aides; MMR: Maternal Mortality Ratio; MoHS: Ministry of Health and Sanitation; SBA: Skilled Birth Attendance; WASSC: West Africa Senior School Certificate Examination

Acknowledgments
The authors would like to acknowledge the approval and support given by the Ministry of Health and Sanitation Sierra Leone for the study.

Funding
The study was funded by UNICEF, Sierra Leone (Grant number 43144788).

Authors' contributions
SJ, SG, CA, NVD, FD, BS, designed the study. SJ, SG, FD, BS, RRL, HK, MM, RK, designed the research tool and carried out acquisition of data; SJ, SG, FD, BS, RRL, HK, MM, RK, NVD, BF analysed the data. SJ, SG, CA, BF, BS, RRL, HK, FD, MM, RK, NVD drafted revised the manuscript and gave approval for the final version.

Competing interests
The authors declare that they have no competing interests.

Author details
[1]School of Human and Health Sciences, University of Huddersfield, Queensgate, Huddersfield HD1 3DH, UK. [2]Centre for Maternal and Newborn Health, Liverpool School of Tropical Medicine, Pembroke Place, Liverpool L3 5QA, UK. [3]Centre for Maternal and Newborn Health, Liverpool School of Tropical Medicine, Wilkinson Road, Freetown, Sierra Leone. [4]Welbodi Partnership, Ola During Children's Hospital, Freetown, Sierra Leone. [5]Ministry of Health and Sanitation, Youi Building, Freetown, Sierra Leone. [6]School of Midwifery, Makeni, Sierra Leone.

References
1. World Health Organization. World health statistics 2016. Geneva: World Health Organization; 2016. Accessed 31/08/2016. http://www.who.int/gho/publications/world_health_statistics/2016/EN_WHS2016_AnnexB.pdf
2. Ministry of Health and Sanitation. Sierra Leone demographic and health survey. Freetown, Sierra Leone: Ministry of Health and Sanitation; 2016.
3. Say L, Chou D, Gemmill A, Tunçalp Ö, Moller AB, Daniels J, et al. 'Global causes of maternal death: a WHO systematic analysis', lancet. Glob Health. 2014;2(6):323–33.
4. Aitken IW, Kargbo TK, Gba-Kamara AM. Planning a community orientate midwifery service for Sierra Leone. World Health Forum. 1985;6(2):110–4.
5. Kargbo TK. Rural maternity care in Sierra Leone. Int J Gynaecol Obstet. 1992; 38(S1):S29–31. https://doi.org/10.1016/0020-7292(92)90026-F.
6. United Nations Development Programme. Human development report, sustaining human progress: reducing vulnerabilities and building resilience. New York: United Nations; 2014.
7. Jones S, Ameh CA, Gopalakrishnan S, Sam B, Bull F, Labicane RR, et al. Building capacity for skilled birth attendance: an evaluation of the maternal and child health aides training programme in Sierra Leone. Midwifery. 2015; 31(2015):1186–92. https://doi.org/10.1016/j.midw.2015.09.011.
8. Ko WH. A study of the relationships among effective learning, professional competence, and learning performance in culinary field. Journal of Hospitality, Leisure, Sport & Tourism Education. 2012;11:12–20. https://doi.org/10.1016/j.jhlste.2012.02.010
9. Liu R, Jung L. The commuter student and student satisfaction. Res High Educ. 1980;12(3):215–26. https://doi.org/10.1007/BF00976093
10. Pike GR. The effects of background, coursework, and involvement on students' grades and satisfaction. Res High Educ. 1991;32(1):15–30. https://doi.org/10.1007/BF00992830
11. Clark SD, Latshaw CA. Effects of learning styles/teaching styles on performance in accounting and marketing courses. World Journal of Management. 2012; 4(1):67–81.
12. Banning M. Approaches to teaching; current opinions and related research. Nurse Educ Today. 2005;25(7):502–8.
13. Fullerton JT, Johnson PG, Thompson JB, Vivio D. Quality considerations in midwifery pre-service education: exemplars from Africa. Midwifery. 2011; 27(3):308–15. https://doi.org/10.1016/j.midw.2010.10.011.
14. Micari M, Light G, Calkins S, Streiwieser B. Assessment beyond performance. Phenomenography in education. Am J Eval. 2007;28(4):458–76.
15. Akerlind GS. A phenomenographical approach to developing academic understanding of the nature of teaching and learning. Teach High Educ. 2008;13(6):633–44.
16. Fasse BB, Kolodner JL. In: Fishman B, O'Connor, Divelbiss S, editors. Evaluating classroom practices using qualitative research methods: defining and refining the process: Proceedings of the Fourth International Conference of the Learning Sciences. New Jersey: Lawrence Erlbaum Associates; 2000. p. 193–8.
17. Duxbury JA, Wright KM, Hart A, Bradley K, Roach P, Harris N, et al. A structured observation of the interaction between nurses and patients during the administration of medication in an acute mental health unit. J Clin Nurs. 2010; 19(17–18):2481–92. https://doi.org/10.1111/j.1365-2702.2010.03291.x.
18. Parahoo K. Nursing research, principles, process and issues. 3rd ed. London: Palgrave Macmillan; 2014.
19. Ward DJ, Furber C, Tierney S, Swallow V. Using framework analysis in nursing research: a worked example. J Adv Nurs. 2013;69(11):2423–31. https://doi.org/10.1111/jan.12127.
20. Gale NK, Heath G, Cameron E, Rashid S, Redwood S. Using the framework method for the analysis of qualitative data in multi-disciplinary health research. BMC Med Res Methodol. 2013;13:117. https://doi.org/10.1186/1471-2288-13-117.
21. McCabe A, O'Connor U. Student centred learning: the role and responsibility of the lecturer. Teach High Educ. 2014;19(4):350–9. https://doi.org/10.1080/13562517.2013.860111.
22. Michel N, Cater JJ, Varela O. Active versus passive teaching styles: an empirical study of learning outcomes. Huma Resour Dev Q. 2009;20(4):397–418. https://doi.org/10.1002/hrdq.20025.
23. Chilemba EB, Bruce JC. Teaching styles used in Malawian BSN programmes: a survey of nurse educator preferences. Nurse Educ Today. 2015;35(2):55–60. https://doi.org/10.1016/j.nedt.2014.12.015.
24. Adegoke A, Utz B, Msuya S, van den Broek N. Skilled birth attendants: who is who? A descriptive study of definitions and roles from nine sub Saharan African countries. PLoS One. 2012;7(7):e40220. https://doi.org/10.1371/journal.pone.0040220.
25. Hassan S, Wium W. Quality lies in the eyes of the beholder: a mismatch between student evaluation and peer observation of teaching. Africa Education Review. 2014;11(4):491–511. https://doi.org/10.1080/18146627.2014.935000.
26. Akyeampong K, Lussier K, Pryor J, Westbrook J. Improving teaching and learning of basic maths and reading in Africa: Does teacher preparation count? Int J Educ Dev. 2013;33(3):72–82. https://doi.org/10.1016/j.ijedudev.2012.09.006.
27. Hardman F, Abd-Kadir J, Tibuhinda A. Reforming teacher education in Tanzania. Int J Educ Dev. 2012;32(6):826–34. https://doi.org/10.1016/j.ijedudev.2012.01.002.
28. G. M. Positive effects of restricting student note-taking in a capstone psychology course: reducing the demands of divided attention in the classroom. Teach Psychol. 2014;41(4):340–4. https://doi.org/10.1177/0098628314549707.
29. Chen P-H. The effects of college students in class and after class lecture note-taking on academic performance. The Asia-Pacific Education Researcher. 2013;22(3):173–80.
30. Barnard A, Nash R, McEvoy K, et al. LeaD-in: a cultural change model for peer review of teaching in higher education. High Educ Res Dev. 2015;34(1):30–44.
31. Wickstrom G, Bendix T. The "Hawthorne effect"–what did the original Hawthorne studies actually show? Scandinavian journal of work. Environ Health. 2000;26:363–7.

Knowledge, attitude, and practice of breast Cancer among nurses in hospitals in Asmara, Eritrea

Amanuel Kidane Andegiorgish[1*], Eyob Azeria Kidane[1] and Merhawi Teklezgi Gebrezgi[2]

Abstract

Background: Breast cancer accounted for 1.03% of all deaths in 2014 in Eritrea. Yet the knowledge, attitude, and practice (KAP) of the population in general or the health personnel in the country in relation to the disease, remains unknown. Hence, this study was designed to assess the KAP regarding breast cancer among female nurses working in ten hospital wards in Asmara, Eritrea.

Methods: This was a cross-sectional study conducted among 414 nurses. Descriptive statistics, t-test, and ANOVA were used to evaluate the KAP of the nurses.

Results: Nurses' knowledge about the possible risk factors of breast cancer was low but the nurses knew the signs and symptoms of breast cancer since each sign or symptom was mentioned by > 50% of them. The practice of breast cancer screening, however, was low (only 30 and 11.3% practiced clinical breast examination and mammography respectively). Respondents' family history of breast cancer, having breast problems, their professional level and unit where they worked were associated with the KAP of nurses about breast cancer.

Conclusion: Training programs could help to increase the nurses' knowledge about the risk factors of breast cancer and practice of breast cancer screening. This could also help to increase the knowledge of the public about breast cancer.

Keywords: Breast cancer, Knowledge, Attitude, Practice, Nurse, Asmara, Eritrea

Background

Breast cancer is a major, life-threatening, public health concern. Long-term increase in the incidence of the disease has been observed in both developed and developing countries [1]. It is the most common cause of cancer mortality among women, accounting for 16% of cancer deaths in adult women [2].

In Eritrea, 370 women died from breast cancer in 2014 accounting for 1.03% of total deaths in that year giving an age-adjusted death rate of 21.40 per 100,000 of population [3]. Other source shows similar figures, with increasing rates in recent years in the country [4]. All malignant neoplasms of the breast in all age groups of women reported from all health facilities in Eritrea in the last 13 years (2004–2016) show a steady growth, with minor fluctuations in 2005 and 2009 (Health Information Management System of the Ministry of Health).

Breast cancer risk factors include increased age, genetic mutation, early menstrual period, late or no pregnancy, starting menopause after age 55, not being physically active, being overweight or obese after menopause, having dense breast, using combination hormone therapy, taking oral contraceptives, personal history of breast cancer, personal history of certain non-cancerous breast diseases, a family history of breast cancer, previous treatment using radiation therapy and drinking alcohol [5]. Adequate knowledge about the signs and symptoms and early breast cancer detection through breast self-examination (BSE) or clinical breast examination (CBE) or mammogram, is crucial to reducing breast cancer-related morbidity and mortality.

* Correspondence: akidane2016@gmail.com
[1]Department of Epidemiology and Biostatistics, Asmara College of Health Sciences, School of Public Health, P.O.Box: 8566, Asmara, Eritrea
Full list of author information is available at the end of the article

Information is needed to identify the underlying factors that might influence nurses' own practice of early detection methods of breast cancer. Empowering nurses with information about early detection methods and their related benefits could help in advancing their skills in performing breast self-examination and expanding their role as client educators [6]. Education and awareness need to be culturally appropriate and targeted towards the relevant population, because this may contribute towards an increase early presentation so that highest benefit can be gained [7, 8]. Health care providers, especially those who come in regular contact with women, can play an important role in providing the information regarding breast cancer [9].

Several cross-sectional studies on Knowledge Attitude and Practice (KAP) of breast cancer have been done among nurses in Nigeria [10–13] Ethiopia [14], Turkey [15] Jordan [16, 17], India [18], United Arab Emirates [19], Saudi Arabia [20] and Singapore [21]. Nurses KAP on breast cancer was ranging from relatively low to as high as 100%. There were varying responses in attitude, knowledge of breast cancer screening methods and practice.

Previously, studies on the clinical aspects of breast cancer have been conducted in Eritrea [22–24]. Yet, no published study is available about the KAP of breast cancer among nurses in the country. The aim of this study was, therefore, to assess the (1) nurses' knowledge of breast cancer risk factors, (2) nurses' knowledge of breast cancer signs and symptoms, and (3) nurses' knowledge and practice of breast cancer examinations among female nurses working in ten hospital wards in Asmara. The information obtained could help to initiate interventions to address the gaps in KAP of nurses towards breast cancer. Ultimately, it is hoped that an improved KAP of nurses will contribute towards educating the public about the risk factors and early detection of breast cancer and, thereby, reduce morbidity and mortality due to breast cancer in the population.

Methods
Study design and study population
This was a cross-sectional study designed to assess the KAP of nurses on breast cancer. It was conducted among nurses whose qualifications included certificate, diploma, and degree and who were working in ten hospital wards in Asmara, the capital of Eritrea. All the nurses in the selected health facilities and wards were invited to participate in the study. Majority of the nurses working in the surveyed hospital wards were females.

Data collection
Knowledge of breast cancer among the participants was assessed based on knowledge on risk factors of breast cancer, signs and symptoms of breast cancer and knowledge on BSE, CBE, and mammography. The assessment was done by scoring breast cancer knowledge computed by giving "1" to the correct answer, and "0" for the wrong and 'do not know' answers. Furthermore, a percent knowledge index (PKI) was calculated for each nurse by summing the number of correct answers for all the variables and calculating the percentage of the correct answers. Furthermore, attitude was assessed by asking respondent about their opinions in regards to whether breast cancer is curable, how they would feel if they develop breast cancer and what they would do if they develop BC. Practice was assessed on what respondents do to detect early symptoms and signs of BC.

Data analysis
Data was collected by a pretested, questionnaire. List of study subjects was obtained initially from the Human Resource Management (HRM) office of the studied hospital wards, and after verbal consent was obtained, an interviewer guided self-administered questionnaire was used to collect the data. Collected data were checked for errors and data entry was completed using census survey processing (CSPro) software. Data were analyzed using the statistical package for social sciences (SPSS version 20) software. Descriptive statistics were used for data presentations. Association between categorical variables were explored using Chi-square. Quantitative analysis was performed using t-test for binary variables and ANOVA for more than two variables. $P < 0.05$ was considered statistically significant.

Ethical approval
The study was approved by the Research and Ethics Committee of Asmara College of Health Sciences and Eritrean National Commission for Higher Education. An official letter was sent to concerned hospital directors and oral informed consent was obtained from the study subjects prior to questionnaire administration.

Results
A total of 427 nurses were approached to participate in this study. The complete response rate was 97% and so a total of 414 nurses' responses were included in the data analysis. The mean age of participants was 33.85 ± 11.60 (min 19 and max 69 years). Nearly half (48.6%) of the participants were associate nurses. Similarly, half of the respondents (51%) were unmarried. More than nine-tenths of study participants had no family history of breast cancer or no personal history of breast problems (Table 1).

Table 1 Socio-demographic characteristics of nurses working in ten health facilities in Asmara, Eritrea

Variable	Frequency	Percent
Age		
19–29	222	53.6
30–39	65	15.7
40–49	63	29.7
>=50	64	31.7
Marital Status		
Single	212	51.2
Ever married	202	48.8
Religion		
Muslim	35	8.5
Christian	379	91.5
Family Hx of Breast Cancer		
Yes	32	7.7
No	382	92.3
Having breast problem		
Yes	20	4.8
No	394	95.2
Professional Level		
Associate Nurse	201	48.6
Registered Nurse	170	41.1
BSN	43	10.4
Unite of Work		
Orotta MCH	38	9.1
Private hospital	44	10.6
Medical wards	162	38.9
Surgical Ward	50	12.0
Community hospitals	82	19.7
Ophthalmic hospital	40	9.6

BSN Bachelors of Science in Nursing, *MCH* Maternity Child Health

Knowledge about risk factors of breast cancer

Table 2 shows the responses of the nurses about the risk factors of breast cancer. About 78% of the participants mentioned that smoking is a risk factor for breast cancer. Similarly, 76% stated that breastfeeding decreases the risk of breast cancer and 62% stated that drinking alcohol is a risk factor. About two thirds (69%) agreed that breast cancer could be hereditary and 66% thought that its risk increases with advancing age. Approximately one-third of the nurses stated that having a first child when over 30 is a possible risk factor for breast cancer.

Attitude towards breast cancer

The attitude of the participants on breast lump was satisfactory, 342 (82.2%) of the participants were willing to be examined by a male doctor for their breast (data not

shown). Similarly, 348 (83.7%) were willing to be examined by a doctor within one week suspecting of developing breast lump.

Regarding the first time diagnosis of breast cancer, the response of the participants was scared (61.8%), 95.7% consult a doctor, 10.1% use traditional medicine and 80.8% agree on Mastectomy (If necessary).

When the nurses were asked about their own overall risk of developing breast cancer, 22% thought that they were not at risk, 21.2% thought that they were at low risk, 11.1% at medium risk and 24% at high risk. The remaining 21.6% stated they don't know.

Nurses were also asked if they had any of the risk factors for developing breast cancer, 51.0% answered they had none of the risk factors, 18.8% mentioned having one risk factor, 8.2% having two risk factors and 4.8% having three or more risk factors. On the potential risk factors of breast cancer,51.0% of the respondents answered none, while 18.8% mentioned are having one risk factor, 8.2% two risk factors and 4.8% three and more than three.

More than half (53.6%) of the participants believed that that breast cancer occurs more commonly in old women. In addition, 235 (56.5%) of the participants have thoughts that breast cancer is a curable disease. The overall understanding of the survival period (more than five years) after clinical diagnosed of having breast cancer was 59.4%.

Knowledge about signs and symptoms of breast cancer

Table 3 shows that swelling or enlargement of the breast was the predominantly mentioned signs of breast cancer followed by pain or soreness of the breast. Similarly, more than 85% of the respondents stated that a lump in the breast, change in the size of the breast and discoloration/dimpling of the breasts are the major signs of breast cancer. Weight loss was the least (58.17%) mentioned sign and symptom of breast cancer.

In addition, 56.5% of the participants thought that breast cancer is a curable disease. The overall understanding on the survival period (more than five years) after clinical diagnosis of having breast cancer was 59.4%.

Knowledge and practice of nurses about screening methods

The knowledge of nurses on the correct age for initiation of breast self-examination was 75.8% and more than three quarters (80%) of them reported that they knew how to perform BSE and less than half of them (42%) knew the recommended frequency of conducting BSE.

Three-quarters (75.5%) of the nurses said they practiced BSE. Of these, 60.6% practiced once a month, 7.2%

Table 2 Knowledge about risk factors of breast cancer among nurses in Asmara, Eritrea

Questions	Yes	Percentage (%)	95% Confidence Interval
Does breast cancer risk increases with advancing age	276	66.35	[61.79–70.90]
Is breast cancer hereditary	287	68.99	[64.53–73.45]
Is high fat diet a risk factor for breast cancer	154	37.02	[32.37–41.67]
Is smoking a risk factor for breast cancer	327	78.61	[74.65–82.56]
Is alcohol consumption a risk factor for breast cancer	261	62.74	[58.08–67.40]
Is first child at age more than 30 a risk factor for breast cancer	144	34.62	[30.03–39.20]
Is menarche below 11 years a risk factor for breast cancer	105	25.24	[21.05–29.43]
Is late menopause a risk factor for breast cancer	144	34.62	[30.03–39.20]
Is stress a risk factor for breast cancer	151	36.30	[31.66–40.93]
Is larger breast a risk factor for breast cancer	57	13.70	[10.39–17.02]
Does breast feeding decrease risk of breast cancer	317	76.20	[72.10–80.31]
Is painless breast lump a risk factor for breast cancer	267	64.18	[59.56–68.80]
Is null parity a risk factor for breast cancer	165	39.66	[34.95–44.38]
Is obesity a risk factor for breast cancer	140	33.65	[29.10–38.21]
Do oral contraceptive pills increase the risk of breast cancer	219	52.64	[47.83–57.46]
Is trauma to breast a risk factor of breast cancer	135	32.45	[27.94–36.96]
Does endogenous estrogen hormone increase the risk of breast cancer	234	56.25	[51.47–61.03]
Do you think giving births > 4 decreases risk of breast cancer	125	30.05	[25.63–34.47]
Does physical activity decrease the risk of breast cancer	158	37.98	[33.30–42.66]

once every three months, 14.5% said they did BSE once a year, and 17.8% did not answer. The reasons given for not practicing BSE were; 'carelessness' (17.1%), 'don't have breast problem' (14.2%), 'unsure about its benefit' (8.2), 'don't know how to do it' (5.3), 'too frequent to practice' (2.9%), 'don't feel comfortable doing it' (1.2%) and 'don't think I need to do it regularly' (1%).

Thirty percent of the nurses practiced CBE. Of these, 14.9% were examined only once and 13.3% three times and above. The majority (55.3%) of those who did not practice CBE stated that they were reluctant because

they had no signs and symptoms of breast cancer. Forty-seven nurses (11.3%) (37% of those aged > 40 years) had undertaken mammography examination in their life and only 8.7% of the overall study participants knew that 40 was the correct age for starting mammography as a screening method.

In this study, age and religious affiliation of respondents were associated with knowledge on signs and symptoms of breast cancer. Marital status was not associated with the KAP of nurses. Having breast problems was associated with the KAP of nurses whereas having a

Table 3 knowledge about the signs and symptoms of breast cancer among nurses in Asmara, Eritrea

Questions (Signs and symptoms mentioned)	Yes	%	95% Confidence Interval
Lump in the breast	358	86.06	[82.72–89.40]
Discharge from the breast	344	82.69	[79.05–86.34]
Pain or Soreness in the breast	368	88.46	[85.38–91.54]
Change in the size of the breast	358	86.06	[82.72–89.40]
Discoloration/dimpling of the breast	355	85.34	[81.93–88.75]
Ulceration of the breast	327	78.61	[74.65–82.56]
Weight loss	242	58.17	[53.42–62.93]
Changes in the shape of the breast	337	81.01	[77.23–84.79]
Inversion/ pulling in of nipple	288	69.23	[64.78–73.68]
Swelling or enlargement of the breast	374	89.90	[87.00–92.81]
Lump under armpit	319	76.68	[72.61–80.76]
Scaling / dry skin on nipple region	273	65.63	[61.05–70.20]

family history of breast cancer was only associated with the knowledge of risk factors. Nurses with bachelor's degree had the highest knowledge compared to registered and associated nurses. The place of work was also significantly associated with the knowledge about breast cancer risk factors and its symptoms; nurses who worked at the Orotta Maternity Hospital had the highest knowledge (Table 4).

Moreover, there was a significant association between the professional level of nurses and BSE practice ($p < 0.001$) in which registered nurses had the highest practice (82.40%), followed by associated nurses (74.4%) and

Table 4 Bivariate analysis of factors associated with KAP of nurses in Asmara, Eritrea

	N	Knowledge of Risk Factors (Mean ± SD)	Knowledge of Symptoms (Mean ± SD)	Knowledge and practice about breast cancer screening (Mean ± SD)
Age				
19–29	222	49.47 ± 19.06	83.68 ± 17.16	69.82 ± 17.06
30–39	65	50.26 ± 20.61	78.46 ± 18.47	69.91 ± 16.04
40–49	63	44.62 ± 23.44	78.52 ± 18.33	69.66 ± 21.23
> =50	66	48.52 ± 17.52	85.00 ± 20.62	68.52 ± 19.35
p value^2		0.333	0.042	0.961
Marital Status				
Single	212	49.32 ± 19.95	84.06 ± 16.91	71.23 ± 14.25
Ever married	202	49.60 ± 19.49	80.45 ± 19.24	68.40 ± 19.77
p value^1		0.889	0.050	0.103
Religion				
Muslim	35	48.71 ± 16.72	72.29 ± 17.17	66.35 ± 15.82
Christian	379	48.73 ± 20.09	83.23 ± 18.08	69.96 ± 13.55
p value^1		0.995	0.001	0.138
Family Hx of Breast Cancer				
Yes	30	61.48 ± 15.64	76.87 ± 23.48	65.65 ± 18.29
No	384	47.71 ± 19.78	82.75 ± 17.69	70.02 ± 17.88
p value^1		0.001	0.080	0.180
Having breast problem				
Yes	20	59.88 ± 8.85	73.00 ± 19.49	58.88 ± 13.54
No	396	48.20 ± 20.03	82.77 ± 18.07	70.14 ± 17.95
P Value^1		0.014	0.019	0.006
Professional Level				
Associate Nurse	203	45.78 ± 20.09	82.36 ± 17.31	66.50 ± 18.23
Registered Nurse	170	49.22 ± 19.57	82.26 ± 20.02	72.22 ± 17.65
BSN	43	60.34 ± 14.73	82.09 ± 15.21	73.90 ± 14.72
P Value^2		0.001	0.996	0.002
Unite of Work				
Orotta MCH	38	63.60 ± 12.50	91.58 ± 10.27	71.35 ± 15.85
Private hospital	44	54.80 ± 20.60	86.59 ± 15.99	73.48 ± 11.55
Medical wards	162	49.06 ± 21.91	80.98 ± 24.09	68.38 ± 13.60
Orotta Medical Surgical	50	36.67 ± 15.71	80.60 ± 16.83	68.57 ± 12.44
Community hospitals	82	45.66 ± 15.42	76.71 ± 20.31	71.54 ± 14.83
Ophthalmic hospital	40	45.97 ± 19.97	75.25 ± 17.54	66.39 ± 13.19
P Value^2		0.001	0.001	0.093

1 = T-test, 2 = ANOVA

bachelor science in Nursing (BSN) (55.80%) (data not shown).

Discussion

There are four important findings in this study. Firstly, nurses' knowledge about the possible risk factors of breast cancer is a concern since many established risk factors of breast cancer were mentioned by less than 50% of them. Secondly, nurses had a good knowledge of the signs and symptoms of breast cancer in which each sign or symptom was mentioned by more than half of them. Thirdly, the practice of breast cancer screening was low and lastly, a family history of breast cancer, having breast problems, the professional level of nurses and the unit where they work predicts the KAP of nurses about breast cancer.

In some studies elsewhere, nurses' knowledge about the risk factors of breast cancer has been found to be low [14, 16, 20] whilst other studies have reported nurses' knowledge about risk factors of breast cancer to be high [13]. The fact that there are many risk factors of breast cancer [5] and new factors have been found to be associated with breast cancer might have affected the knowledge of the nurses. The unit they work may influence their knowledge. In the present study, nurses who worked at Orotta Maternity Hospital had the highest knowledge about the risk factors of breast cancer while nurses who were working at Orotta surgical ward had the lowest knowledge. Therefore, efforts need to be taken to increase the knowledge of nurses about the risk factors of breast cancer. Short on-site courses prioritizing those nurses who work outside maternity units/ wards and nurses with associate level could help to update their knowledge.

In line with other studies [11, 15, 20] nurses in this study were found to have a good knowledge of the signs and symptoms of breast cancer. Nurses who work in the Orotta Maternity Hospital had high (91.6%) knowledge about the signs and symptoms of breast cancer.

Knowledge and attitude should be accompanied by practice. A gap in practice was identified in this study in which nurses were found to practice breast cancer screening infrequently. Nurses in this study reported practicing CBE and mammography less often. Only 30% of the nurses practiced clinical breast examination. This was similar to the findings from one study in Nigeria [11] and lower than a similar study in the same country [13]. Of all the nurses, only (11.3%) had undertaken mammography examination. Mammography is the gold standard for early detection of breast cancer but is not recommended for countries with limited resources due to its cost and technical complexity [25]. The practice of BSE among the nurses in this study was lower than studies conducted elsewhere [16, 19] and higher than some other similar studies [18, 20].

There were some limitations in this study. Firstly, the practice of breast cancer screening was reported, but nurses may not adequately remember whether they have done breast cancer screening or not. Secondly, since our subjects were those nurses working in hospitals only, this result may not reflect the knowledge of nurses who work in health centers and small clinics. Despite these limitations, we discovered important gaps in KAP of hospital nurses about breast cancer.

Conclusion

This was the first study to assess the KAP of nurses' about breast cancer. Nurses were found to have good knowledge of the signs and symptoms of breast cancer but little knowledge about the risk factors of the disease. The practice of breast cancer screening among the nurses was low. Therefore, training programs to update nurses' knowledge about the risk factors of breast cancer and practice of breast cancer screening could potentially help in the practice of healthy habits among the nurses. This, indirectly, could also help to increase the knowledge and practice of the public about breast cancer.

Abbreviations

BSE: Breast Self-Examination; BSN: Bachelor of Science in Nursing; CBE: Clinical Breast Examination; HRM: Human Resource Management; KAP: Knowledge Attitude and Practice

Acknowledgments

The authors gratefully acknowledge the National Commission for Higher Education (NCHE) of Eritrea for financial support for this research. The authors appreciate the support of health facility directorates and head nurses. The authors would like to thank all the nurses who participated in this study for their kind cooperation.

Funding

This research was supported by Eritrea Research Fund (ERF).

Authors' contributions

AKA led, wrote and drafted the manuscript. EAK wrote and drafted the manuscript. MTG reviewed the manuscript. All authors approved the final draft of the manuscript.

Competing interests

The authors declare that they have no competing interests.

Author details

[1]Department of Epidemiology and Biostatistics, Asmara College of Health Sciences, School of Public Health, P.O.Box: 8566, Asmara, Eritrea. [2]Department of Epidemiology, Robert Stempel College of Public Health and Social Work, Florida International University, 11200 SW 8th St, Miami, FL 33199, USA.

References

1. Wadler BM, Judge CM, Prout M, Allen JD, Geller AC. Improving breast Cancer control via the use of community health Workers in South Africa: a critical review. J Oncol 2011;2011:8. Article ID 150423. http://dx.doi.org/10.1155/2011/150423.

2. Anderson BO, Braun S, Lim S, Smith RA, Taplin S, Thomas DB. Early detection of breast cancer in countries with limited resources. Breast J. 2003;9(Suppl 2):S51–9.

3. World Health Ranking. Eritrea, Breast Cancer 2014. Available at: http://www.worldlifeexpectancy.com/eritrea-breast-cancer. Accessed on 5 Aug. 2017.

4. Global health Statistics Bareast cancer in Eritrea. 2017. Available at: http://global-disease-burden.healthgrove.com/l/33029/Breast-Cancer-in-Eritrea. Accessed on 5 Aug. 2017.

5. Center for Diseases Control and Prevention. 2016. Avaliable at: https://www.cdc.gov/cancer/breast/basic_info/risk_factors.htm. Accessed on 7 Aug. 2017.

6. Collaborative Group on Hormonal Factors in Breast Cancer. Familial breast cancer: collaborative reanalysis of individual data from 52 epidemiological studies including 58,209 women with breast cancer and 101,986 women without the disease. Lancet. 2001;358(9291):1389–99.

7. Stockton D, Davies T, Day N, McCann J. Retrospective study of reasons for improved survival in patient with breast cancer in east Anglia: earlier diagnosis or better treatment. BMJ. 1997;314:472–5.

8. Ersumo T. Breast cancer in an Ethiopian population, Addis Ababa. East Africa Journal of Surgery. 2006;11(1):81–6.

9. Thomas DB, Gao DL, Ray RM, Wang WW, Allison CJ, Chen FL, et al. Randomized trial of breast self-examination in shanghai: final results. J Natl Cancer Inst 2002;94(19):1445–1457.

10. Bello TO, Olugbenga-Bello AI, Oguntola AS, Adeoti ML, Ojemakinde OM. Knowledge and practice of breast cancer screening among female nurses and lay women in Osogbo. Nigeria West Afr J Med. 2011;30(4):296–300.

11. Odusanya OO, Tayo OO. Breast cancer knowledge, attitudes and practice among nurses in Lagos, Nigeria. Acta Oncol. 2001;40(7):844–8.

12. Akhigbe AO, Omuemu VO. Knowledge, attitudes and practice of breast cancer screening among female health workers in a Nigerian urban city. BMC Cancer. 2009;9:203.

13. Awodele O, Adeyomoye AA, Oreagba IA, Dolapo DC, Anisu DF, Kolawole SO, et al. Knowledge, attitude and practice of breast cancer screening among nurses in Lagos University teaching hospital, Lagos Nigeria Nig Q J Hosp Med 2009;19(2):114–118.

14. Lemlem SB, Sinishaw W, Hailu M, Abebe M, Aregay A. Assessment of knowledge of breast Cancer and screening methods among nurses in university hospitals in Addis Ababa, Ethiopia, 2011. ISRN Oncol. 2013;2013:470981.

15. Andsoy II, Gul A. Breast, cervix and colorectal cancer knowledge among nurses in Turkey. Asian Pac J Cancer Prev. 2014;15(5):2267–72.

16. Alkhasawneh IM. Knowledge and practice of breast cancer screening among Jordanian nurses. Oncol Nurs Forum. 2007;34(6):1211–7.

17. Madanat H, Merrill RM. Breast cancer risk-factor and screening awareness among women nurses and teachers in Amman, Jordan. Cancer Nurs. 2002;25(4):276–82.

18. Fotedar V, Seam RK, Gupta MK, Gupta M, Vats S, Verma S. Knowledge of risk factors and early detection methods and practices towards breast cancer among nurses in Indira Gandhi medical college, Shimla, Himachal Pradesh, India. Asian Pac J Cancer Prev. 2013;14(1):117–20.

19. Sreedharan J, Muttappallymyalil J, Venkatramana M, Thomas M. Breast self-examination: knowledge and practice among nurses in United Arab Emirates. Asian Pac J Cancer Prev. 2010;11(3):651–4.

20. Yousuf SA, Al Amoudi SM, Nicolas W, Banjar HE, Salem SM. Do Saudi nurses in primary health care centres have breast cancer knowledge to promote breast cancer awareness? Asian Pac J Cancer Prev. 2012;13(9):4459–64.

21. Seah M, Tan SM. Am I breast cancer smart? Assessing breast cancer knowledge among health professionals. Singap Med J. 2007;48(2):158–62.

22. Ghebrehiwet M, Paulos E, Andeberhan T. The role of combined ultrasonography and mammography in the diagnosis of breast cancer in Eritrean women with palpable abnormalities of the breast. J Eritrean Med Assoc. 2007;2(1):2–7.

23. Tesfamariam A, Parilla F, Paulos E, Mufunda J, Gebremichael A. Clinicohistopathological evaluation of breast masses and profle of breast diseases in Eritrea: a case of poor concordance between clinical and histological diagnosis. J Eritrean Med Assoc. 2008;3(1):32–5.

24. Tesfamariam A, Gebremichael A, Mufunda J. Breast cancer clinicopathological presentation, gravity and challenges in Eritrea, East Africa: management practice in a resource-poor setting. S Afr Med J. 2013;103(8):526–8.

25. The International Network for Cancer Treatment and Research. Cancer – a neglected health problem in developing countries. Lancet. 2011;358:1389–99.

Medium-fidelity simulation in clinical readiness: a phenomenological study of student midwives concerning teamwork

Zukiswa Brenda Ntlokonkulu*, Ntombana Mc'deline Rala and Daniel Ter Goon

Abstract

Background: Teamwork during obstetric emergency ensures good outcomes for both the woman and her baby. Effective teams are characterised by mutual respect, support, and cooperation among team members.

Methods: This qualitative, interpretive, phenomenological analysis study was conducted on a purposive sample of five, fourth-year Bachelor of Nursing Science student midwives at the University of Fort Hare (UFH). In-depth semi-structured interviews were conducted. Data analysis applied the interpretative phenomenological analysis method.

Results: Superordinate theme demonstrated teamwork elicited four clustered themes namely delegation of duties, the importance of teamwork, team support, and confident team leader. The participants recognised that there should be a team leader who is capable of delegating duties to other team members in the management of an obstetric emergency, Participants were confident not only to assign duties but to be kept updated of the intervention. They expressed the need to work collaboratively as a team to achieve the desired goal of providing quality care to the woman. The participants maintained that the team must be supportive and be able to help in decision making during simulation of an obstetric emergency. A sense of mutual respect is echoed by some participants in the process of caring for the woman. Some participants were confident at being team leaders and could see themselves as leaders in the real-life clinical situation.

Conclusion: The participants acknowledge the importance of teamwork in resolving obstetric emergencies. The importance of delegating duties to other team members, providing updated progress report ensures better outcomes for the woman.

Keywords: Medium-fidelity simulation, Teamwork, Obstetric emergency, Interpretative phenomenological analysis

Background

Simulation has been used in nursing education to teach both technical and non-technical skills such as teamwork. It is evident that simulation based on teamwork prepares healthcare personnel to manage obstetric emergencies in a practical setting [1]. In midwifery, an obstetric emergency requires teamwork for better outcomes for both the woman and her baby. Apart from the lecture method, which appears to be less attractive in the modern era in terms of applicability and skills acquisition, the experiential learning involving simulation can be used in healthcare team training [2]. Moreover,

simulation is ideal for team training as it is hands-on and can encourage collaboration among participants [3]. Teamwork is imperative in any kind of emergency. During obstetric emergencies, staff members need to consolidate their learning to function as a team for better outcomes such as the safety of the woman and her baby.

Globally, there has been a commendable concern for patient safety in health care settings [4, 5]. The World Health Organisation (WHO) has stressed the importance of educating health-care professionals on the principles and concepts of patient safety [6]. Countries such as Australia and England have made patient safety a priority in government agenda [7, 8]. In South Africa, the Department of Health has made patient safety one of its

* Correspondence: zntlokonkulu@ufh.ac.za
Department of Nursing Science, Faculty of Health Sciences, University of Fort Hare, East London, South Africa

priorities through the implementation of the strategic plan for nurse education, training and practice [9].

The institutions of health care professional training have committed themselves to provide training programmes that are designed for hospital-specific risks. Patient safety has always been part of the nursing curriculum for years but its lack of transferability in practice has been well documented [10]. Cockerham [11] states that patient safety is the ultimate attribute that a newly qualified nurse should possess. Debourgh and Prion [10] assert that the clinical experience of a student in team performances and patient safety is often limited by the student role and scope of practice. However, due to the lack of opportunities for the students to practice during real clinical emergency simulation provides an ideal environment where team processes and behaviour can be learned without putting a patient at risk [12, 13]. The growing interest in simulated learning over the years is born out of concern for patient safety [14, 15]. Patient safety during simulation is further reinforced during the debriefing session allowing the student to assimilate learning [16].

There is a dearth of research on nursing teamwork, despite evidence that many errors committed by nurses are partly due to poor teamwork. Deering et al. [17] assert that complications in health care are not attributed to the individual but to team performance failure. A focus on team performance and training started in the aviation discipline, then proceeded to the army to improve safety [17]. Several studies have shown that strategies to enhance teamwork in health care have been adapted from these high-risk professions [2–4]. Training programmes in obstetric emergencies, such as Managing Obstetrical Emergencies and Trauma (MOET) [18], Multidisciplinary Obstetric-Simulated Emergency Scenarios (MOSES) [19], Practical Obstetric Multi-Professional Training (PROMPT) [20] are used for both clinical and non-clinical skills such as teamwork and woman safety. These training programmes have been adapted to meet the training needs of healthcare workers in developing countries such as South Africa and Zimbabwe [21]. Incorporating PROMPT in the training programme resulted in increased staff confidence in the management of emergencies, improved teamwork and inter-professional relations [20].

In midwifery, midwives work as an interdisciplinary and multi-disciplinary team. This is evident in an obstetric emergency which requires the presence of a multi-disciplinary team; who have different pieces of training and sometimes may not understand the scope of practice of each discipline. Whilst there are studies in obstetrics focusing on interdisciplinary and multi-disciplinary teams during obstetric emergency simulation [19, 22, 23]. There is a paucity of literature on obstetric emergency team simulation tailored mainly

for midwives. Medium-fidelity simulation can be of benefit to training midwives in the management of obstetric emergencies.

Medium fidelity simulation (MFS) is the use of manikins or task trainers that offer breath sound, heart sounds, bowel sound or simulated blood but lack the authenticity of a realistic environment. Medium-fidelity simulation is a cost-effective method to train student midwives in both technical and non-technical skills such as teamwork and leadership obstetric. Medium-fidelity simulation creates a realistic environment where students can learn to manage obstetric emergencies as part of a team. Despite the availability of MFS at UFH, its benefit on the clinical readiness of student midwives is not known. Would student midwives be able to acquire attributes that are needed in team performance during an obstetric emergency?

Aim

The aim of the study was to explore, describe and analyse the views of student midwives concerning teamwork during medium-fidelity obstetric emergency simulation.

Research design

An interpretative phenomenological analysis (IPA) approach was used to explore, describe and analyse the lived experiences of student midwives with regards to teamwork during a medium fidelity obstetric emergency simulation. The student midwives' individual experiences of the post-partum haemorrhage (PPH) simulation demonstrated the diverse experiences of the same phenomenon which are the reflective, interpretative and idiographic premises of IPA [24].

Population

The target population was a fourth-year Bachelor of Nursing Science student midwives at the University of Fort Hare. The inclusion criteria were the fourth-year student midwives who had passed the first semester's midwifery module. A purposive sampling method was used to select five fourth-year student midwives who were the team leaders during the management of post-partum haemorrhage (PPH) using MFS. Fourth-year student midwives were selected because, at the University of Fort Hare, obstetric emergencies are taught in the second year of midwifery. Usually, high-risk midwifery involves emergencies that require teamwork. Ethical approval of the study was obtained from the University of Fort Hare Ethics Committee. Permission to conduct the study was granted by the Head of Department of Nursing Sciences, University of Fort Hare.

Trustworthiness

Trustworthiness of this study was ensured by applying the principles of trustworthiness, namely transferability, credibility, confirmability, and dependability as outlined by Guba [25]. Transferability of the study was ensured by keeping both hard and soft copies of the research steps taken that can be accessed on request. Both the soft and hard copy of the data will be made available on-line at the university repository. The credibility of the findings was determined by taking the research transcripts to a co-coder for data validation. Confirmability was attained by ensuring that there was enough data to support the findings and conclusions. Dependability was ensured by narrating a detailed description of the research design and the steps taken in data collection.

Ethical considerations

Ethical approval of the study was obtained from the University of Fort Hare Ethics Committee. Permission to conduct the study was granted by the Head of Department of Nursing Sciences, University of Fort Hare. Three fundamental ethical principles were applied, namely; the principle of respect for the person, beneficence, and justice [26].

The principle of respect for the person

The student midwives were informed of the right to refuse to participate and to withdraw from the study at any given time without any prejudice or penalty. The nature and aim of the study were explained to the participants, prior to data collection.

Principle of beneficence

The principle of beneficence refers to the individual's right to protection from harm. This study was non-invasive, and the student midwives were informed that the simulation was not for assessment reasons but for exploring their experiences of the simulation.

Principle of justice

The principle of justice refers to how the researcher comes to choose the study population. The student midwives' right to anonymity was maintained. Before the beginning of each interview, permission was sought from each student midwife to use a pseudonym during the interview. Participants were made to understand their right to the privacy of any information provided, and their consent was sought before the use of a tape recorder. Prior to the interview, each student midwife completed an informed consent form with a clear explanation. The participants had the right to ask any question(s) during and after interviews.

Methods

An Essential Steps in Management of Obstetric Emergency (ESMOE) post-partum haemorrhage video which was sent on-line through Blackboard to all fourth-year student midwives in order to demonstrate the process. Management of PPH is one of the contents that are taught in the midwifery abnormal pregnancy, labour and puerperium module. The student midwives had an opportunity to watch the video repeatedly in order to thoroughly comprehend the demonstrated skill. The day before the simulation the six bedded simulation laboratory was prepared for the PPH simulation. Only four-bed spaces were used for the simulation. The advanced OB Susie a Gaumard with an audible foetal and maternal pulse was filled with simulated blood and urine and was positioned in the centre of the bed. Four large dressing trolleys were prepared with all the equipment needed for the management of PPH. Each bed space had an oxygen outlet with an oxygen mask and two drip stands and a blood pressure machine and relevant ward documentation. On the day of the simulation, the standardised patient (SP) was given a scenario. The Nursing Science Department recruit members of the community to pretend to be SPs for some of the undergraduate practical program. The SPs were provided with a scenario. Critical points of the scenario were explained to the SPs such as when to call for the nurse, when to pass out and when to regain consciousness, what question to ask. The SPs clad in a hospital gown was positioned above the OB Susie torso to create a hybrid. The hybrid was draped with green towels. On the day of the simulation, the students were given the simulation scenario to read prior to the simulation. The ESMOE video was played for the group the second time before the demonstration of the simulation. The students decided among themselves which roles to play during the simulation.

Data collection

Fourth-year midwifery students were recruited by the first author (ZN) during their theory block. The 4th year students were approached in class after a lecture. The aim and nature of the study were explained to the students. ZN is the simulation laboratory manager and had no prior relationship with the students. A semi-structured interview guide was used with nine questions. Open-ended questions were used in order to allow the student midwives the opportunity to explore their lived experiences of an obstetric emergency using medium-fidelity simulation. Prompts during the interview centred on the students' experiences of obstetric emergencies using medium-fidelity simulation, for example, how did the participant feel being the team leader? How was the communication between team members? Individual interviews were conducted at the University of Fort Hare's simulation laboratory by the first author (ZN) over a period of 1 month, each interview session lasted between 26 min and 44 min. A Samsung smartphone was used to record the interviews, and a notepad was used to make notes of gestures such as smiles or other facial expressions. After each interview, the recorded interview was transferred onto a laptop and a file was opened for the interviewee, identified by a pseudonym. The interviews were transcribed verbatim as Word documents by the first author.

Data analysis

Data were analysed by the first author following the six steps suggested by Smith et al. [24] namely reading and re-reading, initial noting, developing emergent themes, searching for connections across the emergent themes, moving to the next case and looking for patterns across cases. The transcript was read through twice. The first reading was done whilst listening to the recording. During that time any parts of the transcription that did not make sense were clarified by moving back and forth on the recording. During the second reading, the researcher listened in detail, immersed herself in the words of the participant. The transcript was analysed line by line, to identify three types of exploratory comments, namely; descriptive, linguistic and conceptual, while trying to make sense of each participant's experiences and being consciously aware not to change original meaning. The researcher tried to interpret the exploratory comments. This is the double hermeneutics of IPA. Then the researcher found a connection among emergent themes. Abstraction was used for the clustering of themes, as the superordinate theme was identified. Some differences were identified in some clusters, indicating polarization. Each interview was transcribed and analysed separately before moving on to the next case. Finally, all the themes clustered together and commonalities, differences and individuality were identified.

Results

The superordinate theme demonstrated teamwork elicited the following themes:

Delegation of duties

Participants highlighted that there is a need for someone to assume the leadership role during emergencies. The person who assumes the leadership role should be able to do introspection for his or her capabilities. As team leaders, the five participants all felt responsible to assign duties to other team members. Assigning duties in an emergency are important so as to ensure that tasks are carried out effectively. The effectiveness of assigned tasks needs to be confirmed through continuous mutual updates from team members. In a midwifery unit, every midwife should be competent to assume a leadership role and to direct team members in order to manage the case effectively, at the correct time and in the correct sequence, as affirmed by the following comments:

'I delegated duties to other team members and asked for the updates to ensure that duties are carried out and whether they are effective.' [Thembi].

'As the person who arrived first and assumed the leadership role, I felt I should assign duties to other team members such as taking vital signs, inserting intravenous cannulas and calculating the amount of blood loss.' [Anga].

'You have to delegate specific duties to your team members. If this person is responsible for observations and you want an equipment, you can't ask this person to take an equipment for you.' [Lunga].

'Delegating duties to other team members ensures the duties are carried out. Specific duties were delegated to team members and team members kept me updated on the progress of the woman.' [Zandie].

Importance of teamwork

Some of the participants were not aware that obstetric emergencies require a team effort. Participants acknowledged that the team leader should give out instructions and team members should be co-operative. Some participants felt that working in cooperation with other team members contributed towards the well-being of the woman. Also, most participants acknowledged the importance of teamwork in resolving obstetric emergencies. In a midwifery unit, collective teamwork results in better outcomes. Teamwork is alluded to by the following comments:

'Firstly, I didn't know that when you are managing PPH you need more people. I knew that you call for help and you do some of the things then the person will come and help you.' [Lunga].

'I felt confident because I was able to do it with the help of my team members and it made me value teamwork more. This made me realise that there are certain things you cannot do alone.' [Thembi].

'Teamwork was very good because my team had knowledge about PPH so there was a good teamwork.' [Sino].

'Working with a team that wants to help and that keeps on advising made my job easy. I was a team leader who was unsure of what I was doing, but I knew that my team knows what to do.' [Zandie].

'Teamwork ... I could say that my colleagues cooperated very well with me. They did everything I told them to do and then we managed the woman well.' [Anga].

Team support

Having a supportive team helped the participants rely on fellow team members. The team members were not just a source of support but also help each other with critical thinking and decision making. Team members give advice when necessary, pointing out to the team leader when important steps are missed. In an emergency, every team member can have a positive contribution that could be of great benefit to the team and the emergency. One participant reported that her team demonstrated a sense of serenity and respect, as they were consciously aware that they were having a discussion about the woman and that the woman was present; therefore, they have to be careful speaking negatively about the process and the woman. The team leader needs to acknowledge and value other team members. Team support in the midwifery unit is a significant factor to pay attention to, to ensure positive midwifery outcomes. In a supportive midwifery unit, achievements are not regarded as belonging to any individual but to the whole unit. Team members who work in collaboration with one another avoid the chaos that defines many emergencies, as affirmed by the following comments:

'I just needed someone to reassure me that this is the step that follows after the other one. That's how I did my critical thinking, and with the assistance of others.' [Zandie].

'The team leader was the one giving the instruction but others were just talking because it's an emergency. You can't keep quiet when you see that the team leader is missing something.' [Lunga].

'If another member has forgotten something, the team leader or another colleague will say please do this, not in a harsh way, but in a respectful way, so that even the woman does not sense that something is wrong.' [Sino].

Confident team leader

Participants had varying experiences of the role of a team leader during the simulation. Being able to confidently delegate tasks and making sure that people carried out those tasks increased the student midwives' confidence in being a leader. Participants reported seeing themselves as leaders in the real-life clinical situation. Simply being chosen to be a leader by one's peers has the effect of increasing confidence. Knowing that people see the potential in one to lead has a motivating effect and encourage people to give in their best. Participants reported feeling nervous in the role but found that as they were immersed in the simulation, their capabilities and confidence increases. Assuming a leadership role in a simulation enables the participant to visualise a similar role for her/himself in the clinical setting. However, a lack of knowledge in a team leader about the subject matter can at times make the leader doubt his capabilities. The sense that team members had to take over at certain points made one participant feel less of a leader:

'I was not impressed because the things didn't according to plan, so I'm not happy about being a leader ...Yes, I did the job, but I missed some of the important points during the procedure so you can't be impressed having your team members talking over you because you missed some important points whereas it's your job.' [Lunga].

Others were more positive:

'The whole scenario, it's challenging and when something is challenging, it brings out the best in you. I could see myself delegating to my peers and seeing them carrying out duties without complaints.' [Thembi].

'The fact that they chose me to be the team leader like they have trust and confidence in me that I can to do this, it means I can do this.' [Zandie].

'At first, I was nervous being chosen as a team leader, but I thought OK let me try it, but as time went on I felt proud of myself that I'm able to assign duties to people.' [Anga].

'I feel like I'm competent, even if I can come across PPH in the institution I will be able to take part in saving the woman's life. You gain confidence and more experience when you do things practically.'

Discussion

The present study was undertaken to explore the views of student midwives concerning teamwork during medium-fidelity obstetric emergency simulation. The team working during obstetric emergency provides good outcomes for both the woman and her baby. Most of the participants in this study were confident in delegating duties to team members. The role of the team leader during the emergency is of significance as he/she is the one who gives direction to team members. These findings were consistent with the findings of the studies conducted by Woods; Simkins; Gravlin [27–29] which reported that the participants were comfortable delegating duties. However, the findings of this study were in contrast with the findings of the study conducted by Johnson et al. [30] on Newly Qualified Nurses (NQN). The participants reported that Inadequate delegation skills resulted in an NQN who is stressed, anxious and unable to manage time adequately [30].

The participants of the present study reported that sharing duties among team members is important during emergencies. This is congruent with the findings of the study by Deering et al. [17], that monitoring the actions of others during teamwork ensures that the workload is evenly shared and woman safety is guaranteed. There is a need to clearly share and specify the duties to be performed by each member of the team in order to achieve the group goal. The participants of the present study affirmed that in order to ensure that the delegated work was carried out, the team leader should ask or be provided with regular updates by team members. Receiving updates from team members contributes to the leader's awareness of the woman's condition [17]. One participant felt that delegating people to perform specific functions is important so as to ensure that tasks are performed. However, Johnson et al. [30] point out that poor delegation by NQNs can result in loss of collaboration and a lack of a sense of responsibility by healthcare assistants (HCA).

The participants had good experiences working in a team; only one participant expressed a degree of ignorance about teamwork during obstetric emergencies. Monod et al. 22 found that simulated team training for the management of obstetric emergencies was considered useful. One participant acknowledged the importance of working in a team. Having a confident team ensures good outcomes. In a retrospective study by Siassakos et al. [31] on the effect of team training, good teamwork was deemed necessary for the management of obstetric emergencies. Poor teamwork is one of the causes of adverse events in woman care [2]. Working in close collaboration during emergencies is more likely to result in good outcomes for both the woman and the caregivers [32].

Two participants affirmed that co-operative teamwork brought good results and success. A sense that team members support and respect one another during obstetric emergencies is important. In this study, it was found that one participant recognised that team support enabled her to think better; to apply her critical thinking.

Advice from team members during an emergency benefitted both the woman and the team leader. Phipps et al. [23] study on determining the implementation of labour and delivery team-training programmes with a simulation component stressed the importance of 'shared responsibility' and 'cross monitoring', which equipped team members to be assertive. Supporting each other during an emergency is done in a harmonious manner, demonstrating respect and good teamwork [17, 23]. Collective attributes of individual team members contribute to the performance of the team as a whole and tend to strengthen the confidence of the team leader. Participants had varied experiences of team leadership. One participant found the simulation challenging, thus bringing out the best in her. This is consistent with the findings of other studies, which found that it was the challenging aspect of simulation that enabled students to give of their best [33, 34]. Smith et al. [1] assert that simulation training in obstetric emergencies encourages teamwork and increases confidence in managing such emergencies. This is congruent with the experience of one participant, who felt that having a good team alongside her gave her the confidence to be a good team leader.

One participant felt nervous as a team leader initially but gained confidence as she became immersed in the leader's role. Deering et al. [17] state that the role of the leader in an obstetrical emergency is to ensure that duties are performed effectively without unnecessary delays. Providing the students with an opportunity to practise a skill in a simulated environment increases students' confidence in managing complications [35]. One participant felt that his limited knowledge inhibited his ability as a team leader. This is inconsistent with the other studies [36, 37] which found that the experiential learning pedagogy made possible in high-fidelity simulation (HFS) and root cause analysis facilitated student learning.

By creating a safe learning environment where students are allowed to make mistakes without causing harm to the patient, MFS has the effect of increasing student confidence. This safe learning environment can also be achieved through the use of teaching modalities such as high-fidelity simulation and root cause analysis [25, 26]. The participants asserted that the safe learning environment helped them to learn the necessary skills.

Limitations

Given that the study focused on the lived experiences of fourth-year student midwives utilising simulation laboratories at one university, its findings cannot be generalized to other universities in South Africa. Therefore, exploring the views of the nursing students in other universities is needed.

Conclusion

The participants gained confidence as they assumed leadership roles during the obstetric emergency simulation. The simulation provided the participants with an opportunity to exercise their delegation roles by assigning duties to team members. Student midwives had an opportunity to assume leadership roles and to function as part of a team in resolving an obstetric emergency. Medium–fidelity simulation provided a safe environment where collaborative teamwork can be practised.

Abbreviations

ESMOE: Essential Steps in Management of Obstetrical Emergency; HCA: Health Care Worker; HFS: High-fidelity simulation; IPA: Interpretative phenomenological analysis; MFS: Medium-Fidelity Simulation; MOET: Managing Obstetrical Emergencies and Trauma; MOSES: Multidisciplinary Obstetric-Simulated Emergency Scenarios; NQN: Newly Qualified Nurse; PPH: Post-partum haemorrhage; PROMPT: Practical Obstetric Multi-Professional Training; UFH: University of Fort Hare

Acknowledgements

The authors would like to thank the student midwives who participated in the study.

Authors' contributions

ZN designed the study, collected data, analysed and wrote the first draft. NR and DG provided inputs in the data analysis and writing up of the paper. All authors critically revised and approved the manuscript.

Competing interests

The authors declare that they have no competing interests.

References

1. Smith A, Siassakos D, Crofts J, Draycott T. Simulation : improving patient outcomes. Semin Perinatol. 2013;37:151–6.
2. Guise J, Segel S. Teamwork in obstetric critical care. Best Pract Res Clin Obstet Gynecol. 2008;22(5):937–51.
3. Aggarwal R, Mytton OT, Derbrew M, Hananel D, Heydenburg M, Issenberg B, et al. Training and simulation for patient safety. Qual Saf Health Care. 2010;19:i34–43.
4. Martijn LLM, Jacobs AJE, Maassen IIM, Buitendijk SSE, Wensing MM. Patient safety in midwifery-led care in the Netherlands. Midwifery. 2013;29(1):60–6. Available from: http://dx.doi.org/10.1016/j.midw.2011.10.013
5. Usher K, Woods C, Conway J, Lea J, Parker V, Barrett F, et al. Patient safety content in pre-registration nursing curricula: a national cross-sectional survey study. Nurse Educ today. 2018;66:1–37. Available from: https://doi.org/10.1016/j.nedt.2018.04.013

6. World Health Organisation. Patient safety curriculum guide. multi-professional edition. Geneva: WHO Press; 2011. http://apps.who.int/ins/bitsream10665/44641/1/9789241501958. Accessed 2 May 2018
7. Australian Commission on safety and quality in health. National safety and quality health service standards. 2nd ed. Sydney: ACSQH; 2017. Accessed 02/05/2018
8. Department of Health. A promise to learn-a commitment to act. 2013. http://www.gov.uk/government/uploads/attachment_data/file/226703/Berwick_Report.pdf Accessed 02805/2018.
9. Department of Health. Strategic plan for nurse education, training and practice. 2013. http://www.health-e.org.za/2013/10/06 strategic-plan-nurse Accessed 02/05/2018.
10. Debourgh GA, Prion SK. Using simulation to teach Prelicensure nursing students to minimize patient risk and harm. Clin Simul Nurs. 2011;7(2):e47–56. Available from: https://doi.org/10.1016/j.ecns.2009.12.009
11. Cockerham ME. Effect of faculty training on improving the consistency of student assessment and debriefing in clinical simulation. Clin Simul Nurs. 2015;11(1):64–71. Available from: https://doi.org/10.1016/J.ecns.2014.10.011
12. Ballangrud R, Hall-Lord ML, Persenius M, Hedelin B. Intensive care nurses ' perceptions of simulation-based team training for building patient safety in intensive care : a descriptive qualitative study. Intensive Crit Care Nurs. 2014; 30(4):179–87. Available from: https://doi.org/10.1016/j.iccn.2014.03.002
13. Roh YS, Lee WS, Chung HS, Park YM. The effects of simulation-based resuscitation training on nurses' self-efficacy and satisfaction. Nurse Educ Today. 2013;33(2):123–8. Available from: https://doi.org/10.1016/j.nedt.2011.11.008
14. Argani CH, Eichelberger M, Deering S, Satin AJ. The case for simulation as part of a comprehensive patient safety program. Am J Obstet Gynecol [Internet]. 2012;206(6):451–5. Available from: https://doi.org/10.1016/j.ajog.2011.09.012
15. Tuzer H, Dinc L, Elcin M. The effects of using high- fidelity simulators and standardized patients on the thorax, lung, and cardiac examination skills of undergraduate nursing students. Nurse Educ Today. 2016;45:120–5. Available from: https://doi.org/10.1016/j.nedt.2016.07.002
16. Kim J, Park J, Shin S. Effectiveness of simulation-based nursing education depending on fidelity: a meta-analysis. BMC Med Educ. 2016;16:1–8. Available from: https://doi.org/10.1186/s12909-016-0672-7
17. Deering S, Johnston LC, Colaccio K. Multidisciplinary teamwork and communication training. Semin Perinatol. 2011;35:89–96.
18. Jyothi NK, Cox C, Johanson R. Management of obstetric emergencies and trauma (MOET): regional questionnaire survey of obstetric practice among career obstetricians in the United Kingdom. J Obstet and gynaecology. 2001;21(2):107–11.
19. Freeth D, Berridge EJ, Mackintosh N, Norris B, Sadler C, Strachan A. Multidisciplinary obstetric simulated emergency scenarios (MOSES): promoting patient safety in obstetrics with teamwork-focused. J Contin Educ Heal Care. 2009;29(2):98–104.
20. Crofts J, Teclar M, Murove BT, Mhlanga S, Dube M, Sengurayi E, et al. Onsite training of doctors, midwives, and nurses in obstetric emergencies, Zimbabwe. Bull World Health Organ. 2015;93(August 2014):347–51.
21. Frank K, Lombaard H, Pattison R. Does completion of the essential steps in managing obstetric emergencies (ESMOE) training package result in improved knowledge and skills in managing obstetric emergencies ? South African J Gynecol. 2009;15(3):94–9.
22. Monod C, Voekt CA, Gisin M, Gisin S, Hoesli IM. Optimization of competency in obstetrical emergencies : a role for simulation training. Matern Med. 2014; 289:733–8.
23. Phipps MG, Lindquist DG, McConaughey E, Brien JAO, Raker CA, Paglia MJ. Outcomes from a labour and delivery team training program with simulation component. YMOB. 2012;206(1):3–9. Available from: https://doi.org/10.1016/j.ajog.2011.06.046
24. Smith JA, Flowers P, Larkin M. Interpretative phenomenological analysis. Theory, method and research. London: Sage Publications Ltd; 2009.
25. Guba EG. Criteria for assessing the trustworthiness of naturalistic inquiries. Educ Commun Technol. 1981;29(2):75–91.
26. Brink H, Van der Walt C, Van Rensburg G. Fundamentals of research methodology for healthcare professionals. 3rd ed. Juta: Cape Town; 2012.
27. Woods C, West C, Mills J, Park T, Southern J, Usher K. Undergraduate student nurses ' self-reported preparedness for practice. Collegian. 2015; 22(4):359–68. Available from: https://doi.org/10.1016/j.colegn.2014.05.003
28. Simkins IL, Jaroneski LA. Integrated simulation : a teaching strategy to prepare prelicensure nursing students for professional practice — the students perspective. Teach Learn Nurs. 2016;11:15–9.

29. Gravlin G, Bittner NP. Nurses ' and nursing assistants ' reports of missed care and delegation. J Nurs Adm. 2010;40(7):329–35.

30. Johnson M, Magnusson C, Allan H, Evans K, Ball E, Horton K, et al. " Doing the writing " and " working in parallel " : How " distal nursing " affects delegation and supervision in the emerging role of the newly qualified nurse. Nurse Educ Today. 2015;35(2):e29–33. Available from: http://dx.doi.org/10.1016/j.nedt.2014.11.020

31. Siassakos D, Hasafa Z, Sibanda T, Fox R, Donald F, Winter C, et al. Retrospective cohort study of diagnosis – delivery interval with umbilical cord prolapse : the effect of team training. J Obstet Gynecol (Lahore). 2009; 116:1089–96.

32. Siassakos D, Draycott T, Montague I, Harris M. Content analysis of team communication in an obstetric emergency scenario. J Obstet Gynecol (Lahore). 2009;29:499–503.

33. Reid-Searl K, Happell B, Vieth L, Eaton A. High Fidelity patient silicone Simulation : a qualitative evaluation of nursing students ' experiences. Collegian. 2012;19:77–83.

34. Rush S, Acton L, Tolley K, Marks-Maran D, Burke L. Using simulation in a vocational programme: does the method support the theory? J Vocat Educ Train. 2010;62(4):467–79.

35. Andrighetti TP, Knestrick JM, Marowitz A, Martin C, Engstrom JL. Shoulder dystocia and postpartum hemorrhage Simulations : student confidence in managing these complications. J Midwifery Womens Health. 2011;57:55–60.

36. Pollock C, Biles J. Discovering the lived experience of students learning in immersive simulation. Clin Simul Nurs. 2016;12:313–9.

37. Carter AG, Sidebotham M, Creedy DK, Fenwick J, Gamble J. Using root cause analysis to promote critical thinking in final year bachelor of midwifery students. Nurse Educ Today. 2014;34(6):1018–23.

Birth preparedness and complication readiness among pregnant women in Tehulederie district, Northeast Ethiopia

Demlie Belete Endeshaw[1], Lema Derseh Gezie[2] and Hedija Yenus Yeshita[3*]

Abstract

Background: Motherhood is a time of anticipation of joy for a woman, her family, and her community. In spite of this fact, it is not as enjoyable as it should be because of numerous reasons. Insufficiency or lack of birth preparedness and complication readiness is the most common reason. The aim of this study was to assess the practice of birth preparedness and complication readiness and associated factors among pregnant women in Tehuledere district, northeast Ethiopia.

Methods: A community-based cross-sectional study was conducted in Tehuledere district, northeast Ethiopia. Participants were selected using the multistage sampling technique, and data were analyzed both descriptively and analytically using the binary logistic regression.

Result: Out of the total 507 samples, 500 (response rate 98.6%) pregnant women participated in the study. Less than half (44.6%) and (43.4%) of the respondents had knowledge and practice on birth preparedness and complication readiness, respectively. In the multivariate analysis, knowledge of birth preparedness and complication readiness (AOR = 1.648, 95%CI: 1.073, 2.531), knowledge of danger signs during pregnancy (AOR = 2.802, 95% CI: 1.637, 4.793), gestational age (AOR = 3.379, 95% CI: 2.114, 5.401), and antenatal care follow up starting time (AOR = 2.841, 95% CI: 1.330, 6.068) were significantly associated with the practice of birth preparedness and complication readiness, but pregnant women in rural areas (AOR = 0.442, 95% CI:0.244, 0.803) were less associated with birth preparedness and complication readiness compared to women in urban settlements.

Conclusion: This study identified that poor knowledge, inadequate birth preparedness, and complication readiness were prevalent among mothers in the study area. Government officials, partners, and health care providers working in the areas of maternal and child health should operate together to maximize birth preparedness and complication readiness practices.

Keywords: Birth preparedness, Complication readiness, Knowledge, Danger signs, Northeast Ethiopia

* Correspondence: kedijayenus@gmail.com
[3]Department of Reproductive Health, Institute of Public health, University of Gondar, Gondar, Ethiopia
Full list of author information is available at the end of the article

Background

Motherhood is a time of expectation and joy for a woman, her family, and her community. However, for thousands of women, the experience is not as pleasurable an event as it should be [1].

Each year in Africa 30 million women become pregnant, and about 250,000 of them die from pregnancy-related causes [2]. It is not possible to predict which women will experience life-threatening obstetric complications that lead to maternal mortality. On the whole, 42% of all pregnancies suffer complications – in rich and poor countries alike – and in 15% of all pregnancies, the complications are life-threatening. Scaling up birth preparedness and complication readiness (BPCR) practices and providing care by skilled providers (doctor', nurse' or midwives) during pregnancy, childbirth, and in the immediate postnatal period are fundamental for maternal health [2].

In many societies in the world, cultural beliefs and lack of knowledge of BPCR inhibit in advance preparations for delivery and expected babies. Since no action is taken prior to delivery, the family tries to act only when labor begins. To this end, the utilization of BPCR is the cornerstone for most developing countries, including Ethiopia. It is a strategy to promote a timely use of skilled maternal and neonatal care, especially during pregnancy, childbirth, and through the two-day post-partum period. The role of BPCR is to improve the use and effectiveness of key maternal and neonatal services through reducing the deadly delays (the first two delays) in deciding to seek care. Due to increases in the level of knowledge about complication readiness and the recognition of danger signs, the identification of problems and the delays in seeking health care services have been improved [3–8].

The Ministry of Health (MOH) has designed & initiated the application of BPCR in different maternal and neonatal health interventions to reduce maternal and newborn morbidity and mortality in Ethiopia. Currently, the Maternal Mortality Rate (MMR) of Ethiopia is 420 per 100,000 live births. Only 15% of the births in Ethiopia are at health facilities, 14% at public and 1% at private [9, 10].

Women's BPCR practices were examined by different authors who no doubt used sound methods. For instance, a study conducted in India on BPCR among slum women recognized steps; like identifying a trained birth attendant, selecting a health facility, arranging transport for delivery and obstetric emergency, and saving money for delivery; responding positively to at least three of the four elements was considered as an appropriate preparation [11].

In community-based cross-sectional studies conducted by Mpwapwa district of Tanzania, Plateau district in Nigeria, and a rural district of Ghana on BPCR among women showed that only a few of the women knew three or more obstetric danger signs [12–14].

According to a study conducted in rural Uganda, 52% of women knew at least one key danger sign during pregnancy, 72% during delivery and postpartum periods. Overall, 35% of the respondents who made arrangements in three of the four birth preparedness practices were classified as "well prepared for birth" [15].

A similar study conducted by Ife Central Local Government, Nigeria, on BPCR among pregnant women showed that 158 (39.3%) respondents knew no danger signs of pregnancy, childbirth, and postpartum periods. Only 24 (6.0%) had adequate knowledge of obstetric danger signs without prompting. Three hundred and forty (84.8%) of women identified birthplaces and 312 (78.3%) began saving money for delivery. However, 304 (79.4%) of the women made no arrangements for blood donors [16]. Other studies conducted in Adigrat and Goba districts of Ethiopia showed that only 118 (22.1%) and 128 (29.9%) of the total respondents, respectively, were found to be well prepared ahead of childbirth [17, 18].

A study done in Aleta Wondo district using five measures of BPCR that included identifying health provider, health facility and potential blood donor, the arrangement of transportation, and saving money for costs of delivery and emergency showed that among 743 pregnant women, only 20.5% identified skilled providers. In the same study, only 8.1% identified health facilities for delivery and/or for obstetric emergencies. On the other hand, the majority (87.9%) of the respondents reported that they intended to deliver at home, whereas only 60(8%) planned to deliver at health facilities, and 17% of the pregnant women were well prepared [19].

A study on the elements of BPCR in Jimma, Ethiopia, reported that 12.5%, 65.7%, 81%, 20.2%, and 58.9% of the pregnant women made prior decisions regarding skilled birth attendance, money, place of delivery, mode of transportation, and potential blood donor, respectively. On the whole, the study identified that less than one-third, 106 (29.4%) of the study participants were prepared for BPCR, indicating the prevalence or existence of poor practices or preparedness for birth and its complications in the area [20].

With regard to risk factors, studies done in Adigrate and Goba districts showed that residence, occupation, educational level, family size, ANC follow up, knowledge of danger signs during pregnancy, labor and postnatal period, as well as gravida and parity were found to have statistically significant associations with BPCR [17, 18].

Generally, almost all of the findings in the above studies revealed that BPCR remains almost unutilized to improve maternal and neonatal health in most developing countries, especially in sub-Saharan Africa. Hence, one can clearly understand that among the population studied, BPCR is comparatively low. The findings can also tell us BPCR is very low, especially in Ethiopia, compared to findings in other developing countries. As a result, the majority of the pregnant women did not give birth at health institutions; therefore, it is necessary to further investigate knowledge and practice of BPCR and possible associated factors.

As a matter of fact, not only were studies on BPCR in this particular area scarce but also the studies available varied in terms of time and place of study, geographic location, and population. Most previous studies focused on urban communities and among non- pregnant women [17–21]. In addition, the level of BPCR practice and its associated factors among pregnant women was not clearly examined in the study areas. So, the aim of this study was to assess BPCR practices and associated factors among pregnant women in Tehulederie district, Amhara National Regional State, northeast Ethiopia. Hence, the findings of the study will be crucial for the study woreda health officials, South Wollo zone health departments, the Amhara National Regional Health Bureau, and other maternal and neonatal health program implementers.

Methods

Study design and setting

A community-based cross-sectional study was conducted in Tehulederie district, the Amhara National Regional State, northeast Ethiopia, 2015. The district had 134,131 inhabitants (48% female), of which 31,628 were women in the reproductive age group, and 4520 were expectant pregnant women [22]. Tehulederie has a total of 26 kebeles (the lowest administrative units usually with multiple villages). It had 21 health posts, six small private clinics, three medium private clinics, five public health centers, seven drug stores, and one diagnostic facility [23].

The study was intended to represent all pregnant women who had the chance to be sampled in the district. After orientating about the significance of the study, pregnant women able to give informed consent were included.

Sample size determination and sampling procedure

The required sample size of the study was determined using the single population proportion formula. In determining the sample size, the proportion (p) of BPCR [18], the margin of error or precision (w), and confidence level were assumed to be 29.9%, 5%, and 95%, respectively. Moreover, a design effect of 1.5 and a non-response rate of 5% were applied to the initial sample size to get the final one (507).

In the district, about 4520 women were estimated to be eligible, that is expected to be pregnant. First, the district was stratified into urban and rural in order to deal with the effect of residence. Two of the five urban and eight of the twenty-one rural kebeles were proportionately selected by the simple random sampling technique. Then, the total sample size was allocated proportionally to each kebele according to their proportion of pregnant women. Thus, one hundred and seven participants from the two urban kebeles and four hundred from the eight rural kebeles were included in the study. To prepare the frame of pregnant mothers, Health Extension Workers (HEWs) of each selected kebele updated the identifications of pregnant women registered in the health centers/posts. Finally, every third pregnant mother was selected systematically by tracking them with the updated pregnant women registration location.

Operational definitions

For reasons of clarity and standardization, some concepts were defined operationally. Accordingly, birth preparedness and complication readiness elements included identifying a skilled birth attendant and health facility, arranging means of transport for delivery as well as in case of obstetric emergency, saving money, arranging blood donors in case of obstetric emergency, identifying a birth companion, temporary family caregiver, medical facility in case of obstetric emergency, and decision making in case of emergency.

A woman was considered as "knowledgeable in BPCR" if she identified and mentioned at least six key components of birth preparedness and complication readiness elements [18]. Similarly, a study participant would be considered as "knowledgeable in key danger signs of pregnancy" if she could spontaneously mention at least three key danger signs of pregnancy. On the other hand, a woman would be classified as "knowledgeable in key danger signs of labor" if she could spontaneously mention at least five key danger signs of labor/childbirth. Likewise, a woman would be considered as "knowledgeable in key danger signs of postpartum" if she could spontaneously mention at least five key danger signs of a postpartum period within two days [18].

Data collection procedure

A close-ended structured questionnaire was used to collect data from the participants. The questionnaire was prepared in English and translated to Amharic and retranslated to English by a language expert to check its consistency (Additional files 1 and 2). The questionnaire included Information on socio-demographic and obstetric characteristics, knowledge questions on key obstetric danger signs, birth preparedness, and complication readiness. After evaluation, the final version of the questionnaire was developed. For each of the questions, a participant who had the practice was given a score of "one", and lack of the practice was given a score of "zero". Seven diploma graduated nurses working out of the district, fluent in the local language and familiar with local norms collected the data. The data collectors interviewed participants in person. One BSc. the graduate health officer was assigned to supervise the data collection process. Training was given to both the data collectors and supervisor by the principal investigator for two days.

Data quality control/management

In order to ensure clarity and consistency, the questionnaire was pretested on 10% of the sample in a similar population of a nearby kebele. After that, the necessary modifications were made to the items and evidence-based time was allocated to each respondent. All data collected was checked for completeness by the principal investigator and the supervisor immediately at the end of each data collection day.

Data process and analysis

Data was entered, coded, cleaned and analyzed using SPSS version 20 software. Descriptive statistics such as frequencies and percentages were computed; then, a bivariable analysis was used to examine the crude associations of factors on BPCR. Variables with less than 0.2 p-values in the bivariable analysis were candidates for multivariable logistic regressions. Statistical significance was declared at a p-value of 0.05 and adjusted odds ratios were used to determine the strength of associations.

Result

Socio-demographic characteristics of respondents

Out of the total 507 samples, only five hundred pregnant women participated in the study, giving a response rate of 98.6%. The mean and ± Standard Deviation of respondent age was 28.8 ± 5 years; women's age ranged from 20 to 38 years. Of the total respondents, 472 (94.4%) were married and 4.4% single. Most of the respondents (469 or 93.8%) were housewives, and 391 (78.2%) of the pregnant women were rural dwellers; 338 (67.6%) attended formal school (Table 1).

Obstetric characteristics of respondents

In the assessment of obstetric characteristics, 135 (27%) of the respondents were primigravida, and about 365 (73%) had more than two pregnancies. Regarding gestational age, 185 (37%) respondents were in the first trimester and twenty-five (5%) in the third trimester. About 358 (71.6%) respondents had two and more than two ANC visits (Table 2).

Regarding knowledge of key danger signs during pregnancy, childbirth, and the postpartum period within two days, 492 (98.4%) of the 500 respondents reported that they had information about danger signs during

Table 1 Socio-demographic characteristics of pregnant women in Amhara National Regional State, northeast Ethiopia, 2015

Variables	Category	Frequency	Percentage
Age	15–24	107	21.4
	25–34	308	61.6
	35–44	85	17.0
Marital status	Single	22	4.4
	Married	472	94.4
	Divorce	4	0.8
	Widow	2	0.4
Residence	Urban	109	21.8
	Rural	391	78.2
Occupation	Housewife	469	93.8
	Government employee	9	1.8
	Merchant	15	3.0
	NGO employee	7	1.4
Religion	Orthodox	44	8.8
	Muslim	456	91.2
Family size	1–3	232	46.4
	4–6	244	48.8
	>/=7	24	4.8
Educational status	No formal education	338	67.6
	Primary education	98	19.6
	Secondary education	51	10.2
	College and above college	13	2.6
Monthly income	< 500 ETB	226	45.2
	500–1500 ETB	193	38.6
	> 1500 ETB	81	16.2
Ethnicity	Amhara	500	100.0
Partner education	No formal education	343	68.6
	Primary education	59	11.8
	Secondary education	58	11.6
	College and above College	40	8.0
Partner occupation	Farmer	354	70.8
	Employee	36	7.2
	Merchant	82	16.4
	NGO employee	28	5.6
Distance of HF from home (round trip)	</= one hour	162	33.0
	> one hour	338	67.0

pregnancy, childbirth, and within two days of the postpartum period. About 128 (25.6%), 333 (66.6%), and 321 (64.2%) of the pregnant women were not knowledgeable about danger signs during pregnancy, labor/childbirth and within two days of the postpartum period, respectively. When vaginal bleeding, the most frequently

Table 2 Obstetric characteristics of pregnant women in Tehulederie district, Amhara National Regional State, northeast Ethiopia, 2015

Variables	Category	Frequency	Percentage
Gestational age	1–3 months	185	37.0
	4–6 months	290	58.0
	7–9 months	25	5.0
Starting time for ANC visit	No	4	.8
	Yes	496	99.2
Number of ANC visits	One time	142	28.4
	Two times	168	33.6
	Three times	135	27.0
	Four times	51	10.2
	Five times	4	.8
ANC service was given by	Midwife/clinical nurse	471	94.2
	HEWs	29	5.8
ANC starting time	at < 3 month	54	10.8
	at 3–4 month	310	62.0
	>/= 5 month	136	27.2
Plan of ANC visit	< 4 visits	14	2.8
	4 visits	471	94.2
	> 4 visits	15	3.0
Para	0	135	27.0
	1–3	227	45.4
	>/= 4	138	27.6

Table 3 Knowledge of birth BPCR among pregnant women in Tehuledere district, northeast Ethiopia, 2015

Variable	Response	Frequency	Percentage
Identification of health facility	No	71	14.2
	Yes	429	85.8
Identification of skilled birth attendant	No	358	71.6
	yes	142	28.4
Saving money	No	60	12.0
	Yes	440	88.0
Preparation of transport	No	306	61.2
	Yes	194	38.8
Identification of temporary family caregiver	No	199	39.8
	Yes	301	60.2
Arranging blood donor	No	391	78.2
	Yes	109	21.8
Identification of birth companion	No	206	41.2
	Yes	294	58.8
Identification of decision-maker in case of emergency	No	207	41.4
	Yes	293	58.6
Identification of medical facility in case of emergency	No	88	17.6
	Yes	412	82.4
Knowledge about BPCR knowledgeable	No	277	55.4
	Yes	223	44.6

reported obstetric danger sign was considered, 484 (96.8%) had it during pregnancy, 483 (96.6%) at labor/ childbirth, and 455 (91%) in the postpartum period.

Knowledge of respondents about preparation for birth and its complications

All of the respondents reported that they had information about BPCR. Out of the total respondents, 223 (44.6%) were considered as knowledgeable. Regarding each recommended element which had to be done as BPCR; 440 (88%) said they saved money for delivery and possible obstetric emergency, 429 (85.8%) identified place of delivery, 109 (21.8) arranged potential blood donor, and 142 (28.4) spontaneously chose a skilled birth attendant (Table 3).

Birth preparedness and complication readiness practices of respondents

The majority of the respondents reported making arrangements for some of the recommended elements of BPCR. Out of 500 participants, 391 (78.2%), 175 (35%), 336 (67.2%), 202 (40.4%), and 104 (20.8%) identified health facilities for delivery, skilled birth attendants, financial sources

for delivery and possible obstetric emergencies, modes of transport, and potential blood donors, respectively. Similarly, out of the same number of participants, 352 (70.4%) identified a temporary family caregiver in case of emergency, 348 (69.6%) chose a birth companion, 380 (76%) selected medical facility in case of obstetric emergency, and 346 (69.2%) nominated decision maker in case of obstetric emergency. Overall, 43.4% of the women practiced BPCR.

Maternal socio-demographic and obstetric characteristics associated with their practices of birth preparedness and complication readiness

In the bivariate logistic regression analysis, a statistically significant association ($p < 0.05$) was observed between maternal practices of BPCR and their educational status, gestational age, spouse occupation, knowledge of danger signs during pregnancy and childbirth, number of ANC visits, marital status, residence, spouse education, knowledge of BPCR, monthly income, and starting time of ANC service. In the multivariate logistic regression analysis, a statistically significant association was observed on knowledge of women on BPCR [AOR = 1.648, 95% CI: 1.073, 2.531]. Similarly, women knowledgeable about danger signs during pregnancy were three times more likely to practice BPCR compared to those who had no knowledge about danger signs during pregnancy [AOR

= 2.802, 95% CI: 1.637, 4.793]. Pregnant women with a gestational age of 4–6 months were three times more likely to practice BPCR than women whose gestational age was up to three months [AOR = 3.379, 95% CI: 2.114, 5.401]. In addition, pregnant women who started ANC follow-up within 3–4 months of their pregnancy were three times more likely to practice BPCR compared to with those who started late [AOR = 2.841, 95% CI:1.330, 6.068] (Table 4).

Discussion

The aim of this study was to examine mainly the BPCR practice of pregnant women. Our study revealed that only less than half of the participants were practicing BPCR (217 or 43.4%) and that a nearly equal number of women were knowledgeable about the practice (223 or 44.6%).

The majority of the respondents reported that they made some arrangements on some of the recommended elements of BPCR. Out of five hundred respondents, 391 (78.2%) identified a health facility for delivery, 175 (35%) identified a skilled birth attendant, 336 (67.2%) saved money for delivery and any possible obstetric emergency, 202 (40.4%) determined mode of transport, 104 (20.8%) identified potential blood donor in case of emergency, 352 (70.4%) selected temporary family care giver, 348 (69.6%) nominated birth companion, 380 (76%) identified medical facility in case of obstetric emergency, and 346 (69.2%) selected decision maker in case of obstetric emergency. Generally, only 217 (43.4%) of the participants made BPCR arrangements.

In this study, 391 (78.2%) pregnant women identified health facility for delivery. This is almost comparable with the findings of studies done in Jimma town and Goba woreda, Oromia Region, Ethiopia, which reported 285 (81%) and 432 (76.9%), respectively [18, 20]. However, the finding of this study is lower than that of a study done in Mpwapwa district Tanzania which detected 583 (97.3%) [12]. The likely explanations for this dissimilarity might be differences in study subjects and settings. On the other hand, this finding is higher than those of studies done in Adigrat town, northern Ethiopia, and Aleta wondo, southern Ethiopia, which reported 209 (39.1%) and 59 (8.1%), respectively [17, 19]. This difference might be due to variations in the times of investigations in that currently some more attention is being to the issue by maternal health implementers. Accessing health extension workers nearby in the community might increase the number of ANC attendants and improve decision on the identification of health facility for delivery.

The finding of the current study showed that 175 (35%) of the respondents identified skilled birth attendants. This finding was lower than those of studies done in Indore City, India, which noted 217 (69.6%), Mpwapwa district, Tanzania 436 (86.2%), and Chamwino district, Tanzania 333 (77.8%) [11, 12, 24]. The observed discrepancy might be due to study settings, target populations, and knowledge of women about BPCR and obstetric danger signs during pregnancy, labour, and postpartum period. Conversely, it was higher than the findings of studies conducted in Adigrat and Duguna Fango district, Wolayta

Table 4 Maternal socio-demographic and obstetric characteristics associated with BPCR practices in Tehuledere district, northeast Ethiopia, 2015

Variables		Practices of BPCR			95% C.I. for AOR		P-value
		No	Yes	AOR	Lower	Upper	
Gestational age*	up to 3 month	133	52	1			
	at 4–6 month	132	158	3.379	**2.114**	**5.401**	.000
	at 7–9 month	18	7	1.422	.512	3.948	.500
Residence*	Urban	44	65	1			
	Rural	239	152	.442	**.244**	**.803**	.007
Starting time o ANC*	at < 3 month	38	16	1			
	at 3–4 month	166	144	2.841	**1.330**	**6.068**	.007
	>/= 5 month	79	57	1.278	.555	2.942	.564
Knowledge of BPCR*	Not knowledgeable	177	100	1			
	Knowledgeable	106	117	1.648	**1.073**	**2.531**	.023
Knowledge of danger signs during pregnancy*	Not knowledgeable	101	27	1			
	Knowledgeable	182	190	2.802	**1.637**	**4.793**	.000
Partner occupation	Farmer	229	125	1			
	Employee	12	52	2.259	.891	5.723	.086
	Merchant	32	50	2.280	1.263	4.114	.06

Zone which reported 56 (10.5%) and 62 (10.9%), respectively [17, 25]. The difference could be due to the study period, an increased number of ANC visits which might have increased access to information. The expansion of Health Extension Workers (HEWs) to the rural community might have created an opportunity for raising women's knowledge regarding the role of skilled attendants at birth.

In the present study, saving money for delivery and any possible obstetric emergency was 336 (67.2%). This result was consistent with 388 (69%) of a study conducted in Goba woreda, Oromia Region [18]. However, our finding was lower than those of studies conducted in Indore City, India, Chamwino district, Tanzania, West Bengal, India, Mpwapwa district, Tanzania, and in Plateau State, Nigeria which reported 240 (76.9%), 360 (84.1%), 84.6%, 536 (89.3%), and 209 (83.6%), respectively [11–13, 24, 26]. This could be due to differences in settings, resulting in variations in socio-economic status, culture, and level of female empowerment. If women are empowered educationally and economically, they could have a better understanding of obstetric danger signs or complications and benefit from BPCR and save money for delivery and obstetric complication services. However, the current finding was higher than those of studies conducted in Duguna Fango district, Wolayta Zone 308 (54.1%) and Adigrat 190 (35.6%) [27, 17]. The difference might be due to variations in the study period and knowledge status of women about BPCR. The knowledge level of the respondents about BPCR was higher compared to the above studies. This fact showed that women who knew that money could help them to buy important medical supplies or pay for transportation in case of delivery and obstetrics emergency made better BPCR arrangements.

This study revealed that 202 (40.4%) of the pregnant women arranged the mode of transportation for delivery/obstetric emergency. This finding corroborated a study conducted in Adigrat and noted 40.8% [17]. However, the finding was lower compared with those of studies conducted in Mpwapwa district, Tanzania and Plateau State, Nigeria which reported 494 (82.3%) and 135 (54%), respectively [12, 13]. This could be because of variations in study settings, resulting in differences in socio-economic status and access to transportation. But our finding was higher than the result of a study (103/18.1%) done in Fango district, Wolayta Zone [27]. This could be due to an increase in the number of HEWs and repeated ANC visits which might have created awareness on the benefits of early arrangement for transportation. In cases of geographical inaccessibility or financial problems, our community arranged traditional ways of transportation such as donkeys, horses, or mules and local stretchers. Identifying transportation ahead of childbirth and

improvement in decision-making can reduce maternal and neonatal mortality.

Our study found that 104 (20.8%) of the women identified potential blood donors in cases of emergency. This finding was similar to that of a study done in Plateau State, Nigeria which reported 58 (23.2%) [13]. But it was higher than the results of studies done in Fango district, Wolayta Zone 17 (3.0%), Goba woreda, Oromia Region 51 (9.1%), Robe woreda, Arsi Zone 57 (9.9%) and Adigrat 4 (0.7%) [17, 18, 21, 27]. This might be due to an improvement in the knowledge of pregnant women and their families about the importance of early identification of blood donors. In this study, nearly 100% of the pregnant women attended ANC which created a good opportunity for getting appropriate information on the elements of BPCR by skilled birth attendants. Making arrangements for blood donors is important because women giving birth may need a blood transfusion in the event of hemorrhage or cesarean section.

This study indicated that 352 (70.4%) of the pregnant women identified temporary family caregivers. This finding was lower than that of a study done in Mpwapwa district, Tanzania and documented 548 (91.3%) [12]. This could be due to differences in study settings resulting in variations in the quality of counseling and strength of applying BPCR strategy in order to reduce maternal and child mortality.

In the current study, 380 (76%) of the women identified the medical facility in preparation for the obstetric emergency. The result of this study was higher than the result of a study done in Fango district, Wolayta Zone, Goba woreda, Oromia Region, and Adigrat town, northern Ethiopia, which found out 43.6%, 47.5% and 6.6%, respectively [17, 18, 27]. This could be due to the expansion of the Health Extension Program which might have improved the number of ANC attendants in the health facilities- which probably increased awareness on obstetric danger signs and arrangements for medical facilities to cope with obstetric emergencies.

The finding showed that 346 (69.2%) of the respondents identified decision makers for cases of obstetric emergency. This finding is lower than that of a study conducted in Mpwapwa district, Tanzania, and noted 564 (94.0%) [12]. This difference might be due to variations in the socio-economic and educational status of women and the implementation of BPCR strategies. But the finding was higher than 12 (2.2%) reported from Adigrat, northern Ethiopia [17]. This could be due to differences in study periods. That is, currently the Ethiopian government has given special attention to BPCR integration and implementation at the grassroot levels by each primary health care unit and the emphasis given to male involvement in maternal health care services which might have encouraged women to identify decision-makers in cases of obstetric emergencies.

In this study, 217 (43.4%) respondents practiced BPCR. The finding was lower than the results of studies done in Indore City, India, Chamwino district, central Tanzania, Edo State, Nigeria, and the rural area of Darjeeling West Bengal, India, which reported (47.8%), (58.2%), (87.4%), and (57%), respectively [11, 24–26]. The possible reason could be the differences in study areas as the current study included both rural and urban/city communities. However, it was higher than those of studies done in rural Uganda, Aleta Wondo, southern Ethiopia, Adigrat town, northern Ethiopia, Jimma town southwest Ethiopia, Goba woreda, Oromia Region, Ethiopia, Robe woreda, Arsi zone, Oromia Region, central Ethiopia, and Dugna Fango district, Wolayta Zone, Ethiopia, which found (35%), (17%), (22.1%), (29.4%), (29.9%), (18.3%), and (16.5%), respectively [15, 17–21, 27]. The likely reason for the difference could be that the recommended BPCR elements might have been given more focus in these healthcare setups.

In the multivariate logistic regression analysis, knowledge of BPCR was two times more likely to encourage BPCR practice compared to no knowledge. This finding is inconsistent with that of a study done in Goba woreda [18]. The possible reason for the difference could be the quality of information given to women about BPCR. Increasing the number of ANC attendants and knowledge on the elements of BPCR to pregnant women during each visit might motivate them to prepare for birth and to be ready for obstetric complications.

Participants knowledgeable about danger signs during pregnancy were three times more likely to practice BPCR compared to those who had no knowledge. This finding is similar to those of studies done in Goba and Robe woredas, Ethiopia, but differs from that of a study done in Adigrat [17, 18, 21]. The possible reason could be the study period and the clarity of information on BPCR addressed at times of repeated ANC visits. Besides, their partners might have been involved in BPCR. Knowledge about the danger signs of obstetric complications is important for recognizing complications early and taking immediate actions to access essential emergency obstetric care.

Pregnant women who started their ANC services within three to four months of pregnancy were three times more likely to be prepared to practice BPCR compared with those who started late. This finding was in line with those of studies conducted in Robe woreda, Arsi Zone, Fango district, Wolayta Zone and Goba woreda [18, 21, 27]. This might indicate that there was a better exposure to information on BPCR during the repeated visits.

Rural pregnant women were 0.44 times less likely to be prepared for BPCR. That is, urban dwellers were more likely to be prepared for BPCR. This finding is similar to that of a study done in Goba woreda [18]. The possible reason could be that urban residence improves access to information, service, and BPCR practice.

Limitations of this study were since the design of our work was cross-sectional; it might not have been strong enough to demonstrate the cause and effect relationships between dependent and independent variables. In addition, as the data collectors were health professionals, there was a possibility of social desirability bias in the responses to some of the variables.

Conclusion

The present study identified that there has been poor preparedness for birth and complications. Residence, knowledge about BPCR and danger signs during pregnancy, gestational age, and the starting time of ANC service were significantly associated with BPCR practice.

Health professionals should create awareness on birth preparedness and complication readiness among pregnant mothers, families, or communities. Government officials, partners, and health care providers that are working in areas of maternal and child health should work together to ameliorate factors that influence the low practice of birth preparedness and complication readiness. Researchers need to conduct qualitative studies to explore the main reasons for their poor preparedness of pregnant women for birth and in cases of obstetric complications in order to bring significant changes in the reduction of maternal and neonatal deaths.

Abbreviations

ANC: Antenatal care; BPCR: Birth preparedness and complication readiness; BSc: Bachelor of science; EDHS: Ethiopian demographic health survey; EFMOH: Ethiopian federal ministry of health; ETB: Ethiopian birr; FMOH: Federal ministry of health; HAD: Health development army; HEWs: Health extension workers; MDGs: Millennium development goals; MMR: Maternal mortality ratio; NGOs: Non-governmental organizations; PNC: Postnatal care; SNNP: Southern nations, nationalities, and people; SPSS: Statistical package for social sciences; TBA: Traditional birth attendant; WHO: World Health Organization

Acknowledgements

The authors would like to acknowledge the data collectors and the supervisor for their unreserved work. They also forwarded compliments to the study participants for providing the necessary information.

Funding

The funding body was the University of Gondar for data collection and analysis. However, the funder has no role in manuscript preparation and publication.

Authors' contributions

DB wrote the proposal, implemented the proposal, analyzed the data and drafted the paper. HY participated in revising the proposal and involve on data analysis and the subsequent drafts of the paper. LD worked on the methodology and analysis sections of the study, as well as the discussion section. All authors read and approved the final manuscript.

Authors' information

Principal Investigator: Demlie Belete Endeshaw.

Ethics approval and consent to participate

Ethical approval was obtained from University of Gondar, College of Medicine and Health Science, Institute of Public Health Institutional Review Board (IRB). Letter of permission to conduct the study at the area was collected from Tehulederie Woreda Health Office. Since the authors thought that there was no any potential risk associated on the provision of the data and it is a cross-sectional study, informed verbal consent was considered and obtained from each respondent. The ethics committee also approved the appropriateness of the informed verbal consent for this study. Participants were informed about their rights to decline if they didn't want to continue. The questions were coded instead of using names; so confidentiality was assured throughout the study. Involving the use of any animal or human data or tissue: "Not applicable" in this research section. Data from any individual person in any form (including individual details, images or videos): "Not applicable" in this research.

Competing interests

The authors declare that they have no competing interests.

Author details

[1]Maternal and Child Survival Program (MCSP), Community Based Newborn Care (CBNC) Coordinator, Save the children, Woldia, Ethiopia. [2]Department of Epidemiology and Biostatistics, Institute of Public health, University of Gondar, Gondar, Ethiopia. [3]Department of Reproductive Health, Institute of Public health, University of Gondar, Gondar, Ethiopia.

References

1. World Health Organization (WHO). Preventing maternal deaths. 1989.
2. Luwei P, Margareta L, Vincent F, Judith S. Childbirth care, opportunities for African newborns. 2012.
3. Family Care International London. Women deliver organization partner. 2007.
4. JHPIEGO. Monitoring birth preparedness and complication readiness, tools and indicators for maternal and newborn health. 2004.
5. The White Ribbon Alliance for Safe Motherhood. Saving mothers' lives. India; 2010.
6. Kakaire O, Kaye DK, Osinde MO. Male involvement in birth preparedness and complication readiness for emergency obstetric referrals in rural Uganda. Reprod Health. 2011;8:12.
7. Thaddeus S, Maine D. Too far to walk maternal mortality in context. Soc Sci Med. 1994;38(8):1091–110.
8. Program J-ManhM. Birth preparedness and complication readiness: a matrix of shared responsibilities. 2001.
9. Ethiopia Press materials. No woman should die while giving life, safe motherhood monthly calls for zero home deliveries. 2014.
10. Central Statistical Agency Addis Ababa Ethiopia. Ethiopian mini demography and health survey. 2014.
11. Agarwal S, Sethi V, Srivastava K, Jha PK, Baqui AH. Birth preparedness and complication readiness among slum women, Indore City, India. International center for diarrheal disease research, Bangladesh. J Health Popul Nutr. 2010;28(4):383–91.
12. Urassa DP, Pembe AB, Mganga F. Birth preparedness and complication readiness among women in Mpwapwa district, Tanzania. Tanzania J Health Res. 2012;14(1):42–7.
13. Envuladu EA, Zoakah AI. Assessment of the birth and emergency preparedness level of pregnant women in Jos, plateau state. Nigeria IJBAIR. 2014;3(1):2–7.
14. Kuganab-Lem RB, Dogudugu R, Kanton L. Birth preparedness and complication readiness: a study of postpartum women in a rural district of Ghana. Public Health Research. 2014;4(6):225–33. https://doi.org/10.5923/j.phr.20140406.02.
15. Kabakyenga JK, Östergren P-O, Turyakira E, Pettersson KO. Knowledge of obstetric danger signs and birth preparedness practices among women in rural Uganda. Reprod Health. 2011;8:33.
16. Kuteyi EAA, Kuku JO, Lateef IC, Ogundipe JA, Mogbeyteren T, Banjo MA. Birth preparedness and complication readiness of pregnant women attending the three levels of health facilities in Ife central local government, Nigeria. J Community Med & Prim Health. 2011;23(1-2).
17. Hiluf M, Fantahun M. Birth preparedness and complication readiness among women in Adigrat town, northern Ethiopia. EthiopJHealth Dev. 2007;22(1):14–20.
18. Markos D, Bogale D. Birth preparedness and complication readiness among women of childbearing age group, Goba woreda, Oromia region. Ethiopia BMC Pregnancy and Childbirth. 2014;14:282.
19. Hailu M, Gebremariam A, Alemseged F, Deribe K. Birth preparedness and complication readiness among pregnant women, Aleta Wondo, southern Ethiopia. PLoS One. 2011;6(6):e21432. https://doi.org/10.1371/journal.pone.0021432.
20. Kitila SB, Tebeje B. Predictors of birth preparedness and complication readiness among pregnant women in Jimma town, Southwest Ethiopia. Research. 2014;1:595.
21. Kaso M, Addisse M. Birth preparedness and complication readiness in robe district, Arsi zone, Oromia region, Central Ethiopia. Reprod Health. 2014;11:55.
22. Central Statistics Agency Ethiopia. Census report. 2007.
23. South Wollo Zone Health Department Dessie Ethiopia. Annual key indicators performance report by Woreda. 2013/2014.
24. Bintabara D, Mohamed MA, Mghamba J, Wasswa P, Mpembeni RNM. Birth preparedness and complication readiness among recently delivered women in Chamwino district, Central Tanzania. Reprod Health. 2015;12:44. https://doi.org/10.1186/s12978-015-0041-8.
25. Tobin EA, Ofili AN, Enebeli N, Enueze O. Assessment of birth preparedness and complication readiness among pregnant women attending at primary health care Centres in Edo state. Nigeria Annals of Nigerian Medicine. 2014;8(2):76–81.
26. Mandal T, Biswas R, Bhattacharyya S, Das DK. Birth preparedness and complication readiness among recently delivered women in a rural area of Darjeeling, West Bengal. India AMSRJ. 2015;2(1):14–20.
27. Gebre M, Gebremariam A, Abebe TA. Birth preparedness and complication readiness among pregnant women in Duguna Fango district, Wolayta zone. Ethiopia PLoS ONE. 2015;10(9):e0137570. https://doi.org/10.1371/journal.pone.0137570.

"I see myself as part of the team" – family caregivers' contribution to safety in advanced home care

Christiane Schaepe* [ID] and Michael Ewers

Abstract

Background: The use of medical technology and the various contributing and interdepending human factors in home care have implications for patient safety. Although family caregivers are often involved in the provision of advanced home care, there is little research on their contribution to safety. The study aims to explore family caregivers in Home Mechanical Ventilation (HMV) safety experiences and how safety is perceived by them in this context. Furthermore, it seeks to understand how family caregivers contribute to the patients' and their own safety in HMV and what kind of support they expect from their health care team.

Methods: An explorative, qualitative study was applied using elements from grounded theory methodology. Data were collected through individual interviews with 15 family caregivers to patients receiving HMV in two regions in Germany. The audiotaped interviews were then subject to thematic analysis.

Results: The findings shows that family caregivers contribute to safety in HMV by trying to foster mutual information sharing about the patient and his/her situation, coordinating informally health care services and undertaking compensation of shortcomings in HMV.

Conclusion: Consequently, family caregivers take on considerable responsibility for patient safety in advanced home care by being actively and constantly committed to safety work.
Nurses working in this setting should be clinically and technically skilled and focus on building partnership relations with family caregivers. This especially encompasses negotiation about their role in care and patient safety. Support and education should be offered if needed. Only skilled nurses, who can provide safe care and who can handle critical situations should be appointed to HMV. They should also serve as professional care coordinators and provide educational interventions to strengthen family caregivers' competence.

Keywords: Qualitative research, Family caregivers, Advanced home care, Home mechanical ventilation, Patient safety

Background

Advanced technology for the provision of enteral tube feeding, home-based dialysis, intravenous therapy and home mechanical ventilation (HMV) is widely used in the community in many western countries. Multiple factors have contributed to this converging trend, such as advances in technology, increased availability of 'hospital at home' services, demographic changes paired with an increasing number of people living with chronic conditions or surviving congenital conditions, reduced institutional care and cost savings [1, 2]. These developments enable technologically dependent patients with complex needs to remain at home while receiving intensive nursing care on a comparable level to that provided in the hospital setting [3]. Advanced home care, thus, promises to be a cost-efficient and patient-centered alternative to institutionalized care [4, 5].

This paper will focus on HMV as an example of advanced home care. The latter is a therapeutic option for individuals with various underlying diseases ranging from conditions leading to progressive respiratory failure to unsuccessful weaning after an acute respiratory

* Correspondence: christiane.schaepe@charite.de

Charité – Universitätsmedizin Berlin, corporate member of Freie Universität Berlin, Humboldt-Universität zu Berlin, and Berlin Institute of Health, Institute of Health and Nursing Science, Berlin, Germany failure. The HMV can be delivered noninvasively (via mask) or invasively (via tracheostomy) on a continuous or intermittent basis [6]. Users of HMV represent a vulnerable, heterogeneous, small, but increasing group of technology-dependent individuals in many western countries [7, 8]. Although the number of patients on HMV in Germany is unknown due to a lack of prevalence data, it is estimated that 20,000 individuals are living with HMV in Germany [9]. Caring for an individual receiving HMV is very complex, because it entails the care of a person who is receiving life support due to their critical illness and has substantial care needs. Their condition makes patients dependent on technological assistance and skilled nursing services providing personal care, several daily medical and therapeutic procedures, and educational and psychosocial support for the patients and their family.

The fact that ventilator-dependent patients receive up to 24-h professional nursing services and medical treatment in their private homes funded by the Statutory Health and Nursing Care Insurance in Germany is of particular relevance. The main goal of this form of advanced home care is to guarantee a hospital-like immediate and qualified intervention in life-threatening situations [10]. Thus, providing intensive care in a private home brings challenges for all actors involved, including health professionals, patients and family members [3]. For families, the intrusiveness of medical technology in the private home care setting and the constant presence of nurses, flanked by occasional visits of other health care providers, results in a lack of privacy, which often proves to be a great challenge [11–13].

Furthermore, advanced home care has implications for patient safety. Various contributing and interdependent human factors have an impact on patient safety in home care. The individual characteristics of the patients and their caregivers, the nature of health care tasks, the home and social environment, medical devices and new technology are major components [14, 15]. The home care setting, for example, has distinctive characteristics that are very different from institutional environments and that have an impact on patient safety. Home care nurses work in isolation and their role is rather that of a guest in the family's home [15, 16]. The unique nature of each individual home contributes to home care being viewed as unregulated and uncontrolled [17]. Despite this background, corresponding research is mainly conducted in institutional settings and little attention has been paid to safety in home care [17, 18]. Recent research from Canada has gleaned information that adverse events in home care are not rare [19, 20]. The Pan-Canadian Home Care Safety Study reports that 10.1% of the clients experience adverse events annually and that 56% of these were predictable [21]. Existing studies on safety in home care focus on safety risks and specific adverse events, such as falls, pressure ulcers, unplanned hospital admissions and medication errors, which are reported from the perspective of the health care provider [18, 20, 22, 23]. Very few studies have, however, focused on patient safety in home care from the perspective of the patient and family caregiver [24, 25]. Among these studies, the Pan-Canadian Home Care Safety Study has found that patient safety is strongly influenced by the understanding of family members, caregivers and providers regarding safety [26]. Consistent with these findings, another Canadian study found that safety concerns from the perspective of patients and family caregivers are multidimensional and intersectional, and are influenced by physical, spatial and interpersonal factors [25]. That is also a reason why the general definition of *patient safety* needs to be broadened by incorporating the perspective of all actors involved, including the family caregivers [17, 27].

A recent scoping review found that the compulsory enrollment to take on the caregiver role, the lack of preparedness and support, and loss of control have an impact on family caregiver safety [28]. In addition, psychological and physical health impairments and financial problems create a safety concern for caregivers [28]. Whether this applies to advanced home care is not known. To date, most qualitative research on family caregiving in advanced home care focuses on the perspective of parent caregivers to children. These studies have shown that family caregivers play a pivotal role in advanced home care, providing complex caregiving tasks, including technical procedures in daily care. They advocate for their family members within the health care system, take care of the equipment and coordinate health care services [29–31]. The responsibility for care has been shifted from the personnel to the parents [12, 13, 32]. Consequently, physical and emotional burdens and social isolation among caregivers of technology-dependent children are widely reported throughout the literature [13, 31, 33]. The main concern of family caregivers regarding adult HMV users is the constant struggle with health care services, including the lack of involvement in decision-making processes, the lack of continuity of care and the inadequate professional support [34]. Accordingly, access to psychosocial support was reported as being important to family caregivers [35, 36].

Family caregivers might be the first to witness any safety-related issue in the home setting due to their daily interaction with the care recipient and the formers' often extensive shared life experience, and can, consequently, provide a unique perspective of home health care delivery. Given that the number of patients who require advanced home care in general and HMV specifically will probably increase, there is a need to better understand the role of the various actors involved in patient safety in this context. Nevertheless, the literature on family caregiving and safety remains focused on two aspects. Family caregivers are either referred to as "secondary patients" who need to be protected from physical and emotional harm, or as easily available providers of care with the potential of harming their family members [37]. Family caregivers' own perspective of their role in providing safety in home care has not yet gained attention from the research community. However, a better understanding of family caregivers' perspective of their contribution to safety their perspective could provide health professionals with additional strategies for providing safe, effective and patient-centered care in the home setting. To date, little empirical work has been undertaken to examine family caregivers' perspective of safety [28]. The present study, therefore, aims to fill this research gap by exploring family caregivers in HMV safety experiences and how safety is perceived by them in such a special care arrangement. Furthermore, it seeks to understand how family caregivers contribute to the patients' and their own safety in HMV and what kind of support they expect from their health care team.

Methods

An explorative, qualitative research design using elements of grounded theory methodology [38] has been chosen for this study.

The study was part of a larger, multistage qualitative health services research project called SHAPE ("Safety in Home Care for Ventilated Patients") which aimed at providing impulses for the conceptualization of safety work in advanced home care based on empirical data from the perspective of both users and providers. Partial results of this study, which has been funded by the German Federal Ministry of Education and Research and was performed from 2013 to 2017, have been published elsewhere [39].

Recruitment

Recruitment was facilitated by the staff of nursing care providers (gatekeepers) who are in daily contact with the families. They provided some basic verbal information and distributed an introductory letter about the study to eligible participants. Other ways of approaching participants were through a hospital-based specialized respiratory care center, a health care insurance company, personal contacts and organizations, such as the German Association for Muscular Dystrophy and patient advocacy groups. Those who were interested in participating contacted the research team themselves and or via the nursing care providers and a mutually convenient appointment for the interview was scheduled. Participants were recruited in rural and urban areas in Northeast and South Germany to identify regional differences.

Family caregivers had to be at least 18 years, speak and understand German, and be involved in the care of an adult HMV user in some way to be included in the study. Maximum variation in participant characteristics, for example age, relationship to the care recipient, years of experience of HMV in the home, was used as a sampling strategy. It aims to include a wide spectrum of participants to gain a broad insight into their diverse perspectives and experiences [40].

Data collection

Data was collected on two visits, as part of an iterative process over a period of 12 months (from June 2014 to June 2015). Potential participants were given additional information prior to the onset of the study.

Written and oral informed consent to participation was obtained on the first visit. Participants were asked to provide sociodemographic information (e.g. age, hours of caregiving, income and educational level) and to fill in the Burden Scale for Family Caregivers [41]. In addition, sociodemographic-, disease- and treatment-related information of the patients was collected. It was made clear that participation was voluntary and that they could withdraw from the study at any point in the data collection or analysis. Participants' confidentiality was guaranteed. On the second visit, a pilot tested, semi-structured interview guide with open-ended questions was used to elicit information on the everyday life of caregivers ("I would like to get an idea of how your everyday life looks like and therefore ask you to tell me how your day yesterday looked like") and the role of HMV and their caregiving. They were further asked to give examples of situations where they felt particularly unsafe ("Can you describe a situation where you felt particularly unsafe?"), what they did in this situation, how the professionals reacted and what could have been done better or differently. At the end of the interview, they summed up their meaning of safety in home care. New questions evolved during data analysis and topics became more focused in later interviews.

Apart from a few exceptions, most of the interviews were conducted in the HMV recipient's home. The interviews lasted between 32 and 250 min and were audio-taped (with one exception; permission was refused by one informant and detailed notes were recorded). Two researchers were present during the interviews in most cases. Nonverbal expressions and gestures, potential disruptions, and the topics addressed before and after the interview were recorded in an interview protocol. An additional, detailed observational protocol was written on the home environment.

Data analysis

Although data collection and data analysis were intended to occur concurrently in an iterative process, this could not always be realized due to initial recruitment difficulties. The interviews were transcribed verbatim and identifying information were pseudonymized in this process. The analysis was performed in German and the software MAXQDA 11 (verbi GmbH, Berlin Germany) was used to organize and manage the data. The thematic analysis began after the first interview with repeated reading of the first transcripts in order to become immersed in the data [42–44]. In the next step, the data were coded. Three forms of coding were employed: *Open coding* with in vivo coding was performed. The constant comparison technique was used with codes and concepts and clustered to create preliminary categories. Connections between categories were built in the *axial coding*. In *selective coding*, categories were saturated with data from new interviews. Memos were written throughout the whole analysis process to document ideas and reflections about the emerging codes and categories. After all the data were coded, the categories were sorted and combined into themes. Finally, several relevant themes were defined and named and condensed for reporting.

Trustworthiness

Strategies that were used to evaluate the rigor of the study were based on the concept of trustworthiness by Lincoln and Guba [45]. Credibility was strengthened by the prolonged engagement in the field and by maximum variation sampling [46]. Prolonged engagement means that the researcher spent extended time in the field in order to gain a deeper understanding of the social context of the interviewees' narratives, which helped to gain their trust and thereby facilitated authentic data collection. Dependability was enhanced by performing the analysis as part of a research team. To this end, several discussions and reflections were done throughout the analysis process. The team discussed and reflected for example on alternative ways of approaching participants in order to avoid selection bias, if more variation was needed in the sampling, the next analytical steps that had to be taken, the themes that emerged from the data. A thick description of the sample, setting and data collection, and analysis are presented for the reader's judgment of transferability.

Results

Sample description

A total of 15 relatives of HMV patients gave consent to participate in the study (see Table 1 for participants key characteristics). Nine of them are spouses or partners, three mothers, two children and one sister. The participants' age ranged from 31 to 83 years, with three males and 12 females. Four caregivers were employed, eight retired and three partially retired or unemployed. Eight of the 15 participants were living in a common household with the HMV users and seven were living separately.

The nature of family caregivers' involvement in everyday care varies. While some of them provide 24-h care (including endotracheal suctioning, supervision of the functioning of the technical devices and constant vigilance over the care recipient), others merely visit the patients in their homes on a regular basis. The degree of involvement ranged from 1, 5 to 24 h per day. All but one family were receiving (professional) nursing services. The extent of skilled nursing care offered ranged from 8 to 24 h per day. Despite this variation, the results of the Burden Scale for Family Caregivers in our sample show that most of the participants experience little and moderate burden (see Table 1).

Apart from using HMV, the care recipients are similarly a heterogeneous group. The reasons for HMV dependency varied from neuromuscular diseases, restrictive, thoracic disorders to chronic obstructive pulmonary disease. Average daily ventilation use ranged from 10 to 24 h. A more detailed description of the care recipient's characteristics can be found elsewhere [39].

Contribution of family caregivers to safety in HMV

Several themes emerged from the interview data during analysis exploring the broad spectrum of safety experiences and perspectives of relatives of HMV users. It also became apparent that family caregivers of ventilated patients use several strategies to cope with their specific situation and to guarantee the care recipients' and their own safety. "Fostering mutual information sharing about the patient and his/her situation", "coordinating health care services" and "compensating for shortcomings in HMV" are the most evident contributions family caregivers make to guarantee safety in advanced home care for technologically dependent patients based on our empirical data.

Mutual information sharing

Family caregivers in this study often try to foster mutual information sharing about the patient and his/her situation based on their familiarity and their intimate knowledge about their relatives' needs, wishes and personal preferences. That is particularly the case when the patients themselves have limited communication possibilities due to the ventilation or when they cannot express themselves due to their vulnerable physical or mental status. They not only intend a more personalized care by sharing their information with members of the health care team, but rather to prevent adverse events and promote patient safety. Exemplarily, this strategy is being applied by Ms. Yilmaz, who has been caring for her ventilated and bedbound husband 24-h a day for many years. Due to her long-standing marriage and her

Table 1 Characteristics of family caregivers and care recipients

Caregivers Pseudonym	Age of caregiver	Gender of caregiver	Level of Education	Employment status	Relationship to the care recipient	Living arrangement	Years of experience of HMV in the home	BSFC Results*	Care recipients Disease group	Hours of HMV	Hours of nursing service	IV or NIV
Mrs Becker, Katrin	31	Female	High School	half-time employment	daughter	separated from the patient	1	40	neuromuscular disorder	continuous	24hs	IV
Mrs Wagner, Monika	63	Female	College or University	part-time retirement	wife	together with the patient	2	13	neuromuscular disorder	continuous	24hs	IV
Mrs Yilmaz, Fatma	60	Female	High School	full-time employment	wife	together with the patient	7	23	neuromuscular disorder	continuous	24hs	IV
Mr Meyer, Peter	56	Male	College or University	early retirement	son	separated from the patient	10	27	pulmonary disease	continuous	24hs	IV
Mrs Wolf, Christa	71	Female	Basic	retirement pension	wife	together with the patient	1	16	neuromuscular disorder	> 16hs	24hs	IV
Mr Richter, Karl	79	Male	College or University	retirement pension	husband	separated from the patient	missing	missing	vegetative state	> 16 hs	24hs	IV
Mrs Bauer, Ursula	70	Female	High School	retirement pension	mother	together with the patient	41	19	tetra paresis	< 16 hs	9hs	IV
Mrs Braun, Sabine	56	Female	Basic	early retirement pension	wife	together with the patient	6	21	Tetra paresis	< 16 hs	without nursing service	IV
Mrs Schulz, Angelika	62	Female	Basic	half-time employment	sister	separated from the patient	4	28	metabolic disease	continuous	24hs	IV
Mrs Werner, Gabrielle	54	Female	High School	full-time employment	wife	separated from the patient	3	23	neuromuscular disorder	continuous	24hs	IV
Mrs König, Renate	61	Female	High School	early retirement pension	spouse	separated from the patient	1	37	neuromuscular disorder	continuous	24hs	IV
Mrs Peters, Birgit	59	Female	High School	no gainful employment	mother	together with the patient	41	7	neuromuscular disorder	continuous	8hs	NIV
Mrs Koch, Ingrid	69	Female	Missing	retirement pension	wife	together with the patient	missing	missing	infectious disease	continuous	8hs	IV
Mrs Zimmermann, Andrea	56	Female	Basic	unemployment	mother	together with the patient	15	45	tetra paresis	10hs	11hs	NIV
Mr Hoffmann, Günther	83	Male	High School	retirement pension	husband	together with the patient	14	31	neuromuscular disorder	continuous	24hs	IV

*BSFC Results: no/little burden: 0–24 points, moderate burden: 25–55 points, severe burden: 56–84 points

extensive experience of caring for her technologically dependent husband, she is convinced that she knows his needs, wishes and preferences very well. She wants to share this unique information with the nurses so that they can act accordingly. In exchange, she herself wants to be informed regularly about what happens in everyday care and how her husband reacts to the care services offered. The following quotation illustrations her motivation:

"Well, I see myself as part of the team, I would say, I do other things, but anyway. However, if this exchange happened more often, my husband would be or feel better. If he was better, then that would mean safety for me." (Ms. Yilmaz).

Although Ms. Yilmaz is aware that she is not performing the same duties as the nurses, she perceives herself as a constitutive member of the care team. Regular information exchange between family caregivers and the health care team about the patients' needs, wishes and preferences would, according to her assumption, benefit the patient's health and, thus, promote safety for all parties involved.

Many other family caregivers from our sample wish to be seen as a relevant source of information about the patients and, therefore, get more involved in caring for their loved ones, albeit to a varying extent. Family caregivers wish to be taken seriously so that they can speak for the care recipient and offer insights into their individuality. However, this mutual information sharing is not always valued, and some health professionals make the family caregivers feel like they are an unwanted factor in HMV. In such cases, decisions regarding the patient are made without them, their opinion and experience is deemed insignificant, their perspective is not heard, and information is withheld. Feelings of insecurity on the side of the users, or even worse, near misses and adverse events are consequences that might arise from this disregard of the family caregivers and the information they have to share in advanced home care.

Informal coordination

Family caregivers contribute to safety in HMV by coordinating care. This is not a formal function assigned to them, it is rather imposed on them accidentally. However, this implies a substantial organizational effort and is sometimes a burden for them. They identify what equipment is needed for the provision of care (e.g. wheelchair, second back-up ventilator, consumable materials, care aides) and make sure it is available in time. Occasionally, they have to negotiate with the health insurance company in an attempt to gain access to fully functional replacement devices or other equipment on site. Moreover, family caregivers sometimes perceive the need to link and coordinate the activities of the several

isolated working health professionals involved in HMV. This is demonstrated by the experiences of Ms. Becker. Although she is not living together with her 24-h a day ventilated father, she is still actively involved in his everyday care:

"Well, I am also the link between the therapists, physicians, nurses and suppliers of care equipment. I am often present, so that I know what is being said, so that I can transfer this to everybody. I am part of this." (Ms. Becker).

This citation shows that Ms. Becker takes on the responsibility of bringing together the different health care providers involved in the home care of her father. She is the one who transmits information among them, which otherwise would not have been transmitted, which might cause severe safety problems. This requires her presence when the health professionals are doing home visits and to remember all the appointments of the different parties involved. She also keeps an information diary, where she expects the health professionals to write to her when something unexpected occurred.

This role of an informal care coordinator is not only very responsible, but also an exhausting one for the family caregivers. Sometimes they find themselves between the different sides, especially when some parties are withholding information from them or each other. If the family caregivers are actively excluded from the team, feelings of uncertainty, worry and anger are triggered.

Compensating for shortcomings

Experiences with professional home nursing services differ widely. Those who have positive experiences can rely completely on nurses in terms of safety. Others who have had negative experiences (e.g. when nurses fall asleep during the night shift) put little trust in them and want to be prepared for compensating of shortcomings in HMV.

Some family caregivers seek to expand their knowledge and skills in order to ensure a high degree of safety for the patients using various strategies. Some report having been instructed by nurses, while others have learned by observing nurses performing the tasks. When they are not instructed regarding care and emergency situations, it is not uncommon that they try to acquire skills behind the nurse's back in order to be prepared. The elderly married couple Mr. and Ms. Bauer who are taking care of their ventilated and multi-morbid adult son can be seen as an example of that strategy:

"What I have also done, yes, is that I have changed the cannula myself together with my husband. I said I would simply like to do it, because I have to be able to do it in an emergency." (Ms Bauer).

The context of this citation suggests that neither Ms. nor Mr. Bauer have been taught how to change a tracheostomy tube, although they would like to know how to do it so that they can handle critical situations themselves when the professionals are not observing or available. The Bauers – like other family caregivers in HMV – want to be prepared for handling emergency situations, but are prevented from doing so.

Most of the family caregivers in our study tried to keep control over the home care situation, making sure that the care recipient is well cared for and nothing is overlooked. Some of them reported that they had to remind the nurses of different nursing measures, such as changing the tube or administrating medication. Some family caregivers, such as Ms. Zimmermann, even try to instruct the nurses to ensure the HMV recipient's safety in the absence of a proper initial on-the-job training for new and inexperienced nurses. She cares for her adult son during the daytime, whereas a nurse is on duty and responsible for his care and safety at night when he is mechanically ventilated. However, Ms. Zimmermann is constantly alert.

"I instruct them always. I, I as mother, have to instruct qualified personnel, show them how to catheterize, I have to do it, that isn't my job." (Ms. Zimmermann).

Ms. Zimmermann is well aware that instructing or supervising professional caregivers is not her task as a mother. She must do it anyway and compensate for qualification deficits as well as organizational shortcomings so that her son gets proper help when necessary during the night.

Some family caregivers even feel the need to prepare themselves and the health care team for emergency situations. Exemplarily, Mr. Hoffmann's wife cannot move or breathe by herself because of her advanced neuromuscular disease and so she is completely dependent on the medical devices and human assistance. Mr. Hoffmann simulates critical situations like a power failure and observes the nurses' reactions:

"And you know, my presence is necessary. The women are not able to do it alone. I understand that, nervous, making mistakes and then this and that happens. And you have to have that under control. The more you train, the better it is." (Mr. Hoffmann).

Mr. Hoffman guides the "training" to make sure that everybody on the care team is prepared for a potentially hazardous situation. Thereby, he is the one who tries to gain control in order to prevent potential risks for adverse events. The citation further illustrates the shift of roles: He is in charge, guiding the training and not the nurses, as it should be from a professional point of view.

Not all family caregivers in our study might go as far as Mr. Hoffmann. However, most of them are on alert and constantly on call for supervision. They need to be sure that the ventilated care recipient is monitored closely and that someone can intervene quickly at any time. When nurses perceived as inexperienced or insecure are in charge, relatives feel indispensable and make arrangements to be at home to supervise the care recipient and the functioning of the technical devices themselves. Being present enables family caregivers to intervene if necessary. As a result of their feeling indispensable for the patient's safety, some family caregivers mentioned not having taken time off for many years and being trapped in their own house. However, they are convinced that they make an important contribution to patient safety in advanced home care by undertaking this form of compensation.

Discussion

Moving advanced medical technology from institutional settings to the community equates partially with a shift of responsibility for patient care from professionals to family caregivers [13]. Even if nurses are responsible for advanced home care up to 24 h day, such as in Germany, family members still have an active, complex and demanding part to play. The findings of this study extend previous research by showing that family caregivers take considerable responsibility for patient safety by being actively and constantly committed to safety work. This is in line with the findings of the Pan-Canadian Home Care Safety Study stating that all actors (clients, family members, caregivers and paid providers) in home care are creating and maintaining safety [26]. Moreover, the findings of the present study broaden the body of literature on family caregivers and safety by indicating that in many cases, family members are the ones to ensure patient safety in advanced home care by applying several strategies. Exemplarily, their intimate knowledge of the needs, wishes and preferences of the care recipient is a valuable resource for the health care team and family care givers are acting a guarantor of patient safety by sharing this information. Therefore, a change in focus from considering family caregivers as "secondary patients" or harmful to patients [37] to acknowledging their valuable contribution to patient safety in HMV is needed. Raising awareness about family caregivers valuable contribution to patient safety among nurses and other health professionals and conducting further research on family caregivers' contribution to safety would be ways towards such a change.

However, the study findings illustrate that some of the family caregivers' actions are putting the client at risk, for example, when relatives whose need for preparedness is not met through proper professional instructions execute advanced nursing tasks, such as changing the tracheostomy tube behind the nurse's back or simulating emergency situations. Their intention is certainly not to put the care recipient in danger, but they need to be sure that they can offer immediate assistance in life-threatening situations when professionals cannot. Our findings show that even qualified nurses sometimes lack expertise regarding HMV care, which makes family members feel indispensable and responsible, as reported in previous studies [34, 47]. Therefore, they feel forced to gain knowledge and technical skills regarding HMV therapy to compensate for this lack of professional expertise. It is problematic that family members must take the initiative to (re)gain control, instead of the nurses enabling them to handle critical situations and strengthening their self-management competence through educational interventions.

The partnership approach

The need for family members to participate in the provision of home care has been highlighted before in research on technologically dependent children [12, 13], but has not been discussed previously either in relation to family caregivers of adult patients or to safety. The current findings indicate that family caregivers are involved in care, even if qualified nurses are in charge. Furthermore, they feel responsible and indispensable for the safety of their loved ones, as reported previously [34]. This perceived responsibility also entails supervising and educating nurses in the management of the devices, as seen in previous studies [32]. Family caregivers feel forced to take on these tasks because they do not feel that the nurses in charge are sufficiently prepared to care for the HMV recipient properly. Similar to previous findings [34], they compensate for their health care professionals' perceived lack of competence by being present and constantly alert. However, participation in care should not equate with compensating for health care providers' deficiencies or training professionals, but valued as an important resource. The rationale for their need to participate in the provision of home care is that they see themselves as patients' advocates due to their closeness to their loved ones and due to their long caring experience, which agrees with other studies [31, 48]. This valuable perspective helps to identify issues that professionals may not recognize and, therefore, foster patient safety.

Our study further shows that being involved in HMW means knowing that the loved one is well cared for and makes the family caregivers themselves feel safer. That patient safety is inextricably linked with family caregivers' safety has even been found in previous research [17]. Therefore, advanced home care draws attention to the partnership approach between health professionals and family caregivers. So far, caregiver roles and responsibilities have not been clarified and should, therefore, be openly negotiated between partners and not be imposed upon families against their will [49]. Due to the complex nature of caring for this high-risk population and the numerous professionals involved in advanced home care,

negotiation of roles might be even more relevant in this setting than in usual home care. It also seems important that this role negotiation does not result in an over-reliance on family caregivers to keep the patient safe, this being the key role of contemporary nursing [50].

Family caregivers should be offered support

The results of the Burden Scale for Family Caregivers show that most participants in our sample experience some burden due to their participation in home care provision, although in most cases qualified nurses are in charge up to 24 h a day, which could be expected to ease the burden. One explanation might be that they cannot rely completely on the health professionals providing safe and quality care. As a consequence of their lack of trust in professional care, and mutual information sharing as well as difficulties with health care team coordination, they are concerned about the patients' safety and feel forced to partially take on professional roles and responsibilities which can be burdensome. Thus, it is of utmost importance that they have permanent access to professional problem-solving support along with psychosocial and emotional support, which echoes previous studies about technology-dependent patients' close relatives, emphasizing the importance of the availability of professional support either in-person or by phone [31, 36, 51, 52]. It is imperative that nurses and other health professionals acknowledge the relatives' perception of their own support needs, offer targeted support themselves or refer them to relevant services. The support should be easily available to promote a sense of safety. This support is particularly important at the beginning of HMV [36]. Furthermore, it is equally important that family caregivers are educated on how to handle unexpected situations and properly supervised to protect them from becoming a risk factor for the care recipient. This is a key nursing task, which is apparently not fulfilled sufficiently in HMV in Germany.

Limitations

The strength of this study lies in integrating the family caregivers' voice into home care safety research. At the same time, it is its major limitation that these findings only reflect a single perspective. Future studies triangulating our findings with the perspectives of patients and nurses or other professionals need to be undertaken to provide a holistic understanding of patient safety in home care.

As in all qualitative studies, findings are context-bound. The care provision of HMV in Germany is different to that in other countries and it remains unclear whether family caregivers' contribution to safety is dependent on the qualification of formal caregivers. It is, however, likely that the findings will have some relevance for other family caregivers in advanced home care, which could be investigated in further research.

Furthermore, recruiting participants through nursing service providers can be a disadvantage, because these might have selected relatives who are satisfied with their services. However, further recruitment strategies were used to address this risk of selection bias (see above).

Conclusions

As advanced home care is gaining momentum, there is an increasing need to focus on patient safety in this setting. The perspective of family caregivers presented yields interesting insights into the multiple tasks family caregivers take on to guarantee safety for their loved ones. In conclusion, nurses and other health professionals should meet family caregivers with respect and value their considerable role and the responsibility that they take for patient safety. Given the essential role they play in advanced home care, family caregivers should be seen as important, valuable and trustworthy partners.

However, the fact that family caregivers are performing nursing and medical tasks and even train professionals raises serious concerns. Instead, only competent personnel should be in charge of helping family caregivers feel less indispensable for patient safety. Nurses and other health professionals should act in partnership with family caregivers and allow them to deliberately choose their role in patient care and safety.

Implications for nursing practice

Given family caregivers' enormous commitment to ensure patient safety, nurses need to regain their professional responsibilities and duties from families. Our findings suggest that only skilled nurses who can provide safe care and handle critical situations should be appointed for HMV. Nurses should also serve as professional care coordinators and provide educational interventions to strengthen families' competence. An adequate training should encompass providing concrete instructions on areas in which family caregivers would like to be involved, such as the proper use of the medical equipment or preparedness for emergency situations. Another important family nursing intervention should be the negotiation of roles in advanced home care.

Abbreviation

HMV: Home mechanical ventilation

Acknowledgements

We would like to thank the study participants for their generous contribution to this study. We would also like to thank Armin Hauss for his help in data collection.

authors upon reasonable request and with permission from the official data protection officer at the Charité – Universitätsmedizin Berlin.

Funding

The study received funding (funding code 01GY1315) by the German Federal Ministry of Education and Research under the research priority "Qualitative Health Services Research". The funding body played no role in the design of the study and collection, analysis, and interpretations of data and in writing the manuscript.

Authors' contributions

ME designed the health services research project SHAPE. CS collected data and CS and ME made substantial contributions to the analysis and interpretation of data. CS drafted this manuscript and ME revised it critically. Both authors read and approved on the final manuscript.

Competing interests

The authors declare that they have no competing interests.

References

1. Fex A, Ek AC, Soderhamn O. Self-care among persons using advanced medical technology at home. J Clin Nurs. 2009;18:2809–17.
2. Hazenberg A, Kerstjens HA, Prins SC, Vermeulen KM, Wijkstra PJ. Initiation of home mechanical ventilation at home: a randomised controlled trial of efficacy, feasibility and costs. Respir Med. 2014;108:1387–95.
3. Lehoux P. Patients' perspectives on high-tech home care: a qualitative inquiry into the user-friendliness of four technologies. BMC Health Serv Res. 2004;4:28.
4. Huttmann SE, Windisch W, Storre JH. Invasive home mechanical ventilation: living conditions and health-related quality of life. Respiration. 2015;89:312–21.
5. MacIntyre EJ, Asadi L, McKim DA, Bagshaw SM. Clinical outcomes associated with home mechanical ventilation: a systematic review. Can Respir J. 2016; 2016:6547180.
6. Rose L, McKim DA, Katz SL, Leasa D, Nonoyama M, Pedersen C, Goldstein RS, Road JD, Group CA. Home mechanical ventilation in Canada: a national survey. Respir Care. 2015;60:695–704.
7. Lloyd-Owen SJ, Donaldson GC, Ambrosino N, Escarabill J, Farre R, Fauroux B, Robert D, Schoenhofer B, Simonds AK, Wedzicha JA. Patterns of home mechanical ventilation use in Europe: results from the Eurovent survey. Eur Respir J. 2005;25:1025–31.
8. Stuart M, Weinrich M. Protecting the most vulnerable: home mechanical ventilation as a case study in disability and medical care: report from an NIH conference. Neurorehabil Neural Repair. 2001;15:159–66.
9. Lehmacher-Dubberke C. Krankenpflege auf Rädern [health care on wheels]. Gesundheit + Gesellschaft. 2016;19:30–3. (in German)
10. Windisch W, Walterspacher S, Siemon K, Geiseler J, Sitter H, German Society for P. Guidelines for non-invasive and invasive mechanical ventilation for treatment of chronic respiratory failure. Published by the German Society for Pneumology (DGP). Pneumologie. 2010;64:640–52.
11. Gately C, Rogers A, Kirk S, McNally R. Integration of devices into long-term condition management: a synthesis of qualitative studies. Chronic Illn. 2008;4:135–48.
12. Lindahl B, Liden E, Lindblad BM. A meta-synthesis describing the relationships between patients, informal caregivers and health professionals in home-care settings. J Clin Nurs. 2011;20:454–63.

13. Wang KW, Barnard A. Technology-dependent children and their families: a review. J Adv Nurs. 2004;45:36–46.

14. Henriksen K, Joseph A, Zayas-Caban T. The human factors of home health care: a conceptual model for examining safety and quality concerns. J Patient Saf. 2009;5:229–36.

15. Hignett S, Edmunds Otter M, Keen C. Safety risks associated with physical interactions between patients and caregivers during treatment and care delivery in home care settings: a systematic review. Int J Nurs Stud. 2016;59:1–14.

16. Ellenbecker CH, Samia L, Cushman MJ, Alster K. Chapter 13: patient safety and quality in home health care. In: Hughes RG, editor. Patient safety and quality: an evidence-based handbook for nurses. Rockville: Agency for Healthcare Research and Quality: AHRQ publication no. 08–0043; 2008.

17. Lang A, Edwards N. Safety in home care: broadening the patient safety agenda to include home care services. (Institute TCPS, Capital Health EA eds.). Ottawa: The Canadian Patient Safety Institute; 2006.

18. Doran DM, Hirdes J, Blais R, Ross Baker G, Pickard J, Jantzi M. The nature of safety problems among Canadian homecare clients: evidence from the RAI-HC reporting system. J Nurs Manag. 2009;17:165–74.

19. Madigan EA. A description of adverse events in home healthcare. Home Healthc Nurse. 2007;25:191–7.

20. Sears N, Baker GR, Barnsley J, Shortt S. The incidence of adverse events among home care patients. Int J Qual Health Care. 2013;25:16–28.

21. Doran DM, Blais R. Safety at home. A pan-canadian home care study. (Institute CPS, patients Icplsd eds.). Edmonton, AB Ottawa: Canadian Patient Safety Institute; 2013.

22. Lang A, MacDonald JA, Storch J, Stevenson L, Barber T, Roach S, Toon L, Griffin M, Easty A, Curry CG, et al. Researching triads in home care: perceptions of safety from home care clients, their caregivers, and providers. Home Health Care Manag Pract. 2013;XX:1–13.

23. Masotti P, McColl MA, Green M. Adverse events experienced by homecare patients: a scoping review of the literature. Int J Qual Health Care. 2010;22:115–25.

24. Harrison MB, Keeping-Burke L, Godfrey CM, Ross-White A, McVeety J, Donaldson V, Blais R, Doran DM. Safety in home care: a mapping review of the international literature. Int J Evid Based Healthc. 2013;11:148–60.

25. Tong CE, Sims-Gould J, Martin-Matthews A. Types and patterns of safety concerns in home care: client and family caregiver perspectives. Int J Qual Health Care. 2016;28:214–20.

26. Lang A, Macdonald M, Storch J, Elliott K, Stevenson L, Lacroix H, Donaldson S, Corsini-Munt S, Francis F, Curry CG. Home care safety perspectives from clients, family members, caregivers and paid providers. Healthc Q. 2009;12 Spec No Patient:97–101.

27. Stevenson L, McRae C, Mughal W. Moving to a culture of safety in community home health care. J Health Serv Res Policy. 2008;13(Suppl 1):20–4.

28. Macdonald M, Lang A. Applying risk society theory to findings of a scoping review on caregiver safety. Health Soc Care Community. 2014;22:124–33.

29. Heaton J, Noyes J, Sloper P, Shah R. Families' experiences of caring for technology-dependent children: a temporal perspective. Health Soc Care Community. 2005;13:441–50.

30. Noyes J, Hartmann H, Samuels M, Southall D. The experiences and views of parents who cave for ventilator-dependent children. J Clin Nurs. 1999;8:440–50.

31. Winkler MF, Ross VM, Piamjariyakul U, Gajewski B, Smith CE. Technology dependence in home care: impact on patients and their family caregivers. Nutr Clin Pract. 2006;21:544–56.

32. Lindahl B, Lindblad BM. Family members' experiences of everyday life when a child is dependent on a ventilator: a metasynthesis study. J Fam Nurs. 2011;17:241–69.

33. Baxter SK, Baird WO, Thompson S, Bianchi SM, Walters SJ, Lee E, Ahmedzai SH, Proctor A, Shaw PJ, McDermott CJ. The impact on the family carer of motor neurone disease and intervention with noninvasive ventilation. J Palliat Med. 2013;16:1602–9.

34. Dybwik K, Nielsen EW, Brinchmann BS. Home mechanical ventilation and specialised health care in the community: between a rock and a hard place. BMC Health Serv Res. 2011;11:115.

35. Ingadottir TS, Jonsdottir H. Technological dependency--the experience of using home ventilators and long-term oxygen therapy: patients' and families' perspective. Scand J Caring Sci. 2006;20:18–25.

36. van Kesteren RG, Velthuis B, van Leyden LW. Psychosocial problems arising from home ventilation. Am J Phys Med Rehabil. 2001;80:439–46.

37. Reinhard SC, Given B, Petlick NH. A. B: 14. Supporting family caregivers in providing care. In: Hughes RG, editor. Patient safety and quality: an evidence handbook for nurses. Rockville: Agency for Healthcare Research and Quality: AHRQ publication no; 2008. p. 08–0043.

38. Strauss A, Corbin J. Basics of qualitative research: techniques and procedures for developing grounded theory. Thousands Oaks: Sage; 1998.

39. Schaepe C, Ewers M. I need complete trust in nurses' - home mechanical ventilated patients' perceptions of safety. Scand J Caring Sci. 2017;31:948–56.

40. Polit D, Beck C. Essentials of nursing research : methods, appraisal, and utilization. 7rd ed. Philadelphia: Wolters Kluwer/Lippincott/Williams & Wilkins Health; 2009.

41. Gräßel E. Häusliche-Pflege-Skala HPS zur Erfassung der Belastung bei betreuenden oder pflegenden Personen [Burden Scale for Family Caregivers BSFC for the assessment of subjective burden]. Vless: Ebersberg; 2001.

42. Bong SA. Debunking myths in qualitative data analysis. Forum: Qualitative Social Research. 2002;3(2). http://www.qualitative-research.net/index.php/fqs/article/viewArticle/849/1844.

43. Braun V, Clarke V. Using thematic analysis in psychology. Qual Res Psychol. 2006;3:77–101.

44. Pope C, Ziebland S, Mays N. Qualitative research in health care. Analysing qualitative data. BMJ. 2000;320:114–6.

45. Lincoln YS, Guba EG. Naturalistic Inquiry. Beverly Hills: Sage; 1985.

46. Graneheim UH, Lundman B. Qualitative content analysis in nursing research: concepts, procedures and measures to achieve trustworthiness. Nurse Educ Today. 2004;24:105–12.

47. Fex A, Flensner G, Ek AC, Soderhamn O. Living with an adult family member using advanced medical technology at home. Nurs Inq. 2011;18:336–47.

48. Munck B, Sandgren A, Fridlund B, Martensson J. Next-of-kin's conceptions of medical technology in palliative homecare. J Clin Nurs. 2012;21:1868–77.

49. McDonald J, McKinlay E, Keeling S, Levack W. How family carers engage with technical health procedures in the home: a grounded theory study. BMJ Open. 2015;5:e007761.

50. Kowalski SL, Anthony M. CE: Nursing's evolving role in patient safety. Am J Nurs. 2017;117:34–48.

51. Bjuresater K, Larsson M, Athlin E. Struggling in an inescapable life situation: being a close relative of a person dependent on home enteral tube feeding. J Clin Nurs. 2012;21:1051–9.

52. Dybwik K, Tollali T, Nielsen EW, Brinchmann BS. "Fighting the system": families caring for ventilator-dependent children and adults with complex health care needs at home. BMC Health Serv Res. 2011;11:156.

8

Exploring the perceived factors that affect self-medication among nursing students

Ali Soroush[1], Alireza Abdi[2], Bahare Andayeshgar[1], Afsoon Vahdat[1] and Alireza Khatony[3,4*] (iD)

Abstract

Background: Self-medication is the use of one or more medications without physician's diagnosis, opinion, or prescription and supervision, which includes the use of herbal or chemical drugs. Todays, self-medication is one of the biggest socio-health and economic problems among nursing students of various societies, including Iran, and because this issue can affected by contextual factors, this study aimed to explore the perceived factors that affect self-medication among nursing students.

Methods: In this qualitative study, a semi-structured interview was conducted with 11 nursing students. The transcript of each interview was reviewed several times and classified into main categories and sub-categories by content analysis. To evaluate this study, Guba and Lincoln's four criteria, including credibility, transferability, dependability, and confirmability were considered for trustworthiness.

Results: After analyzing the qualitative content of the interviews, four main categories, including educational backgrounds, nature of the disease, access to the media, and beliefs and personal experiences, and ten subcategories, including contact with clinical environment, relative knowledge about medications, simplicity of the disease, recurrence of the disease, influence of the media, use of the internet, believing in own knowledge, positive experiences of traditional medicine, and using own and others' experiences, were extracted.

Conclusions: It seems that, having a relative awareness about various diseases and medications, which is sometimes associated with taking a few educational courses with an internship, creates a false confidence in student for self-medication and prescribing drugs to others. It would be beneficial if the education system and associated tutors could inform the students about the possible consequences of this issue. By knowing the internal and subjective factors that influence the self-medication, this arbitrary practice can be largely prevented.

Keywords: Self-medication, Student, Nurse, Qualitative study

Background

Self-medication is the use of one or more medications without physician's diagnosis, opinion, or prescription and supervision, which includes the use of herbal or chemical drugs [1]. Today, self-medication is one of the biggest socio-health and economic problems of various societies, including Iran [2]. In some developing countries, many medications are available to public without prescription,

thus, self-medication, due to its lower cost, is a replacement for people who cannot afford medical services [3]. This is why in most developing countries more than 60–80% of health problems are associated with self-medication [4]. It is estimated that, about 83% of Iranian people self-medicate [5]. Arbitrary drug administration is common in many societies and is increasing. The prevalence of self-medication in European countries has been reported to be 68%, in USA is 77%, in Kuwait is 92%, in India is 31%, and in Nepal is 59% [6]. On the other hand, drug use pattern is an important indicator in health evaluation. Having adequate knowledge on these patterns helps to identify and determine the prevalence of illnesses, and provides

* Correspondence: Akhatony@kums.ac.ir; Akhatony@gmail.com
[3]Social Development and Health Promotion Research Center, Kermanshah University of Medical Sciences, Kermanshah, Iran
[4]Nursing Department, School of Nursing and Midwifery, Doolat Abaad, Kermanshah, Iran
Full list of author information is available at the end of the article

information on how to use health resources [7]. It is also expected that, the well-educated community including university students, is more aware of the danger of self-medication than ordinary people [8]. In this regard, the results of Ehigiator et al. study showed that, most nursing students, midwives and dentists were self-medicating and its influential factors included getting advice from pharmacy staff, friends and other healthcare professionals, as well as previous experiences with the disease [9]. Studies have shown that, the field of study is an underlying factor for self-medication among nursing, midwifery and medical students [10–13]. The simplicity and recurrence of the disease were among other factors of self-medication mentioned in other studies [13–15]. Since most of the factors contributing to self-medication are related to context-based and internal and subjective factors, identifying these factors can help to take interventional measures that are necessary to reduce or eliminate them. As qualitative studies on the perceived factors that affect self-medication in the world are limited, and no qualitative study in this regard has also been conducted in Iran, therefore, this study was conducted to explore the perceived factors of self-medication among nursing students.

Methods

The present study is a qualitative study with content analysis approach that aimed to explore the perceived factors that affect self-medication among nursing students, which was conducted in 2017. Content analysis is considered as a useful research approach. In this approach, the components or important parts of the content of the existing data are identified and considered [16]. The study population consisted of all nursing students of Kermanshah University of Medical Sciences (KUMS). The samples included nursing students who were self-medicating and had been identified during the previous quantitative study. Hence, in the previous quantitative study entitled: "The prevalence of self-medication among students", we asked the students to write their phone number and email address in the questionnaire if they are interested to participate in another qualitative study on self-medication. Those students who agreed and had experience of self-medication were recruited for the current study by purposeful sampling.

Data collection method

Semi-structured interviews were used in this study. The interview questions included: Why do you do self-medication? How and in what cases do you do self-medication? What are the perceived factors that affect self-medication? In order to clarify the concepts, probing questions were also asked, including "Please explain more", why and how?

After obtaining the approval of Ethics Committee of Kermanshah University of Medical Sciences (Kums.rec.1396.25),

and explaining the aims of study to the participants and obtaining written consent to record their voices, interviews were conducted at the convenient place agreed by the researcher and the participants. Every interview was recorded by a tape recorder. Each interview lasted between 30 and 50 min. After each interview, the recorded interview content was carefully reviewed several times, and then typed verbatim. This was done to increase the accuracy of the information transferred to paper and to further control the information.

Data analysis

Data analysis was done simultaneously with data collection. The data resulted from the interviews were analyzed simultaneously using qualitative content analysis. In content analysis, information units are identified in response to each question. These units, which present as codes, may include concepts, phrases or words that are clearly, understandably and systematically classified in different categories according to the content and, on the basis of their theoretical significance [17].

Among the Mayring's processes of qualitative content analysis, two main approaches are considered for the expansion and classification of appropriate text components, which include inductive and deductive methods. Inductive content analysis is a process that is used to extract classes or themes from raw data based on valid conclusion and interpretation. Deductive content analysis is used when the analysis structure is operational based on previous knowledge and the purpose of study is to examine the theory [18]. Inductive content analysis method was used in the present study, because there was little information on the perception of nursing students about self-medication. The transcripts of each interview were reviewed several times and a general understanding of the participants' statements was obtained. Then, the semantic units were shaped and initial codes were extracted. The codes that were conceptually similar were categorized into a group, thus categories and subcategories were determined. The data saturation was reached at the eighth interview, but further interviews were conducted with three other students to ensure the saturation. The data saturation criteria vary according to sample variety, participant selection method, data collection method, budget, and available resources, but saturation of data occurs when no new code is obtained during data collection and analysis, according to at least two researchers specializing in qualitative research [19].

Trustworthiness

Guba and Lincoln have proposed four criteria for the evaluation of interpretive research, including credibility, transferability, dependability and confirmability [20].

A. **Credibility:** The credibility of a study is the degree to which the findings of the study are true, and reflect the purpose of the research and social reality of the participants [16]. In this study, to enhance the credibility of the qualitative content analysis, methods such as continuous and long-term engagement with samples, control of interpretations against raw data, peer review, and review of the participants were used.

B. **Transferability:** The main goal of qualitative research is not to generalize the findings, as in quantitative research. It is not the duty of researcher to provide guidance for generalizability, but the researcher is required to provide a set of data and a description that is sufficiently rich for other researchers, to enables them to make informed decision about the generalization of the findings in other fields and conditions [18]. In this study, the perceived factors that affect self-medication among nursing students were examined carefully and all cultural and background characteristics of the samples were explained. Finally, findings of the study were given to three nursing students, beyond our participants, who have been self-medicating, and their personal experiences were compared with the results of the study; thus the students' experiences were in line with our participants' results, which confirm transferability.

C. **Dependability:** Dependability indicates the degree to which the researcher has been non-biased and to what extent the findings of the study are in accordance with the responses of the participants and not influenced by the researcher's bias or interests. In this study, all stages of the study were described step-by-step to be properly judged during the external audit.

D. **Confirmability:** The confirmability is the degree of agreement between several independent individuals about the accuracy and relevance of the meanings of the data. In this regard, some of the interviews and transcripts, along with coding, were provided to two other research colleagues who were specialized in qualitative research and confirmed the accuracy of coding.

To manage the data, Maxqda software version 10 was used.

Results

In this study, 11 nursing students with the age of 21–34 years old were enrolled, including 4 males and 7 females from whom, six were graduate students and five were undergraduate (Table 1). After analyzing the

Table 1 Participants' characteristics

Participants	Age range(yrs.)	Grade
First	30–35	MSc.
Second	20–25	BSc.
Third	25–30	MSc.
Fourth	20–25	MSc.
Fifth	20–25	MSc.
Sixth	25–30	MSc.
Seventh	25–30	BSc.
Eighth	25–30	BSc.
Ninth	25–30	BSc.
Tenth	20–25	BSc.
Eleventh	30–35	MSc.

qualitative content of the interviews, four main categories and nine subcategories were extracted. The main categories included "educational background", "nature of the illness", "access to the media" and "personal beliefs and experiences", which also contained 10 subcategories (Table 2) (Fig. 1).

Educational background

During the interview process, all students stated that, the educational background could lead to self-medication. In this regard, two sub-categories, including "contact with clinical environment" and "relative knowledge about drugs" were formed, which are subsequently explained.

Contact with clinical environment

Students with a history of nursing work in a clinical setting believed that, working in the clinic and with patients, as well as being aware of prescribed drugs for various diseases, could help them to treat non-complicated diseases. They stated that, they have adequate ability to treat simple illnesses. In the first interview, a 34-year-old woman who was an MSc nursing student and had ten years of experience at the clinical settings stated: "Considering the work experience and the knowledge that I have about drugs and diseases ... I try to treat simple illnesses myself". In another

Table 2 Classes and sub-classes

Classes	Sub-Classes
1. Educational background	1. Contact with clinical environment 2. Relative knowledge about drugs
2. The nature of the disease	1. Simplicity of the disease 2. Recurrence of the disease
3. Access to the media	1. Use of the Internet 2. Influence of the media
4. Personal beliefs and experiences	1. Believing in own knowledge 2. Positive experiences of traditional medicine 3. Using own and others' experiences

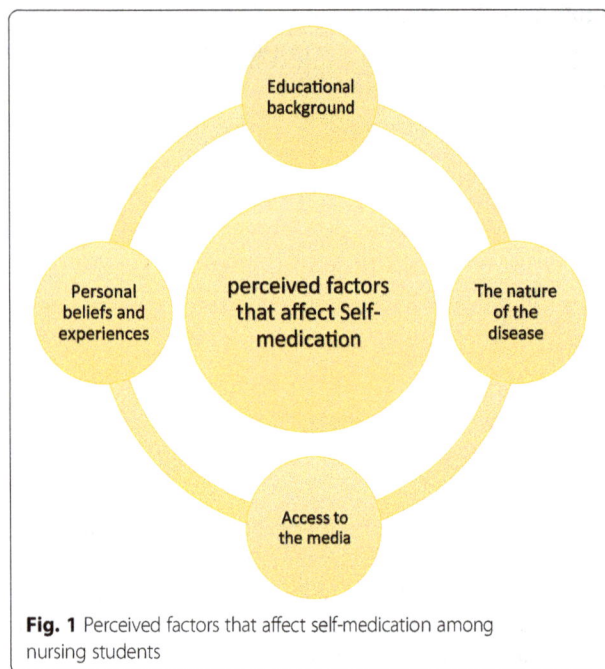

Fig. 1 Perceived factors that affect self-medication among nursing students

interview, another 27-year-old female student pointed out:" For example, in cases where I feel that, the disease is similar to the previous illness I have seen at my workplace, I use the same prescription". (Eighth Interview, a 27 years old female MSc nursing student).

Some students also referred to the access to experienced physicians and colleagues as factor for self-medication. They indicated that, this issue is an obstacle to physician visit for non-complicated illnesses. Moreover, asking the physicians to prescribe medication in the health insurance booklet and physicians' acceptance was another perceived factor for self-medication. In this regard, a nursing student said: "As I work in the ward, I ask the physicians to write and prescribe medication in my insurance booklet and stamp it, or I write medication myself and ask the doctor to stamp it." (First interview, a 34 years old, female post-graduate student).

Relative knowledge about drugs

All participants believed that, they were familiar with many medications because of their pharmacological modules, and some participants believed that, they were somewhat familiar with the complications of the drugs they were taking and could use this information for self-medication. Also, two postgraduate students stated that, the expectation of others, because of their field of study, could be another perceived factor for self-medication and giving medication advice to others.

In the ninth interview, a student stated that "passing a pharmacology module is very effective in self-medication, for example, I used propranolol tablets to reduce the anxiety. During my bachelor's degree study, I began

self-medicating as soon as I became aware of it, and I am still continuing it; I also know its complications". (Ninth interview, a 27 years old, male MSc student).

Another student stated that, she uses simpler medications to prevent side effects: "For example, someone who uses antibiotics that is not suitable for his/her infection due to ignorance, in addition to developing resistant to antibiotics, he/she will not get any better and when it comes to a bigger problem, antibiotic is no longer effective". "I use simpler and less risky drugs when I self-medicate, and I do not buy a dangerous drug from the pharmacy." (Third interview, a 27 years old, female MSc student).

One student, in regard to her own and others' expectation stated: "For example, when I feel that I have a problem and I need to go to doctor, people say that, you are a nurse and do not need to go to doctor. You want to go to doctor to say what. You know, they induce that, because you study and work in this field, you must be aware of such knowledge and it is not good if you to say you don't know. I sometimes have to give medical advice to others unwillingly, as I don't want to put myself under the question, or stop people saying that, she is a nurse but doesn't know anything, or she ignores us". (Eighth interview, a 27 year old, female MSc student).

The nature of the disease

Another perceived factor for self-medication that was suggested by the participants was the nature of the disease. This category consisted of two sub-categories, including "simplicity of the disease" and "recurrence of the disease".

Simplicity of the disease

Participants stated that, they self-medicate because of the type of disease, and do not visit physician for simple illnesses, for example for illnesses such as common cold. A 27-year-old MSc nursing student believed that in some cases, the illness is not that serious to require doctor visit, and said: "For simple illnesses like headaches and stomachache I take drug .... Sometimes someone says the illness is not serious, for example, why should I go to doctor for constipation. It is both laziness, and you think that this is a simple illness and does not require a doctor visit". Another student stated that, he would self-medicate for non-complex diseases and would prefer prevention to treatment: "It depends on the type of disease, if it is simple, I can do something about it, but if it is diabetes for example, I cannot. I think prevention is much better than treatment ... In minor cases, such as a cold or a toothache, I know what to use."(Fourth interview, a 21 years old, male undergraduate student).

Recurrence of the disease

Most students believed that, they did not need to spend time and money on their recurring illness because of their previous knowledge about the treatment, and they could self-medicate. They believed that, if they go to the doctor, they will get the same prescription. In this regard, an undergraduate student stated: "If it is a routine problem that has happened ten times before, and the same medications are being prescribed in every visit, this leads to self-medication." (Seventh interview, a 28 years old, female undergraduate student).

Another student said: "Well, I have had the same problem in the past and the doctor wrote certain drugs for me. So, I do not pay any money, nor I pay MRI or CT scan money, this repetition makes you feel that you know what to do, and what to use and recommend to others." (Eighth interview, a 27 years old, female MSc student).

Access to the media
Most students, who were self-medicating, used internet for information on medications and considered it as the source of information. Also, some of them considered the media, especially national television, to be effective in self-medication.

Use of the internet
Participants considered the availability and affordability of the internet as a reason for self-medication, although some students believed that most websites were unreliable. In this regard, an undergraduate student stated: "The internet can be a source of information, but not all websites ... If I want to do some search, I'll go to Latin and up to date websites, and by studying them, I will be a head and neck above my friends and even university tutors." (Tenth interview, a 21 year old, female undergraduate student).

Another student also said: "I use the internet and pharmacology books for self-medication, but I use internet more often. Although, sometimes I see there are many contradictory information sources, I try to consider a summary of them."(Fifth interview, a 22 years old, male undergraduate student).

Influence of the media
One of the culture-building practices in any field is the use of public media. In regard to self-medication, the media is certainly an influential factor, and can be used properly with control and planning. Some nursing students stated that, giving information about medication and treatment through the media may leads to blind self-medication in some people. In the seventh interview, a 28-year-old female undergraduate student stated: "The programs in which a doctor is talking on television are often harmful, because ordinary people do not properly understand the message, or they take some parts of the message they like and think they know everything about that disease, so they prescribe medication for themselves and others."

Personal beliefs and experiences
Nursing students are influenced by their field of study, work environment, beliefs and experiences that lead to self-medication. Surely, part of these beliefs and experiences come from the society, and many ordinary people in the community also believe them. This category consisted of 3 subcategories, including "believing in own knowledge", "positive experiences of traditional medicine," and "using own and others' experiences".

Believing in own knowledge
Participants believed that, their knowledge was at such level that they could treat themselves in simple diseases and do not need to go to doctor. In this regard, a postgraduate student stated: "At times, I think doctors do not know more than us, and I do not really trust them. Because when I look at their prescription, sometimes I see it is wrong and I know how to correct that mistake, but since I cannot prescribe drugs, my hands are tied. However, when it comes to my own case, I can prescribe drugs for myself." (Ninth interview, a 27 years old, male MSc student).

Positive experiences of traditional medicine
Some students felt that herbal remedies are a good substitute for some chemical drugs because of their low side effects. Part of this issue also seemed to be related to the advice of elderly for using herbal medicines. Also, the positive experiences of peers in the use of herbal medicines were effective in the students' self-medication.

In this regard, one student said: "Self-medication is more likely to go under the complementary medicine, because people think it does not really have any negative consequences. Therefore, they use complementary medicine and their friends and relatives also advise them to take herbal remedy and say; take that herbal remedy and you'll be fine ... I mean, I'd rather mix honey and tea and drink it than take diphenhydramine syrup." (Ninth interview, a 27 years old, male MSc student).

Using own and others' experiences
Some students stated that, the use of medications and knowing about their complications and side effects helped them to self-medicate in some cases. Also, in cases where they have been satisfied with the use of a drug to treat a disease, and were aware of its relative safety, they have been advising it to others and close people.

In the fifth interview, a 22-year-old male student who was doing bachelor's degree in nursing, in regard to others' experiences in similar diseases, stated: "I was trying to get help from those who had similar disease and had gone to visit a doctor for it. I think everyone is doing it and self-medicating."

A 27-year-old female MSc nursing student talked about testing and drug errors and believed that, after using a drug, she could notice its effect, and if it was effective, continued to use it. In this regard she stated: "I did not know there were other medications that are good for headaches before I become nursing student. I took them couples of times and then I realized they are good. It was like trial and error. I had migraine, so I tried ergotamine and I became well."

Discussion

The purpose of this study was to explore the perceived factors of self-medication among nursing students. The results showed that, one of the factors contributing to self-medication was educational background from the perspective of nursing students, so that having contact with the clinical environment and having relative knowledge of diseases was contributing to this behavior of the nursing students. Evidence suggests that, the work environment, getting advice from colleagues and having pharmacological knowledge are effective in self-medication of medical science students [9, 12–14]. For people who have sufficient knowledge about self-medication in simple diseases, the self-medication in addition to being safe it could also be beneficial. According to the World Health Organization (WHO), self-medication is part of the self-care process and can reduce the pressure on the health system and lead to optimal use of facilities, especially in low-income health care settings [21, 22].

The nature of the disease was another cause of self-medication among nursing students. The simplicity and recurrence of illnesses were important factors for self-medication among nursing students. Evidence suggests that, the highest level of self-medication among medical science students is related to simplicity of the diseases, and one of the effective factors in self-medication in these students is the insignificance and non-complexity of the diseases [11, 13–15, 21, 23–25]. From nursing students' point of view, simple illnesses such as colds and headaches can be cured by relying on previous knowledge and experiences. In our opinion, self-medication can be dangerous even for simple illnesses, if is done with insufficient knowledge.

Another perceived factor behind self-medication was the access to media and internet. In a study, 17.6% of nursing students referred to the internet as one of the reasons for self-medication [13]. Results of another study indicated that, paper and electronic media advertisement is effective in the self-medication of students [26]. Medical information on the internet is incomplete and often invalid, which can be dangerous. Among the potential dangers arising from information available on the internet and the mass media, we can refer to false self-belief in illness, false diagnosis, and false self-confidence.

Beliefs and experiences were another cause of self-medication in nursing students. This category consisted of several subcategories including; believing in own knowledge, own and others' previous experiences, and positive experiences of traditional medicine. The results of a study indicated that, medical students intend to have an active role in their health care due to their high level of trust in their own knowledge [12]. In another study, one of the causes of self-medication in medical students was having confidence in own knowledge [14]. Due to having a pharmacological module and attending clinical setting, medical students have an incomplete knowledge that enhances their confidence in the diagnosis and treatment of the diseases, which can endanger their health.

Another perceived factor of self-medication was the use of own and others' experiences. In this regard, the results of a study showed that, previous history of personal use of medications and counseling was one of the main factors behind self-medication in medical students [15]. In another study, 38% of medical students used the experiences of the elderly and classmates as sources of information on self-medication, and 63.6% of them prescribed drug to others, especially family members, friends and peers [25]. Results of another study showed that, more than half of the medical students used their old prescription to treat the same illness [13]. Using others' experiences can be highly hazardous and lead to exacerbation of the disease and drug resistance, as individuals may have inadequate knowledge about drugs and their complications. Symptoms and illnesses may also be similar and differential diagnosis of them is only possible by a valid physician.

We found that, some nursing students used herbal medicines for self-medication, because of the relatively low side effects of herbal drugs compared to chemical drugs. Evidence suggests that, students also use herbal medicines for self-medication in other countries [7, 27–30]. In our opinion, the use of herbal medicines with knowledge and awareness can be beneficial otherwise it may cause serious risks. Traditional medicine can be used to deal with such problems.

One of the limitations in this study was the limitation of the generalizability of the findings, which is the nature of the qualitative research. Our study was conducted on nursing students, so due to the high prevalence of self-medication among different medical science students, it is suggested to assess and compare the perceived factors of self-medication among students of different medical science disciplines.

Conclusions

The factors of self-medication included the educational backgrounds, nature of the disease, access to the media, and personal beliefs and experiences. It seems that, having relative awareness about various illnesses and medications, which is sometimes associated with passing a few lessons and modules with internship, creates a false trust in the student for self-medication and prescribing drugs to others. It would be beneficial if the consequences of this problem could be taught to students by the education system and related university tutors. By knowing the internal and subjective perceived factors that affect self-medication, we can largely prevent this arbitrarily practice.

Acknowledgments
The authors would like to thank all the participants who patiently participated in our study. We also extend our thanks to clinical research development center of Imam Reza Hospital affiliated to Kermanshah University of Medical Sciences for their kind help.

Funding
The study was funded by Kermanshah University of Medical Sciences. Grant number is 96052.

Authors' contributions
AS, AK, AV, AA and BA contributed in designing the study, AV and BA collected the data, and analyzed by BA, AK, AS and AA, the final report and article were written by BA, AK, AV, AS and AA and they were read and approved by all the authors. All authors read and approved the final manuscript.

Competing interests
The authors declare there are no competing interests.

Author details
[1]Clinical Research Development Center of Imam Reza Hospital, Kermanshah University of Medical Sciences, Kermanshah, Iran. [2]Students Research Committee, School of Nursing and Midwifery, Kermanshah University of Medical Sciences, Kermanshah, Iran. [3]Social Development and Health Promotion Research Center, Kermanshah University of Medical Sciences, Kermanshah, Iran. [4]Nursing Department, School of Nursing and Midwifery, Doolat Abaad, Kermanshah, Iran.

References
1. Asefzadeh S, Barkhordari F. Moghadam F.Self – medication among cardiovascular patients of Bu-Ali hospital. J Qazvin Univ of Med Sci. 2003;26,91–4. persian
2. Jafari F, Khatony A, Rahmani E. Prevalence of self-medication among the elderly in Kermanshah-Iran. Glob J Health Sci. 2015;7(2):360.
3. Kumari R, Kiran KD, Bahl R, Gupta R. Study of knowledge and practices of self-medication among medical students at Jammu. J Med Sci. 2012;15(2):141–4.
4. Awad AI, Eltayeb IB. Self-medication practices with antibiotics and antimalarials among Sudanese undergraduate university students. Ann Pharmacother. 2007;41(7–8):1249–55.
5. Ershadpour R, Marzouni HZ, Kalani N. Review survey of the reasons of the prevalence of self-medication among the people of Iran. J Mashhad Univ Med Sci. 2015;18(60):16–23. persian
6. Tabiei S, Farajzadeh Z, Eizadpanah A. Self-medication with drug amongst university students of Birjand. Mod Care J. 2012;9(4):371–8.
7. da Silva MGC, Soares MCF, Muccillo-Baisch AL. Self-medication in university students from the city of Rio Grande. Braz BMC Public Health. 2012;12:339.
8. Ahmadi SM, Jamshidi K, Sadeghi K, Abdi A, Vahid MP. The prevalence and affecting factors on self-medication among students of Kermanshah University of Medical Science in 2014. JCDR. 2016;10(5):IC01.
9. Ehigiator O, Azodo CC, Ehizele AO, Ezeja EB, Ehigiator L, Madukwe IU. Self-medication practices among dental, midwifery and nursing students. Eur J Gen Dent. 2013;2(1):54.
10. De Borrajo Lama C, Arribas Arribas A. Self medication in nursing. Rev Enferm. 2004;27(7–8):6–10.
11. Abay S, Amelo W. Assessment of self-medication practices among medical, pharmacy, health science students in Gondar University. Ethiop J Young Pharm. 2010;2(3):306–10.
12. Alam N, Saffoon N, Uddin R. Self-medication among medical and pharmacy students in Bangladesh. BMC Res notes. 2015;8(1):763.
13. Kumar N, Kanchan T, Unnikrishnan B, Rekha T, Mithra P, Kulkarni V, et al. Perceptions and practices of self-medication among medical students in coastal South India. PLoS One. 2013;8(8):e72247.
14. Badiger S, Kundapur R, Jain A, Kumar A, Pattanshetty S, Thakolkaran N, et al. Self-medication patterns among medical students in South India. Australas Med J. 2012;5(4):217–20.
15. Ibrahim NK, Alamoudi BM, Baamer WO, Al-Raddadi RM. Self-medication with analgesics among medical students and interns in king Abdulaziz University, Jeddah. Saudi Arab Pak J Med Scl. 2015;31(1):14.
16. Rakhshan M, Hassani P, Ashktorab T. Lived experiences of cardiac pacemaker patients. J Qual Res Health Sci. 2013;2(1):33–45.
17. Zohoor A, karimi Monaghi H. Data analysis in qualitative studies. Q J Fundam Ment Health. 2003;6:107–13. persian
18. Graneheim UH, Lundman B. Qualitative content analysis in nursing research: concepts, procedures and measures to achieve trustworthiness. Nurse educ today. 2004;24(2):105–12.
19. Houghton C, Murphy K, Shaw D, Casey D. Qualitative case study data analysis: an example from practice. Nurse Res. 2015;22(5):8–12.
20. Denzin NK, Lincoln YS. The Sage handbook of qualitative research. Los Angeles: S. Lincoln.4, editor; SAGE publication, Inc. 2011.
21. Mumtaz Y, Jahangeer S, Mujtaba T, Zafar S, Adnan S. Self medication among university students of Karachi. Jlumhs. 2011;10(03):102–5.
22. Zafar SN, Syed R, Waqar S, Zubairi AJ, Vaqar T, Shaikh M, et al. Self-medication amongst university students of Karachi: prevalence, knowledge and attitudes. J Pak Med Assoc. 2008;58(4):214.
23. Gutema GB, Gadisa DA, Kidanemariam ZA, Berhe DF, Berhe AH, Hadera MG, et al. Self-medication practices among health sciences students: the case of Mekelle University. J Appl Pharm Sci. 2011;01(10):183–9.
24. Kasulkar AA, Gupta M. Self medication practices among medical students of a private institute. Indian J Pharm Sci. 2015;77(2):178.
25. Banerjee I, Bhadury T. Self-medication practice among undergraduate medical students in a tertiary care medical college. West Bengal J Postgrad Med. 2012;58(2):127.
26. Almalak H, Aal A, Alkhelb DA, Alsaleh HM, Khan TM, MAA H, et al. Students' attitude toward use of over the counter medicines during exams in Saudi Arabia. Saudi Pharm J. 2014;22(2):107–12.
27. Ali SE, Ibrahim MI, Palaian S. Medication storage and self-medication behaviour amongst female students in Malaysia. Pharm Pract (Granada). 2010;8(4):226–32. Epub 2010 Mar 15
28. Klemenc-Ketis Z, Hladnik Z, Kersnik J. Self-medication among healthcare and non-healthcare students at University of Ljubljana, Slovenia. Med Princ Pract. 2010;19(5):395–401.
29. Lau GS, Lee KK, Luk MC. Self-medication among university students in Hong KongAsia Pac. J Public Health. 1995;8(3):153–7.
30. Shankar P, Partha P, Shenoy N. Self-medication and non-doctor prescription practices in Pokhara valley, western Nepal: a questionnaire-based study. BMC Fam Pract. 2002;3(1):17.

9

Voluntary stopping of eating and drinking (VSED) as an unknown challenge in a long-term care institution

Nadine Saladin[1], Wilfried Schnepp[2] and André Fringer[3]* (iD)

Abstract

Background: Chronically ill persons experience conditions of life that can become unbearable, resulting in the wish to end their life prematurely. Relatives confronted with this wish experience ambivalence between loyalty to the person's desire to die and the fear of losing this person. Caring for a person during the premature dying process can be morally challenging for nurses. One way to end one's life prematurely is Voluntary Stopping of Eating and Drinking (VSED).

Methods: This embedded single case study explored the experiences of registered nurses (embedded units of analysis: ward manager, nursing manager, nursing expert) and relatives who accompanied a 49-year-old woman suffering from multiple sclerosis during VSED in a Swiss long-term care institution (main unit of analysis). By means of a within-analysis, we performed an in-depth analysis of every embedded unit of analysis and elaborated a central phenomenon for each unit. Afterwards, we searched for common patterns in a cross-analysis of the embedded units of analysis in order to develop a central model.

Results: The following central concept emerged from cross-analysis of the embedded units of analysis: As a way of ending one's life prematurely, VSED represents an unfamiliar challenge to nurses and relatives in the field of tension between one's personal attitude and the agents' concerns, fears and uncertainties. Particularly significant is the personal attitude, influenced on the one hand by one's own experiences, prior knowledge, role and faith, on the other hand by the VSED-performing person's age, disease and deliberate communication of the decision. Depending on the intention of VSED as either suicide or natural dying, an accepting or dismissing attitude evolves on an institutional and personal level.

Conclusions: To deal professionally with VSED in an institution, it is necessary to develop an attitude on the institutional and personal level. Educational measures and quality controls are required to ensure that VSED systematically becomes an option to hasten death. As VSED is a complex phenomenon, it is necessary to include palliative care in practice development early on and comprehensively. There is a high need of further research on this topic. Particularly, qualitative studies and hypothesis-testing approaches are required.

Keywords: Embedded single case study, Voluntary stopping of eating and drinking (VSED), Hastened death, Unbearable suffering, Long-term care, Palliative care, Nurses, Relatives

* Correspondence: andre.fringer@zhaw.ch
[3]Institute of Nursing, School of Health Professions, ZHAW Zurich University of Applied Sciences, Technikumstr. 81, CH-8400 Winterthur, Switzerland
Full list of author information is available at the end of the article

Background

Persons suffering from chronical diseases, e.g. multiple sclerosis, experience conditions of life which can become unbearable [1]. This may result in the wish to end one's life prematurely [2, 3]. There a several options. One of them is assisted suicide which is legal in Switzerland, in contrast to many other countries [4]. Switzerland can be called a "right-to-die society" [5]. In 2014, 742 persons in Switzerland died by assisted suicide [6], accounting for 1.2% of all deaths [6]. 94% of these persons were older than 55 years, most of them suffering from a chronic disease [6].

Another way of ending one's life prematurely is Voluntary Stopping of Eating and Drinking (VSED) [7–10]. This concerns cognitively unimpaired persons deliberately renouncing food and fluid with the aim to hasten death [7–10]. The definition of VSED applies only to persons being physically capable of oral food/fluid intake and digestion [7]. Additionally, it is important to distinguish VSED from declining interest in food and fluid in persons at the end of life [10, 11]. VSED is characterized by the discipline and endurance of the performing person [12]. Therefore, it is an volitional act, extended over a long time and not a situational impulse [12]. If chronically ill persons decide to end their life prematurely, mental, social and spiritual factors are relevant [13]. Nurses having cared for persons during VSED described various motives for deciding in favor of VSED [10]. They mentioned that the affected persons were willing to die, considered it senseless to go on living, had a low quality of life and wished to control the circumstances of dying [10]. As reasons for wishing a hastened death, affected persons named a deterioration of health status and progression of the disease [11, 14–16]. Furthermore, the burdens of life prevailed over reasons for continuing to live [11, 14–16]. They mentioned to be "tired of life" or to have done everything they wanted [11, 14–16]. Reasons for choosing VSED instead of other methods were related to the possibility of controlling the circumstances of one's death and to act in a self-determined way [11, 14–16]. In planning to fulfill the intention to hasten death, persons often involve their relatives [17]. Attending persons can take over the task of arranging the process of dying as comfortable as possible [18]. This comprises symptom management, taking care of "last things" and saying goodbye [18]. A challenging situations occurs if the person performing VSED suffers from a delirium and wishes to drink [9]. In this case, Quill and Byock (2000) recommend to fulfill this wish [9]. If this is a recurrent problem, VSED should be reconsidered [9]. Chabot (2011) proposes to discuss this scenario in advance with the affected person and to determine how to proceed in this case [18]. Moreover, sedation should be taken into account [18]. Presumably, the accompanying symptom of thirst refers rather to xerostomia than to the desire to drink [18, 19]. Xerostomia can be treated by means of oral care [18, 19]. Due to oral care, persons having ceased to drink take in about 50 ml of fluid per day [20]. It is possible that persons withdraw from the decision for VSED [10]. Reasons for resuming food intake can be various [10]. Ganzini et al. (2003) mention, for example, pressure on the part of relatives, encouragement to resume food-intake, discomfort and hunger, diminished depression or alleviation of concerns [10]. During VSED, tiredness occurs and in a later stage loss of consciousness caused by an increased blood urea level [20]. Continuing to take in small amounts of fluid stimulates urea elimination via the kidneys [20]. This results in a prolonged dying process, however, it also allows intermittent periods of clear consciousness until shortly before death [20]. According to Chabot (2011), VSED lasts seven to 15 days until death occurs if fluid and food are stopped simultaneously [20]. In persons stopping only eating and reducing fluid-intake during several days or weeks, death is to be expected after 16 to 30 days [20]. According to Chabot and Goedhart (2009), death during seven days after stopping drinking can be attributed to the underlying disease or to medication [17]. Usually, persons die from VSED in deep-sleep, mostly caused by circulatory arrest due to dehydration or complications like pneumonia [7, 17, 20]. Attending persons describe death by VSED as peaceful and soft, without suffering or pain and with a pleased expression before death [10, 16, 21]. Nurses having cared for persons requesting premature death reported fears of offending the law. Thus, it seems important to clarify the legal situation [22]. From a legal point of view, VSED is an act of self-killing, although it does not consist of an action but an omission [23]. VSED is positioned between the personal freedom of every human being to decide how and when to end life and the duty of the state and every person to protect another human being´s life [24]. In case of withholding life-sustaining measures in a person willing to die, the right to autonomy is rated higher than the duty to sustain life [24].

The decision to end one's life prematurely can release several emotions in relatives, e.g. rejection, futility, co-responsibility and excessive demand [25]. Furthermore, thinking of an agonizing death caused by thirst can provoke fears [26]. Chabot (2011) describes the ambivalence experienced by relatives [18]. On the one hand, they want to stay loyal towards the affected person. On the other hand, they defend themselves against the fear of separation [18]. Feelings of guilt and anger towards the person wanting to die can also arise [18]. Eating means participating in social life [19]. Thus, relatives can misunderstand VSED as a rejection directed against them personally and as a decision against social participation [19]. According to Walther (2011), relatives respond to a person's decision to die by feeling accountable with regard to insufficient support on their part [25]. This can lead either to more intensive support from relatives or to relieving relatives from support if they are already over-burdened [25]. In contrast to other ways of self-killing, VSED allows relatives to mentally prepare for the forth-coming dying process [11, 21]. This offers the chance to clarify relationships possibly impacted by misunderstand-ings, disputes or conflicts [21]. Relatives' attitudes towards VSED have rarely been a subject of research. According to Chabot und Goedhart (2009), most relatives experience a family member's death by VSED as dignified [17]. VSED has been the subject of publications for a long time. As the literature shows, health care professionals are chal-lenged in dealing with VSED [22]. For nurses, caring for persons during VSED comprises palliative care, informing and counselling [9]. Accompanying persons who decided to hasten death can be morally irritating for health care professionals [22]. They find themselves in the field of ten-sion between a person's right to choose a hastened death and social, moral as well as mental aspects of valuable life [22]. Reflecting the implications of VSED and their own role proves to be important for them [17, 27]. Further-more, nurses should be able to demarcate VSED from assisted suicide [17, 27].

Although nurses have no legal responsibility [9], Harvath et al. (2006) indicate that some of them feel personally responsible for the affected persons and their relatives [22]. A nurse reported that she had the feeling of having failed if patients decided for assisted suicide, since this expressed that they did not feel comfortable [22]. So far, nurses' attitudes towards VSED have been rarely researched. Harvath et al. (2006) described that nurses´ experience of caring for persons with VSED is less challenging than in the case of assisted suicide [22]. Nurses perceive VSED as a natural process, causing less emotional burden for relatives [22]. They also describe VSED as "letting go of life" [22]. In contrast, assisted suicide is an active, temporally limited action from the nurses' point of view [22]. However, health care profes-sionals also express fear of enlarging suffering by means of VSED and thereby causing additional burden [19].

In 2015, the following incident happened in a Swiss long-term care institution. A 49-year old resident suffer-ing from multiple sclerosis decided to end her life by VSED due to progressing mobility impairments and de-pendency for bowel voiding after an incurable exacerba-tion. In view of lacking professional experience with this method, the institution contacted an expert (AF) for VSED. In agreement with the institution (general man-ager, responsible for institutional business as well as for the public representation of the long-term care institu-tion and project commission and the nurse manager, responsible for the staffed nurses as well as for quality and safety of nursing care), the expert team provided external support for the VSED process (especially for the nursing expert, who is responsible for the scientific

questions of nursing practice). Against this background, the necessity of an in-depth investigation of this case arose (including the ward nurse, who is responsible for management of the ward, as well as nurses involved in the care of the resident). So far, there are only several case reports concerning VSED and a few studies explor-ing nurses' attitudes towards VSED. However, up to now, there is no qualitative comprehensive *case study research*, investigating a case from multiple perspectives. Additionally, individual suffering of chronically ill per-sons in the context of VSED also has hardly been researched so far.

Aim

This study intended to comprehensively investigate the complexity of the VSED phenomenon from different perspectives. This is possible by means of an embedded single case study allowing to investigate various pro-cesses, attitudes and approaches, found to be necessary in the current case to explore the experiences of the persons involved [28].

Research questions

Against this background, we derived the following re-search questions: What are the experiences of registered nurses, nurse managers, nurse experts and relatives in caring for a resident suffering from multiple sclerosis – from the first intention to choose VSED until death? What is the common pattern underlying the different embedded units of analysis within the case in dealing with the situation?

Methods

Since this study investigates subjective experiences, we chose a qualitative design allowingto answer the research questions in a circular way [29].

Design

To explore how the persons involved experienced the given situation, an embedded single case study is best suited [28, 30]. The origin of qualitative case studies lies in anthropology and sociology [29]. Merriam (1991) and Yin (2003) define a case study as an in-depth empirical inquiry of a contemporary phenomenon within its real-life context [30, 31]. Based on the given situation, it is possible to investigate the complexity of the VSED phenomenon from different perspectives aiming at a comprehensive understanding [32]. Individuals, groups or social interactions are defined for instance as units of analysis [33]. In the current study, the long-term care in-stitution in which the 49-year-old woman suffering from multiple sclerosis and performed VSED represents the main unit of analysis. To this end, we assigned the persons involved into four groups and explored their experiences. This resulted in an embedded single case study design allowing to compile several units of analysis into one case [29, 33]. A unit lesser than the main unit of analysis is defined as an "embedded unit of analysis" [33]. In the current study, we identified four embedded units of analysis, analysed each unit (within-analysis) and then compared all embedded units of analysis in a cross-analysis. The embedded units of analysis of this study consist of the attending registered nurses, the ward manager, the nursing manager and the nursing expert as well as the relatives of the patient. The *bounded system* defining a case can consist of temporal or spatial aspects [29]. On a temporal level, the case in the current study includes the time between the idea of performing VSED until death. The case is temporally limited by the woman's death one year ago. The spatial limitation of the case relates to the long-term care institution where the woman lived, and she performed VSED.

Sample

This study is based on a convenience sample since the initiative came from the long-term care institution (general manager and nurse manager). In the context of the given situation, we identified four criteria-related embedded units of analysis. The first unit consisted of eight nurses, the second of the ward nurse, the third of the nursing manager and the nursing expert and the fourth of the woman's husband and son. They were also included as a unit of analysis because they were strongly affected by the decision for VSED and influenced the personal attitude of the nurses. In the end, the relatives were even more vulnerable than the person concerned and therefore had a strong impact on the nurses' experiences with the VSED situation. The nursing expert with the gatekeeping function informed the nurses, the ward manager and the nursing manager about the study. Prior to the interviews, all participants received oral information about the significance, the scope and the consequences of participating in this study. We received oral informed consent and recorded it digitally. The gatekeeper also requested the relatives' interest in participation. After a positive response, the author contacted them by phone and explained the significance of the study as well as the implications of participating. Afterwards they received written information and an informed-consent formula.

Data collection

According to Yin (2014), interviews are the primary data source of case studies [33]. Due to the explorative character of the research question, the interviews should rather have the form of a guided conversation than of a structured interview [33]. For this reason, we chose a narrative-generating approach for all four units of analysis. The interviews took place between February 2016 and December 2016.

Data-collection with registered nurses occurred by means of focus group interviews, representing the most recent form of interviews for a moderate group range [34]. Focus group interviews are appropriate to explore group experiences (coping process, dealing with the team, attitude of the team towards the topic of discussion). They are of interest as a method if several persons share similar experiences [34].

We performed a single interview with the ward manager and a group interview with the nursing manager and the nursing expert. Group interviews are suitable for two to three persons [34]. Finally, we conducted single interviews by phone with the husband and the son. We digitally recorded all interviews and transcribed them verbatim from Swiss dialect into German standard language, using transcription principles according to Flick (2009) in an adapted way [35]. During the whole research process we took field notes and wrote memos concerning methodological, personal and case-related issues. They serve to fix spontaneous thoughts and allow to fill the codes with meaning. By means of memos it is possible to grade and weigh the results [36].

Data analysis

Data analysis occurred in two stages. First, we comprehensively analyzed every embedded unit of analysis (within-analysis) and afterwards performed a comparative analysis (cross-analysis). For within-analysis, Baker (2011) recommends to interpret data in a grounded theory style [37], i.e. in three steps [36]. The first step consists of open coding to disaggregate the text analytically [36]. This means that the interviews were read line by line and with constant comparison. The emerging open codes and in-vivo-codes were then bundled and allocated into broader generic codings. Afterwards, axial coding serves to refine and differentiate open codes [36] that were grouped into inductively developed sub-categories. The emerging category is positioned in the center, surrounded by a network of connections which have to be elaborated [36]. As a supporting instrument for the stages of axial and selective coding, a coding paradigm has to be developed. For the within-analysis, we identified the following axial categories: nursing and physician support during VSED, impact of VSED on the family, dimensions of VSED, and contextual factors. In the final stage of selective coding, we elaborated the central phenomenon of each embedded unit of analysis [36]. To this end, we re-worked existing codes, categories, memos and field notes until the central phenomenon emerged [36, 38]. Parts of the within-analysis are to be found again in the case description. At the same time, within-analysis represents the point of departure for cross-analysis of the embedded units of analysis.

We synthesized the results of the embedded units of analysis in the cross-analysis into one result [28]. As a supporting instrument, we used the word-table recommended by Yin (2014) to present axial codes of within-analysis in a homogeneous structure [33]. Finally, we analyzed all tables, searched for patterns and differences and drew conclusions for the units of analysis [33]. By comparing axial codes of the unit of nurses, the ward nurse, the nurse expert and the nurse manager, it was possible to elaborate the central phenomena for the individual axes of the coding paradigm. At this stage, the relatives served to understand the situation, decision and attitudes but were not involved in the cross-analysis. Therefore, the central phenomenon represents the professional situation in the case. On this basis, we developed a central model covering the central phenomenon of the professional units of analysis. Conclusively, all participants validated the results of our study by member-check. For data transcription, analysis and organisation we used MAXQDA 12 [39]. The presentation of the results follows a proposition from Cresswell (2013) [29].

Trustworthiness

To ensure the trustworthiness of this study, we observed the quality criteria of credibility, transferability, reliability, transparency and authenticity [40]. We fulfilled these criteria by means of discussions within the research group (credibility), thick descriptions of all embedded units of analysis (transferability), review of the study by the second and last author (reliability and transparency) and by the embedded-single-case-study design, allowing in-depth exploration of experiences in the real-life-context (authenticity). The relatives of the person who chose VSED were also involved in the study to ensure a "convincing account" as one aspect of trustworthiness [41]. This was carried out by interviewing the relatives during the study process. The relatives and all other units of analysis (encompassing involved nurses, the ward nurse, the nursing expert and the nurse manager) were informed about the results after analysis completion – in form of a "member check".

Ethical aspects

The ethics committee of the canton St. Gallen reviewed the harmlessness of the study (EKSG16/016). All participants gave their written informed consent. In addition, also the oral informed consent was recorded digitally prior to data collection. Due to the risk of vulnerable situations emerging during the interviews, we informed participants about the possibility to end or interrupt the interview at any given time.

We irreversibly pseudonymised names of persons and places preventing conclusions with regard to institutions or persons. All participants received information about the aims, the procedure and a possible publication of the study. Additionally, we informed them about the possibility of withdrawing from the study at any time without consequences. The last author preserves the digital recordings.

Results

In this section, we present the results of the qualitative data analysis, beginning with a description of the given situation. Afterwards, we outline all four embedded units of analysis and finally present the results of the cross-analysis.

Situation

The affected person fell ill with multiple sclerosis 30 years ago. She had been living in the long-term care institution for three years. After an incurable exacerbation, she suffered from progressing mobility impairments. Transfers were possible but only by means of a patient lifter. Additionally, she experienced loss of strength in her hands, leading to impairments concerning eating and leisure activities as well as progressing dependency concerning intimate care and bowel voiding. These restrictions prevented her from continuing her usual visits at home during the weekend. She suffered from pain all over her body. Thus, she was confronted with a crisis and reflected her situation. Her suffering reached a point where she took the possibility into account of dying prematurely.

"I think, she was not tired of life but simply tired of suffering." (NS&AF15022016_2 Z46, nurses)

The woman deliberately and voluntarily decided to stop eating in order to die prematurely and informed her relatives. This wish was not unexpected for them because she had thought about this option previously. The family accepted her wish, hoping she would choose assisted suicide. However, experiencing a dying process as consciously as possible was important for her. Hence, the family finally supported her request for VSED. In the middle of July, the family informed the nursing staff about the wish for VSED. The woman slowly started to reduce food and fluid intake. The nurses informed their superiors (ward manager and nursing expert) about the request for VSED and received the permission to start. When the nursing manager learned about VSED, she informed the general manager. In a conversation, the general manager told the family that VSED is not allowed in the institution. However, they would offer the possibility to organize outpatient care for performing VSED at home. The family did not understand why VSED was suddenly not allowed after obtaining the approval from the nursing expert. The option of performing VSED at home was not realistic for the woman. She preferred to be cared for by the nurses in the center. From the family's point of view, VSED was not an act of self-killing. Therefore, they could not understand the interdiction and the general manager's argumentation. Also for the nurses, the interdiction was incomprehensible. They accepted the woman's wish and were able to understand it due to her long history of suffering and the progression of her illness. The ward manager, the nursing manager, the nursing expert and the nurses continued to advocate for the woman and supported her wish for VSED. They took measures in order to act against the interdiction, e.g. by submitting an application to the ethics committee or by writing a living will. The general manager on her part initiated to investigate the legal situation with regard to VSED. Finally, the nursing manager received the permission after having diagnosed urinary tract infection potentially leading to urosepsis with a probably fatal outcome. In view of this further deterioration and a psychiatric report excluding a depression, the general manager permitted to perform VSED in the centre. The nursing expert elaborated a plan to reduce food and fluid intake. To maintain "normality", the woman regularly attended all meals in the dining room and asked the nurses to remove beverages and meals without commentary. Every day she went to the cafeteria to drink an espresso with her husband. She had informed only one resident about performing VSED. In the further course, the nurses told all other residents that the woman's condition had deteriorated further. The nurses described that the woman had changed after having made the decision. Prior to the decision, she often had been dissatisfied, whereas now she appeared to be relaxed and happy.

"I did not know what to expect. I entered the room and I can still see it before my eyes: she was so radiant, as if...Yes, I was slightly irritated to see her so relaxed, happy and satisfied ..." (NS&AF15022016_2 Z158, nurses)

While performing VSED, the woman deliberately expressed what she wanted to eat. At the beginning, it was a berry or a plum. At the end, she particularly liked flavoured ice cubes. She accurately controlled fluid-intake. While regarding how her body changed, she seemed to hope that the dying process would proceed faster. According to the nurses and her husband, she was impatient and could hardly await her death. She used the time to say goodbye to persons who were important to her. She visited them for the last time without telling them about VSED. Even a reconciliation with her daughter was possible after a conflict. According to the nurses, the terminal stage began approximately two

weeks before her death. She became bedridden and refused fluid except for flavoured ice cubes. Until about ten days before her death she could clearly communicate, afterwards she used facial and vocal expression. During VSED, she received analgesics against headache and antiemetics against nausea. In the terminal stage, she additionally received morphine and lorazepam due to unrest. The nurses reported that at the end they had the impression of an inner struggle as she was very restless, and the terminal stage took a long time. She died in the middle of September, eight weeks after reducing food.

Case description

In the following sections, we describe the identified embedded four units of analysis of this case study.

Nurses

The participants consisted of nurses in training and registered nurses aged between 35 and 61 years with three to 33 years of professional experience. They worked on a ward for younger persons in need of care and had already accompanied the affected woman for three years before her decision for VSED. The woman herself had informed them about her wish and they cared for her until she died.

The nurses felt obliged to fulfill the woman's request and advocated for her:

"...It is her will. We know her. So far, we have always cared for her. It was clear for us that she is completely competent. For me it is not a matter of judging what I personally think about this. It is her will and it is my task to support her" (NS&AF15022016_1 Z49, nurses)

The nurses could not understand the attitude of the general manager since she barely knew the woman. Therefore, they tried to take action against the interdiction. Caring for the affected person during VSED was coherent for the nurses. Providing palliative care for her was not different from caring for persons dying naturally. The nurses reported that it was easy for them to care for the woman since she seemed to be happy.

The central phenomenon of the within-analysis is: *Struggling for the affected person in opposition to the management: respecting her request to die and being obliged to her wish.* This unit of analysis is significant to answer the research question since the nurses cared for the affected person during VSED and supported her request for VSED.

Ward manager

The ward manager was a 61-year-old registered nurse with 33 years of professional experience. She also had cared for the woman for three years before the decision. During the performance of VSED, the ward manager accompanied the woman and her family and was the main contact person. During the whole time, she advocated for the woman, her family and the nurses. She represented their interests towards the management. In her eyes, VSED was something normal and legal. She did not understand the interdiction, considered the approach of the management to be non-transparent and felt uncomfortable with this situation. Caring for the woman during VSED was also coherent for her and she described the woman's death as dignified. The central phenomenon of the within-analysis is: *Being "in-between": ambivalence between promise and duty.* The ward manager´s experience is important to answer the research question because she represented the interests of the affected person, the family and the nurses toward the management and at the same time felt responsibility towards the institution.

Nursing manager and nursing expert

The nursing manager, 48 years, had 25 years of professional experience. The nursing expert, 51 years, possessed 30 years professional experience. The nursing expert was the first person involved in the case. She assumed the responsibility for professionally supporting the nurses. The nursing manager directly communicated with the general manager and mediated between her and the nurses. The nursing manager and the nursing expert ensured that the woman could perform VSED in the institution. However, they could also understand the concern and fear of the general manager. They tried to find a way that was possible and acceptable for all. The central phenomenon of the within-analysis of this unit of analysis is: *Moderating the situation and weighing the interests of persons involved: supporting the nurses and the family members to reach the aim to allow VSED in the institution.* This unit of analysis is important to answer the research question since both persons represent connecting links towards the management and tried to advocate for the interests of the affected woman and her relatives.

Relatives (husband and son)

The family consists of the husband (62 years), the son (30 years) and the daughter (28 years). They accepted the mother's request for VSED and supported her. Every day, the husband spent time with his wife. Accompanying her was coherent for him and he described her death as beautiful and dignified. Although he suffered from the loss of his wife, he could understand her wish. The last time spent together during VSED and the death of his wife welded the family together. Accordingly, his relationship with his children had become very close. The son also visited his mother regularly during VSED. From his point of view, death relieved her from suffering. However, he would have wished for another way for his mother. Watching how her body changed during VSED was hardly bearable for him:

> *"This was the most terrible moment, seeing her lying in bed, very emaciated and nearly irresponsive. This was a very, very terrible moment"* (NS12122016 Z12, relatives)

In his eyes, VSED is one of the most challenging ways of hastening death. However, he mentioned that his mother was a very willful woman doing everything to reach her aim and to have her will. The central phenomenon of the within-analysis of this unit of analysis is: *Caring and understanding: Respecting the request in spite of suffering due to illness and the wish to die.* This unit is meaningful to answer the research question since the relatives' experiences broaden the scope of the professional context, thereby offering a more comprehensive picture.

Cross-analysis of embedded units of analysis

By means of a cross-analysis, it was possible to deduce a central model to answer the research question. The central concept summarizing the complexity of all units of analysis is presented in Fig. 1 and may be formulated this way: *VSED as an option of prematurely ending one's*

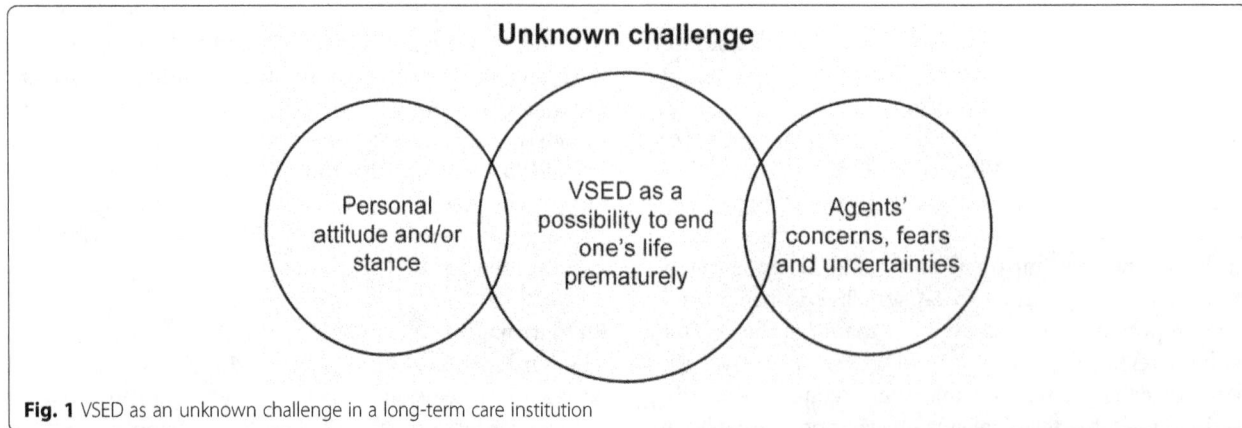

Fig. 1 VSED as an unknown challenge in a long-term care institution

life represents an unknown challenge in the field of tension between one's personal attitude and the concerns, fears and uncertainties of the agents.

As the figure shows, VSED is at the centre as an option to end one's life. For all persons involved, VSED is unknown since there is rarely previous knowledge about this phenomenon and experience is lacking. Dealing with VSED is influenced by the personal attitude of every individual agent. Additionally, dealing with VSED as an unknown phenomenon evokes concerns, fears and uncertainties in all agents. The personal attitude towards VSED depends on the age of the performing person, as visible in Fig. 2.

This figure illustrates that the negative attitude towards VSED diminishes with increasing age of the performing person. With a certain age of the performing person, the acceptance rises. In younger persons, rejection of VSED seems to be highest. VSED is more accepted and perceived as a natural trajectory if the person is older.

"In older persons you don't want to think about the question if it is suicide or deliberate killing in this sense." (NS&AF15022016 Z92, nursing manager and nursing expert)

As this figure shows, the attitude and culture of an institution is decisive for the way it deals with VSED. If VSED is interpreted as suicide, it is not allowed. Perceiving it as natural dying leads to acceptance and permission. This is also true on the personal level. A person interpreting VSED as suicide rejects it. Persons perceiving it as natural dying accept it. A combination of both models in Figs. 2 and 3 shows that implicit VSED in older persons is classified as natural dying and therefore accepted. In younger persons, however, VSED is interpreted as suicide resulting in rejection.

Aside of the age and the way of communicating VSED, other factors contribute to forming a personal attitude towards VSED: one's own experiences, prior knowledge, faith and role as well as the disease of the performing person. The attitude of the agents and the institution is particularly significant for dealing with VSED, as visible in Fig. 3.

The cross-analysis resulted in the model depicted in Fig. 4.

The decision of the woman and her relatives had an influence on all units of analysis and the general manager. In all agents, the process of developing an attitude began as described in Figs. 2 and 3. Due to different attitudes on the personal and institutional level, a conflict happened in the given situation. Against this background, there is a retroactive effect on the central phenomena of the units of analysis in the within-analysis. The result of this process was a form of caring for the affected woman that was perceived as coherent by all persons involved, allowing a dignified death, as expressed in the following quote:

"Finally, a beautiful dying process. She found peace with her daughter and with herself and she was able to choose this process, to bring an end to this. And somehow was given a chance to leave this world as a human being. I'm still touched when I am thinking of her. Yes, I found it very beautiful that she chose this way and followed it so beautifully. So I personally think that it was a beautiful process."
(NS&AF15022016_1 Z133, nurses)

Discussion

For the first time, this embedded case study comprehensively investigated a situation of VSED from different perspectives of each of the group of caregivers and relatives. Based on the experiences of the participating persons, it was possible to elaborate a first model of dealing with VSED in a long-term care institution. The focus of this model reflects the major concept of this study: *VSED as an option of ending one's life prematurely represents an unknown challenge in the field of tension between one's personal attitude and the concerns, fears and uncertainties of the agents.*

Furthermore, it became obvious that the age of the affected person directly influences the attitudes of the agents. Permission and performance of VSED in an institution significantly depend on the attitude towards VSED on the part of the individual agents and the institution. In the subsequent sections, we discuss the following central aspects: options of premature dying, challenges in caring for chronically ill persons, significance of personal attitude and coping with concerns and fears in a professional manner.

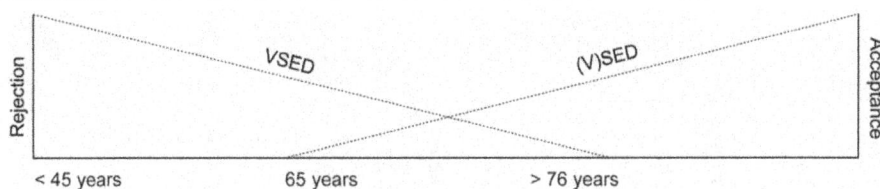

Fig. 2 Development of an attitude towards VSED, depending on the age of the performing person

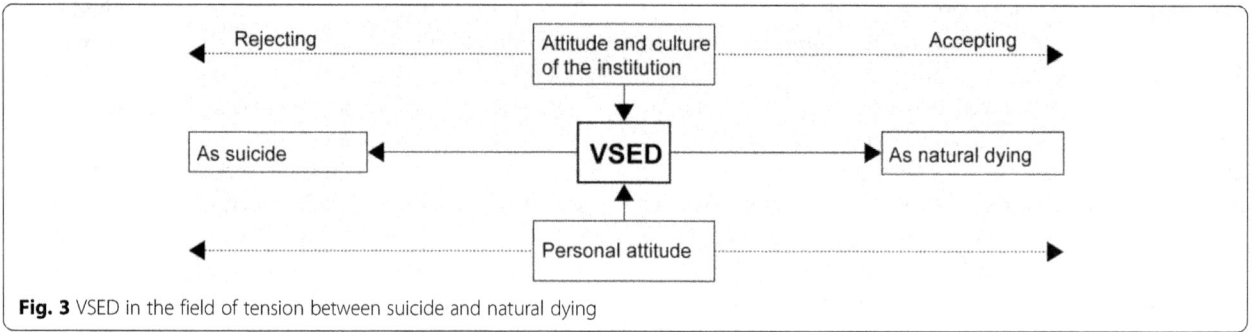

Fig. 3 VSED in the field of tension between suicide and natural dying

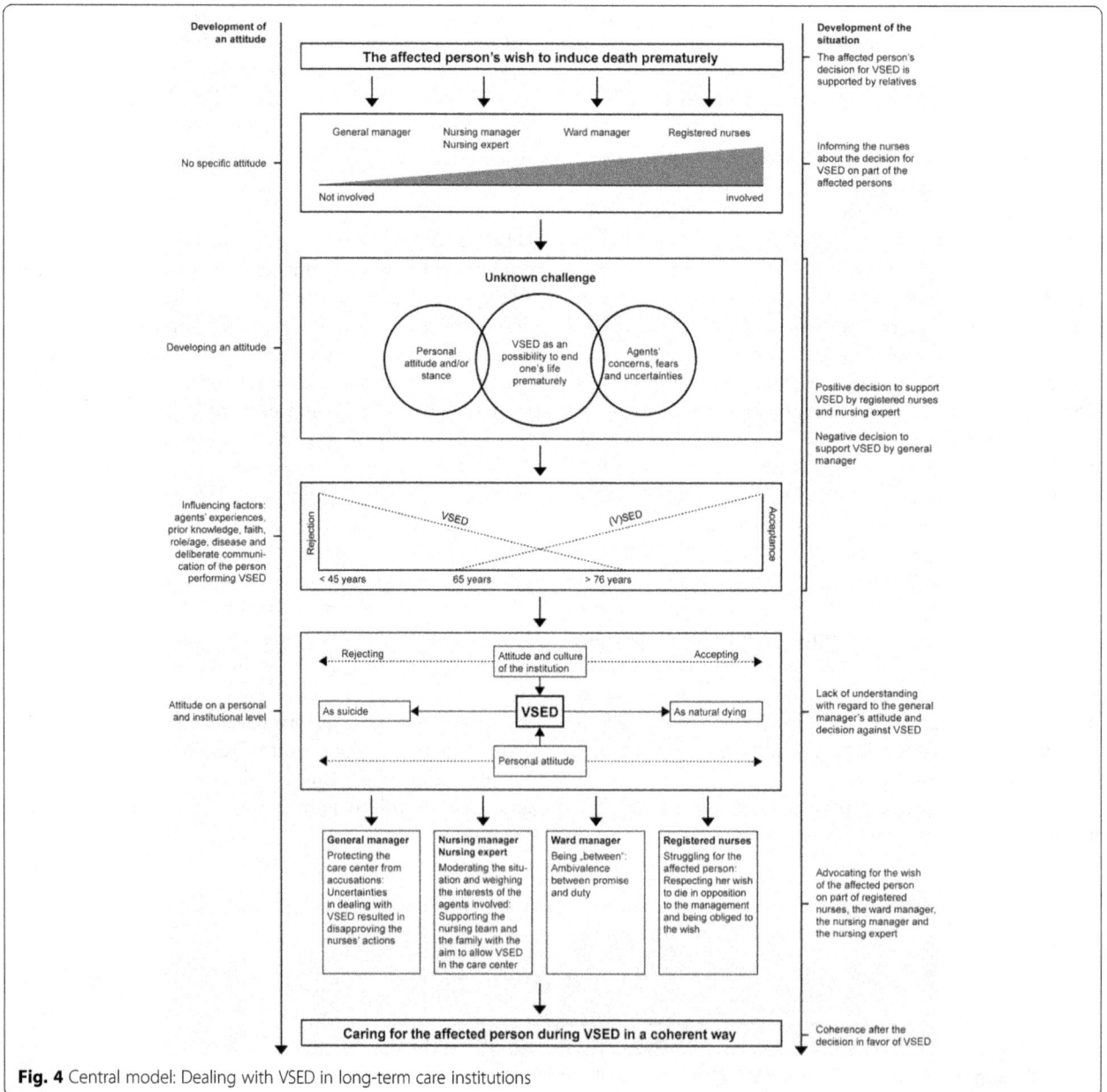

Fig. 4 Central model: Dealing with VSED in long-term care institutions

Options of premature dying

Besides VSED, the literature describes three further methods of prematurely ending one´s life. The first is withholding life-sustaining interventions [21], the second death-accelerating analgesics and sedatives [20]. It is important to demarcate both methods from the killing on request since it is illegal in Switzerland [20]. Only nursing and palliative medical interventions leading to an accelerated dying process as a side effect are in accordance with the law [42, 43]. The third option consists of assisted suicide [20]. Persons who decided to end their life receive a lethal drug on medical prescription [20]. This method is not illegal in Switzerland and is offered by organisations like DIGNITAS or EXIT [20]. Although assisted suicide is legal, this was no option for the affected person as she wanted to ensure a natural dying process. Her son presumed that her faith might have played a role in this decision. In the woman's eyes, the drug prescribed for assisted suicide was poison. Poisoning herself was no option for her.

Classifying VSED proves to be difficult. Depending on the perspective, it can be regarded as withholding treatment, natural death or suicide [7]. Interpreted as an omission causing death, VSED can also be regarded as withholding treatment and therefore is a human right [7, 44]. Focusing on the deliberateness of the action, VSED can be classified rather as suicide [45, 46]. Wolfersdorf (1995) defines suicide as a self-induced action aiming to kill oneself [47]. This action is performed with the expectation and in the faith of achieving this aim by means of the chosen method [47].

However, VSED can be distinguished from suicide as the decision is reversible during the first days [16, 20]. To classify the wish to die, the person's current situation is significant [25, 48]. Is the person alive only by means of medical treatment, withholding treatment is not considered as suicide because it allows a natural death [25]. In this perspective, VSED can also be regarded as a form of withholding treatment [25]. In this context, Schwarz (2007) mentions that persons who are about to die from their disease, do not have the option to decide for life. As a consequence, VSED cannot be regarded as a decision against life [7].

The literature (clinical, philosophical, ethical and discipline-specific) offers heterogeneous answers to the question if VSED should be regarded as natural dying or suicide [49]. Concerning the woman's argument of not wanting to poison or kill herself, it can be assumed that from her point of view, VSED is not an act of self-killing.

The dying process in VSED corresponds to a natural dying process [20]. This distinguishes VSED from other forms of suicide [20]. The participating nurses confirm this view by comparing the dying process in VSED with the natural dying process.

For relatives, the difference between characterizing VSED as withholding treatment, natural death or suicide seems to be relevant on an emotional level [7]. Interpreting VSED as suicide can evoke pain, grief or anger and may negatively affect the bereavement process [7].

The elaborated model shows that classifying VSED as suicide or natural dying is important with regard to the way an institution deals with VSED. To ensure a professional way of dealing with VSED, the aim could consist in positioning VSED in the middle of a continuum ranging from suicide to natural dying. This may allow a reflected handling of VSED for all agents. Regarding VSED as suicide on a personal and institutional level leads to an interdiction of VSED without reflection. On the contrary, interpreting VSED as natural dying on the personal and institutional level, entails the danger of allowing VSED without reflection. This probably results in trivializing it since critical voices are absent. The results show that VSED in young persons is classified rather as a form of suicide, in contrast to implicitly renouncing eating and drinking in older persons. This indicates that institutions tend to reject VSED in younger persons, while implicit renouncement of eating and drinking in older persons is accepted and admitted without reflection. With regard to age-associated changes of food-intake, e.g. reduced appetite and feeling of thirst, swallowing problems, delirium or manual impairments [50], a non-reflected accepting attitude towards VSED can have potentially serious consequences, since the distinction between age-associated changes of food-intake and implicit renouncement of eating and drinking are not always clearly perceptible.

Challenges in caring for chronically ill persons

Caring for chronically ill persons is marked by challenges [51]. It is not comparable with caring for acutely ill persons due to specific features of the nurse-patient-interaction. The aim does not consist in healing but in enabling persons to live with their illness and to preserve their quality of life [52]. The nursing role is extended by supporting, counselling and developing tasks [52]. The long-term patient-nurse-relationship leads to proximity [51]. This entails the danger of intermingling the professional and the everyday view [51]. In the situation described in this study it cannot be dismissed that the nurses' proximity to the affected woman had an influence on their personal view concerning VSED. The closer agents were to the affected woman, the greater was their endeavour to fulfil the woman's request. The nurses argued that they already had known the affected person for a long time and so they could comprehend her wish. The general manager was accused of deciding without knowing the woman and her situation.

Achieving a professional balance between proximity and distance is described as a significant part of in-patient nursing care [53]. This balance allows nurses to act in a professional way [54]. Therefore, they should be able to establish a close relationship with the person and at the same time look at this relationship from a distance [54].

Chronically ill persons are not only in need of functional nursing interventions but also require support for the work of coping and adjusting during the entire course of disease [51]. This poses an additional challenge. Furthermore, it is important that nursing care for chronically ill persons is focused on the entire course of disease and addresses the complexity of a chronic disease [51]. With regard to the situation examined in this study, this requires adjusting care to the progressing course of multiple sclerosis. There is a high need of support for the coping process, particularly after an exacerbation. The exacerbation caused a change from a stable stage to a deteriorating stage of chronic illness [55]. Symptoms were no longer controllable, and the affected person lost physical abilities. It was necessary to adjust activities of daily living to a new situation [55]. As the woman was confronted with progressing physical impairments and therefore became increasingly dependent on nursing support, she experienced a crisis. During this time, the need for support and for adjusting to the new situation was high. However, the woman failed to adapt to this situation and to return to stability [55]. So, she decided to prematurely end her life.

The particular role of chronically ill persons in society can also be challenging for nursing care [51]. Nurses must be aware that chronically ill persons experience an ambivalence between being ill and being healthy. It is necessary to pay increased attention to this ambivalence [51]. Additionally, this ambivalence is associated with the desire for autonomy [51]. Thus, nurses should be able to concentrate not only on patients´ deficits but also on their resources [51]. Schaeffer and Moers (2000) describe the necessity of this rethinking as "accompanying and supporting persons on *their* way to resuming and maintaining wellbeing and an autonomous way of living "(S. 476) [51]. In the situation described in the current study, the affected person's will for self-determination was of central importance. For the nurses, the wish of the affected woman was paramount, and they regarded it as their task to support her on her way, irrespective of their personal attitude. This is in accordance with a study by Mattiasson and Andersson (1994). The authors came to the conclusion that nurses caring for persons with the wish for premature dying respect the patient's will for autonomy even if this is challenging for them [56]. However, to respect patient autonomy, an accordance of nurses' and patients' aims is not necessary, as Boppert (2002) emphasizes [57].

It is evident that caring for chronically ill persons in general entails many challenges [51]. In the current study, VSED posed an additional challenge since the agents were unfamiliar with this method [58]. According to Knight (1921), uncertainty arises in situations in which behavior cannot be traced back to a person's own opinion or to scientific information [59]. Related to the given situation, Knight's statement can be confirmed. The behaviour of all agents was characterized by uncertainty since they had neither experience nor expertise concerning VSED.

Significance of personal attitude

In the professional context, a personal attitude results from a habitus [60]. A person's habitus represents her or his patterns of perceiving, thinking and acting [60]. All experiences of a person are expressed in the habitus which is imprinted by the position a person holds in society [60]. Bourdieu's description of habitus allows to explain why the opinions of various professions and relatives are different. All agents have various experiences and hold different positions in society. This has probably resulted in developing different personal attitudes towards VSED. The results lay bare that the following aspects are relevant for adopting a personal attitude: one's own experience, prior knowledge, faith and role as well as the performing person's age, disease and deliberate communication of VSED. A study by Harvath et al. (2004) revealed that nurses mainly adopt an approving attitude towards VSED and are willing to accompany persons during VSED [61]. In the current study, nurses also showed an affirming attitude towards VSED. Therefore, it could be concluded that the nursing role is associated with an affirmative attitude towards VSED.

A person's attitude towards death is influenced by personal, cultural, philosophical and social belief systems [62, 63]. This is in accordance with the statements of the participating nurses in the current study, expressing that their attitude towards VSED is associated more with culture and faith than with the age and education of a nurse.

Dealing with concerns and fears in a professional way

All agents expressed that VSED as an unknown challenge induced fears and concerns. In the literature caring for dying persons is described not as a professional but a personal challenge [64]. Nurses must reflect their emotions concerning their own mortality and at the same time they have to take over the care for dying persons in their professional life [64]. In the current study, nurses already were experienced in caring for dying persons. However, VSED was unknown to them and raised fears and concerns. These fears were related to interventions against the sensation of hunger and thirst as well as to the following questions: What would happen if the affected person decided to resume food-intake? Is the dying process in VSED different form the normal dying process? How should nurses communicate VSED towards external persons?

Harvath et al. (2006) reported that several nurses caring for persons with a wish for premature dying felt personally responsible for this wish and tried to dissuade them from the way they had chosen [22]. The present study cannot confirm this result. Participating nurses were able to distance themselves clearly from the woman's wish and assigned the responsibility to her. Additionally, Harvath et al. (2006) mentioned that nurses expressed fears about offending the law by caring for persons with the request for premature dying [22]. In our study, fears concerning the legal situation also arose. Nurses reported being uncertain since the general manager accused them of doing something illegal. Another fear-inducing factor in this context are imaginations of letting somebody die of thirst in an excruciating way [26]. The participating nurses shared this fear.

To cope with situations causing uncertainties, fears and concerns, nurses have to achieve a balance between their personal and professional ethics and patient autonomy [22]. In that respect, the participating nurses expressed the need for expertise and a professional contact person for VSED-related issues. Furthermore, knowledge about the legal situation is also important to reduce fears. Having gained positive experiences with caring for a person with VSED also proved to be helpful for the nurses in order to reduce fears in the future.

Limitations

For the first time, this study proposed a central model of caring for a person during VSED in a long-term care institution. We derived this model from the case underlying this study. Due to the degree of abstraction, it might be assumed that the theoretical model generated in this study can be transferred to the in-patient setting. However, this should be tested.

Implications for practice and research

This study reveals the need of professionally embedding VSED into practice. To ensure that VSED can be systematically available as an additional option to prematurely induce death, educative interventions and quality controls are necessary. Since VSED is a complex phenomenon, it is required to involve palliative care into practice development early on and comprehensively. Furthermore, it is necessary to distinguish between accepting VSED and respecting the wish for it. With regard to performing VSED, the study lays bare that consensus, information and moderation are indispensable for the team. To facilitate dealing with VSED in practice, this method and its possible complications require further research. This study offers a conceptual model that should be verified by means of a hypothesis-testing approach. Further research ought to consider different situations for performing theory-generating studies. It is recommended to use lifeworld approaches to investigate experiences of the agents involved. Based on the results, interventions for health care professionals and relatives should be elaborated. Additionally, clinical guidelines ought to be developed to professionalize dealing with VSED in institutions.

Conclusions

The elaborated model of caring for a person during VSED in a long-term care institution allows health care professionals to reflect VSED in an in-depth and professional way. The results show that the problem in institutions does not consist of caring for a person during VSED. It is rather associated with different attitudes towards VSED probably resulting in conflicts.

The personal attitude towards VSED is influenced by one's own experiences, previous knowledge, role and faith as well as by the performing persons´ age, disease and deliberate communication of VSED. If the agents involved are conscious about these influencing factors, they are able to reflect their attitude and to deal with VSED in a professional way. Developing an attitude towards VSED in an institutional and personal way is indispensable.

Thus, it seems to be important that long-term care institutions get acquainted with the option of VSED and explain their position towards it. This comprises obtaining information concerning scientific knowledge and the legal situation. In this way, the institution and every employee can develop a professional attitude towards options of premature dying. If a resident requests VSED, the institution is prepared to meet this wish in a professional way and to offer advice. Relatives may also benefit from a professional attitude towards VSED since they experience a challenging time. They are confronted with the physical decay of their family member and have to cope with fears. Professionally handling VSED paves the way for a dignity-preserving final lifetime for the affected person and the relatives.

Abbreviations

DIGNITAS and EXIT: Swiss legal assisted suicide organizations; EKSG: Ethics committee of the canton St. Gallen; MAXQDA: Software for analysis qualitative data; VSED: voluntary stopping of eating and drinking

Acknowledgements

The authors would like to thank Marie-Claire Baumann and Eleonore Arrer for editing this manuscript. We would also like to thank the nursing director, the nursing expert and all nurses for their willingness to participate in this study. Finally, we would like to thank the husband and son for their willingness to participate.

Authors' contributions

Conception: NS, AF, WS. Interviews: NS, AF. Data analysis: NS, AF. Manuscript: NS, AF. Support for data analysis and manuscript: AF. Review of the manuscript: WS, AF. All authors read and approved the final manuscript.

Competing interests

The authors declare that they have no competing interests.

Author details

[1]Institute of Applied Nursing Science IPW-FHS, FHS St.Gallen, University of Applied Sciences, Rosenbergstrasse 59, 9001 St. Gallen, Switzerland. [2]Faculty of Health, Department of Nursing Science, Chair of Family Oriented and Community Based Care, Witten/Herdecke University, Stockumer Strasse 12, 58453 Witten, Germany. [3]Institute of Nursing, School of Health Professions, ZHAW Zurich University of Applied Sciences, Technikumstr. 81, CH-8400 Winterthur, Switzerland.

References

1. Sprangers MA, de REB, Andries F, van Agt HM, Bijl RV, de BJB, et al. Which chronic conditions are associated with better or poorer quality of life? J Clin Epidemiol. 2000;53:895–907. https://doi.org/10.1016/S0895-4356(00)00204-3.

2. Meier DE, Emmons C, Litke A, Wallenstein S, Morrison RS. Characteristics of patients requesting and receiving physician-assisted death. Arch Intern Med. 2003;163:1537–42. https://doi.org/10.1001/archinte.163.13.1537.

3. Chochinov HM, Wilson KG, Enns M, Mowchun N, Lander S, Levitt M, Clinch JJ. Desire for death in the terminally ill. Am J Psychiatry. 1995;152:1185–91. https://doi.org/10.1176/ajp.152.8.1185.

4. Hurst SA, Mauron A. Assisted suicide and euthanasia in Switzerland: allowing a role for non-physicians. BMJ. 2003;326:271–3.

5. Frei A, Schenker TA, Finzen A, Krauchi K, Dittmann V, Hoffmann-Richter U. Assisted suicide as conducted by a "right-to-die"-society in Switzerland: a descriptive analysis of 43 consecutive cases. Swiss Med Wkly. 2001;131:375–80.

6. Assistierter JC. Suizid (Sterbehilfe) und Suizidin der Schweiz. Neuenburg: Todesursachenstatistik 2014; 2016.

7. Schwarz J. Exploring the option of voluntarily stopping eating and drinking within the context of a suffering patient's request for a hastened death. J Palliat Med. 2007;10:1288–97. https://doi.org/10.1089/jpm.2007.0027.

8. Quill TE, Lo B, Brock DW. Palliative options of last resort: a comparison of voluntarily stopping eating and drinking, terminal sedation, physician-assisted suicide, and voluntary active euthanasia. JAMA. 1997;278:2099–104.

9. Quill TE, Byock IR. Responding to intractable terminal suffering: the role of terminal sedation and voluntary refusal of food and fluids. ACP-ASIM end-of-life care consensus panel. American College of Physicians-American Society of internal medicine. Ann Intern Med. 2000;132:408–14.

10. Ganzini L, Goy ER, Miller LL, Harvath TA, Jackson A, Delorit MA. Nurses' experiences with hospice patients who refuse food and fluids to hasten death. N Engl J Med. 2003;349:359–65. https://doi.org/10.1056/NEJMsa035086.

11. Schwarz JK. Stopping eating and drinking. Am J Nurs. 2009;109:52–61; quiz 62. https://doi.org/10.1097/01.NAJ.0000360314.69620.43.

12. Jansen LA. No safe harbor: the principle of complicity and the practice of voluntary stopping of eating and drinking. J Med Philos. 2004;29:61–74. https://doi.org/10.1076/jmep.29.1.61.30413.

13. Monforte-Royo C, Villavicencio-Chávez C, Tomás-Sábado J, Balaguer A. The wish to hasten death: a review of clinical studies. Psychooncology. 2011;20: 795–804. https://doi.org/10.1002/pon.1839.

14. Schwarz JK. Death by voluntary dehydration: suicide or right to refuse a life-prolonging measure? Widener Law Rev. 2011;17:351–61.

15. Quill TE, Lee BC, Nunn S. Palliative treatments of last resort: choosing the least harmful alternative. University of Pennsylvania Center for bioethics assisted suicide consensus panel. Ann Intern Med. 2000;132:488–93.

16. Berry ZS. Responding to suffering: providing options and respecting choice. J Pain Symptom Manag. 2009;38:797–800. https://doi.org/10.1016/j.jpainsymman.2009.09.001.

17. Chabot BE, Goedhart A. A survey of self-directed dying attended by proxies in the Dutch population. Soc Sci Med. 2009;68:1745–51. https://doi.org/10.1016/j.socscimed.2009.03.005.

18. Chabot B. Informationen zum freiwilligen Verzicht auf Nahrung und Flüssigkeit: Was zu tun ist. In: Chabot B, Walther C, editors. Ausweg am Lebensende: Selbstbestimmt sterben durch freiwilligen Verzicht auf Essen und Trinken. 2nd ed. München: Reinhardt; 2011. p. 59–80.

19. Byock I. Patient refusal of nutrition and hydration: walking the ever-finer line. Am J Hosp Palliat Care. 1995;12:8, 9–13.

20. Chabot B. Information zum freiwilligen Verzicht auf Nahrung und Flüssigkeit: Was man darüber wissen sollte. In: Chabot B, Walther C, editors. Ausweg am Lebensende: Selbstbestimmt sterben durch freiwilligen Verzicht auf Essen und Trinken. 2nd ed. München: Reinhardt; 2011. p. 42–58.

21. Bernat JL, Gert B, Mogielnicki RP. Patient refusal of hydration and nutrition. An alternative to physician-assisted suicide or voluntary active euthanasia. Arch Intern Med. 1993;153:2723–8.

22. Harvath T, Miller L, Smith K, Clark L, Jackson A, Ganzini L. Dilemmas encountered by HospiceWorkers when patients wish to hasten death. J Hosp Palliat Nurs. 2006;8:200–9.

23. Walther C. Rechtliche Fragen zum beabsichtigten, vorzeitigen Versterben durch Verzicht auf Nahrung und Flüssigkeit. In: Chabot B, Walther C, editors. Ausweg am Lebensende: Selbstbestimmt sterben durch freiwilligen Verzicht auf Essen und Trinken. 2nd ed. München: Reinhardt; 2011. p. 101–24.

24. Brunner A, Thommen M. Rechtliche Aspekte von Sterben und Tod. In: Wyler D, editor. Sterben und Tod: Eine interprofessionelle Auseinandersetzung. 1st ed. Zürich: Careum; 2009. p. 87–93.

25. Walther C. Ethische Aspekte des freiwilligen Verzichts auf Nahrung und Flüssigkeit. In: Chabot B, Walther C, editors. Ausweg am Lebensende: Selbstbestimmt sterben durch freiwilligen Verzicht auf Essen und Trinken. 2nd ed. München: Reinhardt; 2011. p. 125–44.

26. Spittler JF. Flussigkeitsverzicht. Ethische Massstabsfindung in der gesellschaftlichen Kontroverse. Dtsch Med Wochenschr. 2005;130:171–4. https://doi.org/10.1055/s-2005-837391.

27. Yale SL. Dying patients who refuse nutrition and hydration: holistic nursing Care at the end of life. Alternative and Complementary Therapies. 2005;11: 100–2. https://doi.org/10.1089/act.2005.11.100.

28. Gerring J. Case study research: principles and practices. New York: Cambridge University Press; 2007.

29. Creswell JW. Qualitative inquiry & research design: choosing among five approaches. 3rd ed. Los Angeles CA u.A: SAGE; 2013.

30. Merriam SB. Case study research in education: a qualitative approach. San Francisco: Jossey-Bass; 1991.

31. Yin RK. Applications of case study research. 2nd ed. Thousand Oaks: Sage Publications; 2003.

32. Stake RE. The art of case study research. Thousand Oaks: Sage Publ; 1995.

33. Yin RK. Case study research: design and methods. 5th ed. Los Angeles, London, New Delhi, Singapore. Washington, DC: SAGE; 2014.

34. Yin RK. Qualitative research from start to finish. New York: The Guilford Press; 2011.

35. Flick U. An introduction to qualitative research. 4th ed. Los Angeles: Sage Publications; 2009.

36. Böhm A. Theoretisches Codieren: Textanalyse in der grounded theory. In: Flick U, Ev K, Steinke I, editors. Qualitative Forschung: Ein Handbuch. 10th ed. Reinbek bei Hamburg: rowohlts enzyklopädie im Rowohlt Taschenbuch Verlag; 2013. p. 475–85.

37. Baker GR. The contribution of case study research to knowledge of how to improve quality of care. BMJ Qual Saf. 2011;20(Suppl 1):i30–5. https://doi.org/10.1136/bmjqs.2010.046490.

38. Saldaña J. The coding manual for qualitative researchers. London, thousand oaks, calif: SAGE; 2009.

39. Kuckartz U. Qualitative Inhaltsanalyse. Methoden, Praxis, Computerunterstützung. 1st ed. Weinheim, Bergstr: Juventa; 2012.
40. Guba EG, Lincoln YS. Guidelines and checklist for constructivist (a.k.a. Fourth generatioxn) evaluation. 2001. http://dmeforpeace.org/sites/default/files/Guba%20and%20Lincoln_Constructivist%20Evaluation.pdf. Accessed 28 Aug 2018.
41. Seale C. The quality of qualitative research. London: Sage; 1999.
42. Stratenwerth G, Wohlers W. Schweizerisches Strafgesetzbuch: Handkommentar. 3rd ed. Stämpfli: Bern; 2013.
43. Aebi-Müller R. Freiwilliger Verzicht auf Nahrung undFlüssigkeit (FVNF). Die Perspektive des Rechts. In: Schweizerische Gesellschaft für Biomedizinische Ethik, editor. Freiwilliger Verzicht auf Nahrung und Flüssigkeit (FVNF); 2015. p. 27–46.
44. Eddy DM. A piece of my mind. A conversation with my mother. JAMA. 1994;272:179–81.
45. Birnbacher D. Ist Sterbefasten eine Form von Suizid? Ethik Med. 2015;27: 315–24. https://doi.org/10.1007/s00481-015-0337-9.
46. Klein RU, Fringer A. Voluntary refusal of food and fluid in palliative care: a mapping literature review. Pflege. 2013;26:411–20. https://doi.org/10.1024/1012-5302/a000329.
47. In the situation dpt?>Wolfersdorf M. Suizidalität –Begriffsbestimmung und Entwicklungsmodellesuizidalen Verhaltens. In: Wolfersdorf M, Kaschka WP, editors. Suizidalität: die biologische dimension. Berlin [u.a]: Springer; 1995. p. 1–16.
48. Anderson F, Downing GM, Hill J, Casorso L, Lerch N. Palliative performance scale (PPS): a new tool. Jourcnal of palliative care. 1996;12(1):5–11.
49. Fringer A, Fehn S, Bueche D, Haeuptle C, Schnepp W. Freiwiller Verzicht auf Nahrung und Flüssigkeit (FVNF): Suizid oder natürliche Entscheidung am Lebensende? Pflegerecht. 2018;02:76–83.
50. Heseker H, Stehle P. Ernährung älterer Menschen in stationären Einrichtungen. In: Ernährungsbericht: 2008. Bonn: deutsche Gesellschaft für Ernährung; 2008. p. 157–204.
51. Schaeffer D, Moers M. Bewältigung chronischer Krankheiten - Herausforderungen für die Pflege. In: Rennen-Allhoff B, Schaeffer D, editors. Handbuch Pflegewissenschaft. Weinheim: Juventa; 2000. p. 447–84.
52. Corbin JM, Strauss AL. Ein Pflegemodell zur Bewältigung chronischer Krankheit. In: Woog P, editor. Chronisch Kranke pflegen: das Corbin-und-Strauss-Pflegemodell. Wiesbaden: Ullstein medical; 1998. p. 1–30.
53. Hofmann I. Schwierigkeiten im interprofessionellen Dialog zwischen arztlichem und pflegerischem Kollegium. Pflege. 2001;14:207–13. https://doi.org/10.1024/1012-5302.14.3.207.
54. Duppel S. Nähe und Distanz als gesellschaftliche Grundlegung in der ambulanten Pflege. Hannover: Schlütersche. 2005;
55. Corbin JM, Strauss AL. Weiterleben lernen: Verlauf und Bewältigung chronischer Krankheit. 2nd ed. Bern, Göttingen, Toronto, Seattle: Huber; 2004.
56. Mattiasson AC, Andersson L. Staff attitude and experience in dealing with rational nursing home patients who refuse to eat and drink. J Adv Nurs. 1994;20:822–7.
57. Bobbert M. Patientenautonomie und Pflege: Begründung und Anwendung eines moralischen Rechts. Frankfurt [u.a.]: Campus-Verl; 2002.
58. Jacobs S. Death by voluntary dehydration--what the caregivers say. N Engl J Med. 2003;349:325–6. https://doi.org/10.1056/NEJMp038115.
59. Knight FH. Risk, uncertainty and profit. Boston Mass. u.a: Houghton Mifflin; 1921.
60. Bourdieu P. Sozialer Sinn: Kritik der theoretischen Vernunft. Frankfurt a.M: Suhrkamp; 1993.
61. Harvath TA, Miller LL, Goy E, Jackson A, Delorit M, Ganzini L. Voluntary refusal of food and fluids: attitudes of Oregon hospice nurses and social workers. Int J Palliat Nurs 2004;10:236–41; discussion 242–3. https://doi.org/10.12968/ijpn.2004.10.5.13072.
62. Rooda LA, Clements R, Jordan ML. Nurses' attitudes toward death and caring for dying patients. Oncol Nurs Forum. 1999;26:1683–7.
63. Braun M, Gordon D, Uziely B. Associations between oncology nurses' attitudes toward death and caring for dying patients. Oncol Nurs Forum. 2010;37:E43–9. https://doi.org/10.1188/10.ONF.E43-E49.
64. Payne SA, Dean SJ, Kalus C. A comparative study of death anxiety in hospice and emergency nurses. J Adv Nurs. 1998;28:700–6.

10

Predictors of organizational commitment among university nursing Faculty of Kathmandu Valley, Nepal

Rekha Timalsina[1*], Sarala K.C.[1], Nilam Rai[2] and Anita Chhantyal[3]

Abstract

Background: Increasing work efficiency, improving psychological health, decreasing turnover, turnover intention, and absenteeism may be dependent on organizational commitment of an employee. This study was carried out to identify the predictors of organizational commitment among university nursing faculty within Kathmandu Valley, Nepal.

Methods: A cross-sectional analytical study was conducted based on a sample of 197 nursing faculty selected from 18 nursing colleges affiliated to 5 universities in Kathmandu Valley by using a proportionate stratified random sampling technique. Structured questionnaires regarding socio-demographic information, perceived faculty developmental opportunity, job satisfaction, perceived organizational support, and organizational commitment were used for data collection. Double data entry and data cleaning were done by using Epi-data software; and data analysis was carried out with SPSS version 16 software. Binary regression analysis was used to identify the predictors of organizational commitment and the adjusted odds ratio (AOR) was also calculated.

Results: The findings of this study showed that a majority of respondents had moderate level of organizational commitment (68%) followed by high level (29%) and low level (3%). This study also revealed that the nursing faculty who had a master's degree in nursing, a permanent appointment, and job satisfaction had a high level of organizational commitment. On the contrary, this study also revealed that the nursing faculty who were in the position of assistant instructor to assistant lecturer level and more than 5 years of work experience within same organization were less likely to have a high level of organizational commitment.

Conclusions: Nursing faculty within Kathmandu Valley have a moderate level of organizational commitment. The predictors of organizational commitment are higher education in nursing, position, type of appointment, current organizational tenure, and job satisfaction. Therefore, an organizational authority must pay attention to the modifiable predictors of organizational commitment to enhance organizational commitment of its nursing faculty. This will help to reduce faculty turnover, increase quality of teaching and student's satisfaction.

Keywords: Nursing faculty, organizational commitment, Predictors

Background

Organizational commitment refers to employee commitment to an organization regarding desire-based (affective commitment), obligation based (normative commitment) and cost-based (continuance commitment) [1]. These form an ecosystem that encourage an employee to voluntarily continue working in an organization [2]. Organizations often try to foster commitment in their employees, which provides an impetus to work harder and be more enterprising to achieve organizational objectives. A combination of these factors ensures that an organization attains stability and reduces costly employee turnover [1]. Therefore, the faculty's commitment to their organization, students, teaching activities, occupation, and colleagues has a positive influence on the effectiveness of an academic institution [3]. Universities worldwide are aiming to retain committed faculty in their system [4].

---

* Correspondence: rekha.timalsina@gmail.com
[1]Patan Academy of Health Sciences, School of Nursing and Midwifery, Lalitpur Nursing Campus, Lalitpur, Nepal
Full list of author information is available at the end of the article

Job satisfaction is the most dominant factor in organizational commitment [5] and a previous study on predictors of nursing faculty members' organizational commitment in governmental universities in Jordan showed that age, job satisfaction, and perceived organizational support were significantly related to faculty members' commitment [6]. Similarly, ex post-facto type descriptive study of private universities' faculty and staff in Nigeria highlighted that marital status, job type, and job tenure significantly predicted organizational commitment and turnover intention [7]. A comparative study on qualification and organizational commitment among the faculty of private universities in Pakistan revealed that faculty members with a master's degree were more dedicated than those with either an MPhil or PhD degree [8]. In Nepal's context, based on available literature, there has been only one study on factors associated with organizational commitment among nurses. This study revealed that 34% of nurses had a high level of organizational commitment, and perceived organizational support was associated with organizational commitment [9]. A qualified and committed nursing faculty is essential to sustain a nursing institution and deliver high quality education. However, there is no rigorous academic inquiry into organizational commitment among nursing faculty and its associated factors. This study was aimed to determine the predictors of organizational commitment among university nursing faculty within Kathmandu Valley, Nepal so that it can help the nursing administrators and managers of various universities to find ways to improve organizational commitment.

Methods
Study design
A cross-sectional analytical study was conducted to identify the predictors of organizational commitment among university nursing faculty of Kathmandu Valley.

Population and sample
The study population consisted of 279 nursing faculty who had completed at least six months of a full-time teaching in a bachelor program or higher level of 18 nursing colleges affiliated to 5 universities (i.e., Tribhuvan University (TU), Purbanchal University (PU), Pokhara University (PokU), Kathmandu University (KU) and National Academy for Medical Sciences (NAMS) of Kathmandu Valley). But, nursing faculty on long leave were excluded from the study. The campus chief, assistant campus chiefs, heads of departments, and visiting professors were excluded from the study population. The sample size was calculated by using the formula [10]:

$$\mathbf{n} = \left[(z^2pq) + ME2/ME2 + z^2pq/N \right]$$

where.

Z = 1.96 for 95% confidence level,
p = 68% [3], q = 1-p,
ME (Margin of Error) = 5%,
n = Sample Size.
N = Population Size (i.e., 279).

The required sample size was 152 nursing faculty for 95% confidence level. Allowing non-response rate of 10% and maintaining the power of test (i.e., n'/0.8), the final sample size was estimated to be 209 nursing faculty. The proportionate stratified random sampling technique was used to divide the population into 5 strata of affiliated universities (See Figure 1). Sample size for each stratum was determined by using following equation [11]: n_h = $(N_h/N) \times n^*$, where, n_h: sample size for stratum h, N_h: population size for stratum h, N: total population size, n^*: total sample size.

After stratification, the sample of 209 nursing faculty were selected with simple random sampling technique from each stratum using random numbers from a random number generator [12].

Research instruments
The instruments used in this study were composed of five parts. Part one was related to structured questionnaire on socio-demographic and personal information.

Part two consisted of 15 items of perceived faculty developmental opportunities measured on a 5-point Likert scale ranging from 1 (strongly disagree) to 5 (strongly agree) with 5 negatively worded items. The minimum and maximum scores of this scale were 15 and 75 respectively. The perception level was categorized into five categories as Most Favorable Perception (75 score), Favorable Perception (46–74 score), Neutral Perception (45 score), Unfavorable Perception (16–44 score) and Most Unfavorable Perception (15 score) [13].

Part three consisted of 36 items of job satisfaction survey (JSS) of nursing faculty measured on 6-point Likert scale ranging from 1 (Strongly disagree) to 6 (Strongly agree) with 19 negatively worded items. The minimum and maximum scores were 36 and 216 respectively. The level of job satisfaction was determined by the score of respondents. A mean item response ≥4 represented satisfaction, whereas mean response ≤3 represented dissatisfaction, and mean scores between 3 and 4 represented as ambivalence [14].

Part four consisted of 8 items of perceived organizational support (POS) [15] of nursing faculty measured on 7-point Likert scale ranging from 0 (strongly disagree) to 6 (strongly agree) with 4 negatively worded items. The minimum and maximum scores were 0 and 48 respectively. The level of POS was determined by the score of the respondents. The scores with 1 standard deviation above mean represented as high POS, whereas 1 standard deviation below mean represented as low POS [16].

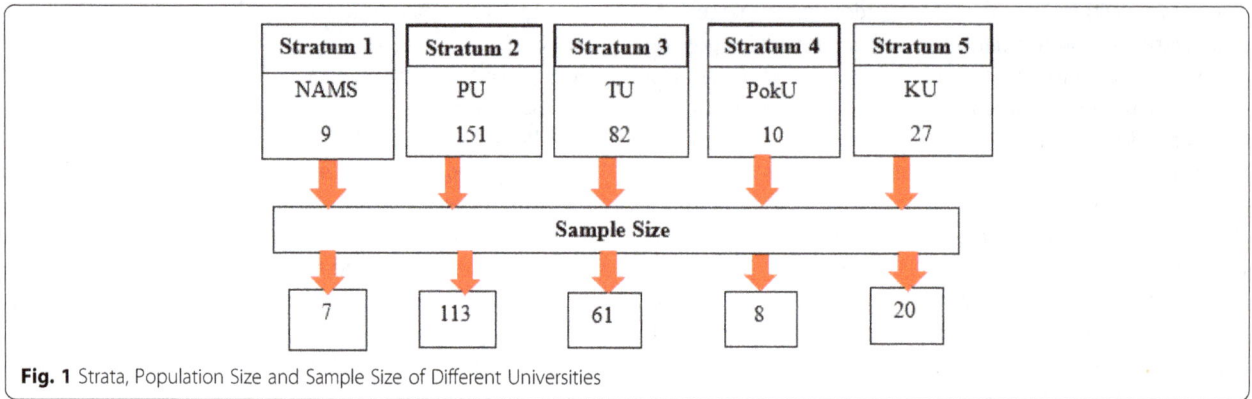

Fig. 1 Strata, Population Size and Sample Size of Different Universities

Part five consisted of 18 items of organizational commitment questionnaire (OCQ) - affective, continuance, and normative [1], measured on 7-point Likert scale ranging from 1 (strongly disagree) to 7 (strongly agree) with 4 negatively worded items. The minimum and maximum scores were 18 and 126 respectively. The level of organizational commitment was determined by score of the respondent. Thus, the scores fell in of the following ranges: 1.00–3.00: Low Commitment, 3.01–5.00: Moderate Commitment and 5.01: 7.00: High Commitment [17]. Negatively worded items of these instruments were reversed before analysis.

The OCQ tool has been already validated in the Nepalese context [18]. To ensure content validity for current study, OCQ along with other instruments were further evaluated by experienced professional nursing faculty, human resource managers, and academics in nursing in order to determine if the instrument reflects the known content area. The OCQ, JSS and POS had already been translated and back translated and used in previous study conducted among nurses in 2015 [9]. Reverse translation of perceived faculty developmental opportunity scale was done for assuring semantic equivalence of this instrument. Pretesting of those instruments was done among 22 nursing faculty from three nursing colleges who were similar in characteristics with actual samples of this study and these colleges were excluded in actual study. This was done for establishing the conceptual/linguistic and functional equivalence. Reliability coefficient based on Cronbach alpha was 0.72, 0.70, 0.85 and 0.81 for perceived faculty developmental opportunity, OCQ, JSS and SPOS respectively.

Data collection procedure

Written permission was taken from the authors for using OCQ and SPOS. JSS is a free tool for educational purposes. Data was collected from 23 January 2017 to 13 March 2017 by applying ethical procedure. The questionnaires were distributed to 209 nursing faculty selected in sample for self-response with provision of sufficient time as requested by the respondents (average 3 days' time) and regular follow-up. Within time frame of data collection period allocated for the study, 197 nursing faculty returned the completed questionnaire and 12 questionnaires were not returned. Thus, a valid response rate for this study was 94.3% and the data analysis was carried out using 197 completed questionnaires.

Questionnaire editing for completeness and consistency of responses was done at field and central level. Double data entry as well as data cleaning was done using Epi Data software and data analysis was done using SPSS software version 16. Descriptive statistics was used to describe the sample characteristics and binary logistic regression analysis was used to identify the predictors of organizational commitment and adjusted odds ratio was also calculated. Logistic regression adjusted for age, marital status, higher education in nursing, higher education besides nursing, position, type of appointment, positional tenure, professional tenure, current organizational tenure, family structure, perceived faculty developmental opportunity, job satisfaction and perceived organizational support. Variables were entered simultaneously in the model and significant results were denoted by an asterisk in the table. For each test, significance was considered at $p \leq .05$ for 95% confidence level.

Results

In this study, the nursing faculty were aged from 24 to 73 years ($M = 36$ years, $SD = 8.3$); 86.8% were married; 54.8% had a master's degree in nursing; 40.1% received education besides nursing; 49.7% had economically dependent family members; 46.2% had a permanent type of appointment; and 48.7% were lecturers. Majority of respondents had less than five years of positional tenure (76.6%) and organizational tenure (64.5%), and ≥ 9 years of professional tenure (74.1%).

Table 1 reveals that 29% of respondents had a high level of organizational commitment (M = 4.63, SD = 0.71).

Table 2 shows that a higher education in nursing ($p = .031$, AOR: 3.743, CI: 1.129, 12.410), and type of appointment ($p = .000$, AOR: 4.542, CI: 1.960, 10.525) contributed significantly to the prediction of a high level

Table 1 Respondent's Level of Organizational Commitment

Level of Organizational Commitment	Frequency	Percent	Min-Max	M ± SD
Low	6	3		
Moderate	134	68	2.72–6.22	4.63 ± 0.71
High	57	29		

n = 197

Note. Mean scores 1.00–3.00: Low Commitment, Mean scores 3.01–5.00: Moderate Commitment and Mean scores 5.01–7.00: High Commitment [17]

of organizational commitment, whereas position ($p = .022$, AOR: 0.242, CI: 0.072, 0.816) contributed significantly to the prediction of a low to moderate level of organizational commitment. The contribution of other socio-demographic factors- age, marital status, and higher education besides nursing were not significant. However, the adjusted odds ratio reveals that respondents who were above 30 years old, unmarried, and had higher education besides nursing were 1.861, 1.598 and 1.348 times more likely to have a higher level of organizational commitment respectively. On the other hand, the respondents with position of Assistant Instructor to Assistant Lecturer were less likely to have higher level of organizational commitment than lecturer to Professor.

Table 3 highlights that current organizational tenure ($p = .044$, AOR = 0.039, CI = 0.098, 0.967) contributed significantly to the prediction of a low to moderate level of organizational commitment, but, positional tenure and professional tenure did not. However, the adjusted odds ratio reveals that respondents with greater than 5 years of experience were 0.039 times less likely to have high level of organizational commitment than others; and respondents with more than 5 years of positional tenure were 1.632 times more likely to have high level of organizational commitment than others.

Table 4 shows that job satisfaction ($p = .032$, AOR: 2.608, CI: 1.087, 6.255) contributed significantly to the prediction of high level of organizational commitment, but contribution of other variables – having economically dependent family members, perceived faculty developmental opportunity, and perceived organizational support were not significant. However, the adjusted odd ratio reveals that the respondents who did not have economically dependent family members, who had a favorable perception towards faculty developmental opportunity, and a high level of perceived organizational support had 2.001, 1.713, and 1.189 times more likely to have high level of organizational commitment than others.

Discussion

This study reveals that a majority of respondents had a moderate level of organizational commitment (68%) and

Table 2 Analysis of Respondent's Socio-demographic Characteristics as a Predictors of Organizational Commitment

Socio- demographic Characteristics	Organizational Commitment		p-value [a]	AOR	95% CI
	Low and Moderate Level N (%)	High Level N (%)			
Age Group					
Up to 30 years [b]	48 (82.8)	10 (17.2)			
> 30 years	92 (66.2)	47 (33.8)	.278	1.861	[0.606, 5.714]
Marital Status					
Married[b]	22 (84.6)	4 (15.4)			
Unmarried	118 (69.0)	53 (31.0)	.482	1.598	[0.432, 5.905]
Higher Education in Nursing					
Bachelor [b]	67 (75.3)	22 (24.7)			
Master	73 (67.6)	35 (32.4)	.031[c]	3.743	[1.129, 12.410]
Higher Education Besides Nursing					
No[b]	88 (74.6)	30 (25.4)			
Yes	52 (65.8)	27 (34.2)	.465	1.348	[0.605, 3.004]
Position					
Assistant Instructor to Assistant Lecturer	54 (70.1)	23 (29.9)	.022[c]	0.242	[0.072, 0.816]
Lecturer to Professor Level[b]	86 (71.7)	34 (28.3)			
Type of Appointment					
Temporary/Contract [b]	89 (84.0)	17 (16.0)			
Permanent	51 (56.0)	40 (44.0)	.000[c]	4.542	[1.960, 10.525]

n = 197

Note. [a]: *p*-value obtained from binary logistic regression. [b] = reference category. [c] = *p*-value significant at ≤0.05 level. *AOR* Adjusted Odds Ratio

Table 3 Analysis of Respondent's Work Experience as a Predictors of Organizational Commitment

Work Experience	Organizational Commitment		p-value [a]	AOR	n = 197 95% CI
	Low and Moderate Level No. (%)	High Level No. (%)			
Positional Tenure					
≤ 5 Years [b]	110 (72.8)	41 (27.2)			
> 5 Years	30 (65.2)	16 (34.8)	.402	1.632	[0.519, 5.128]
Professional Tenure					
≤ 5 Years [b]	14 (77.8)	4 (22.2)			
> 5 Years	126 (70.4)	53 (29.6)	.424	0.524	[0.108, 2.553]
Current Organizational Tenure					
≤ 5 Years [b]	93 (73.2)	34 (26.8)			
> 5 Years	47 (67.1)	23 (32.9)	.044[c]	0.039	[0.098, 0.967]

Note. [a]: p-value obtained from binary logistic regression. [b] = reference category. [c] = p-value significant at ≤0.05 level. *AOR* Adjusted Odds Ratio

29% had high level. The findings of a previous study on effect of organizational climate on organizational commitment among faculty of nursing in Egypt indicated that most faculty had a moderate level of organizational commitment [19]. The findings of the current study are dissimilar with the findings of an empirical investigation of faculty members' organizational commitment in Saudi Arabia, which revealed that faculty had high level (73.4%) and moderate level (26.0%) of commitment for overall organizational commitment [20]. Another study on assessment of work environment and employee's commitment in college of nursing in Saudi Arabia also revealed that the respondents had high commitment

scores (61.2%), and moderate commitment scores (38.8%) [21]. Similarly, a study on organizational commitment among faculty of an educational institute in India also revealed that there was a high level of organizational commitment among the faculty members of the university [3]. The dissimilarities in results from countries might be due to variation in geography, available opportunities, and facilities in each organization.

Regarding predictors of organizational commitment among respondents, the current study reveals that age did not contribute significantly to the prediction of a high level of organizational commitment. This finding is supported by a previous study on determinants of

Table 4 Respondent's Having Economically Dependent Family Members, Perceived Faculty Developmental Opportunity, JS and POS as Predictors of OC

Variables	Organizational Commitment		p-value[a]	AOR	n = 197 95% CI
	Low and Moderate Level No. (%)	High Level No. (%)			
Having Economically Dependent Family Members					
Yes[b]	78 (77.2)	23 (22.8)			
No	62 (64.6)	34 (35.4)	.080	2.001	[0.921, 4.345]
Perceived Faculty Developmental Opportunity					
Neutral and Unfavorable Perception[b]	73 (84.9)	13 (15.1)			
Having Favorable Perception	67 (60.4)	44 (39.6)	.270	1.713	[0.658, 4.457]
Job Satisfaction (JS)					
Dissatisfaction and Ambivalence[b]	105 (80.8)	25 (19.2)			
Satisfaction	35 (52.2)	32 (47.8)	.032[c]	2.608	[1.087, 6.255]
Perceived Organizational Support (POS)					
Low[b]	84 (80.0)	21 (20.0)			
High	56 (60.9)	36 (39.1)	.481	1.189	[0.735, 1.922]

Note. [a] = p-value obtained from binary logistic regression. [b] = reference category. [c] = p-value significant at ≤0.05 level. *AOR* Adjusted Odds Ratio organizational commitment among the faculty of private tertiary institutions in the Philippines which showed that age did not significantly affect organizational commitment [22]. A similar finding from a study on impact of personal attributes on the commitment level among faculty of educational institutions in Pakistan revealed that age was not a good predictor of commitment [23]. The supportive argument related to association between age and organizational commitment is that older employees may assume that they have accumulated personal capital in the organization such as self-identity, friends and social relationships, seniority or retirement benefits which they would not want to lose by leaving an organization. Therefore, they might be more committed to their organization.

The present study shows that marital status did not contribute significantly to the prediction of high level of organizational commitment. The finding of the current study is inconsistent with the finding of a previous study on organizational commitment and turnover intention among private universities' employees in Nigeria, which revealed that marital status significantly predicted organizational commitment and turnover intention [8]. The supportive argument related to the association between marital status and organizational commitment is that married employees are more committed, since they have more financial responsibilities to their families. The contradictory result of the current study might be due to the changing life style and equal sharing responsibilities between couples. Both single and married employees might have same level of financial needs to meet the high living expenses and higher demands for a better living standard.

The recent study highlights that higher education in nursing contributed significantly to the prediction of high level of organizational commitment. The finding is consistent with a comparative study on qualification and organizational commitment among the faculty of private universities in Pakistan, which revealed that faculty holding a Master's degree were more dedicated than those holding MPhil and PhD degrees [7]. The supportive argument for the current study concerning the association between education and organizational commitment is that employees with a higher level of education are likely to leave their current organization. The search for a more fulfilling and dignified job in spite of the type of job, which they are doing, or numbers of years they have put into their current job. The opposite result might occur due to feeling of inadequacy related to opportunity at their current job despite their qualifications.

The current study also revealed that position contributed significantly to the prediction of low to moderate level of organizational commitment. The finding of the current study is consistent a previous study of Saudi Arabia which showed that academic rank was found to be significantly related to organizational commitment [20]. The supportive argument related to association between position and organizational commitment is that at a higher position, opportunities and responsibilities also increase. Therefore, the opportunity and fulfilled responsibilities made employees feel more responsible in decision making and are better integrated into workplace.

The current study shows that permanent type of appointment contributed significantly to the prediction of a high level of organizational commitment. This finding is inconsistent with the finding of a previous study conducted among nurses in Nepal, which did not reveal type of appointment as a predictor of organizational commitment [9]. The supportive argument related to association between type of appointment and organizational commitment is that permanent employees are more committed, since they have a sense of greater job security and job fulfillment.

The current study highlights that respondents with more than 5 years of work experience in current organization were less likely to have a high level of organizational commitment. However, positional tenure and professional tenure did not contribute significantly to the prediction of high level of organizational commitment. A previous study done among nurses in Nepal did not reveal work experience as a predictor of organizational commitment [9]. The supportive argument related to association between work experience and organizational commitment is that employees that have more years of work experience are likely to stay with their existing organization, since they have invested much time and effort, attained seniority and are connected to the organization.

The present study shows that having economically dependent family members did not contribute significantly to the prediction of high level of organizational commitment. This finding is consistent with the previous study conducted among nurses in Nepal, which did not reveal economically dependent family members as a significant predictor of organizational commitment [9]. The supportive argument related to association between having financially dependent family members and organizational commitment is that employees who have economically dependent family members might have higher level of economic needs to meet the high living expenses and basic needs of their dependent members. Therefore, they are more likely to be committed to their organization.

The current study shows that perceived faculty developmental opportunities did not contribute significantly to the prediction of high level of organizational commitment. This finding is similar to a previous study among nurses, which did not reveal staff developmental opportunity as a predictor of organizational commitment [9]. The supportive argument related to association between perceived faculty developmental opportunity and organizational commitment is that each employee might desire to further develop their potential and achieve professional growth and self-actualization. If they feel a favorable perception towards faculty developmental opportunities, they are more likely to be committed.

The present study shows that job satisfaction contributed significantly to the prediction of high level of organizational commitment. The previous study conducted in Jordan showed that job satisfaction was significantly related to faculty members' commitment [6]. The supportive argument related to association between job satisfaction and organizational commitment is that satisfied employees are more likely to be creative, innovative, motivated for increasing their job performance and are more likely to be committed towards their organization. Therefore, effective measures should be taken by relevant authorities at each university to improve job satisfaction among university nursing faculty and enhance organizational commitment.

The present study demonstrates that perceived organizational support did not contribute significantly to the prediction of high level of organizational commitment. This finding is different from previous findings on structural relationships between organizational commitment, job satisfaction, developmental experiences, work values, organizational support, and person-organization fit among nursing faculty in USA. That study revealed that perceived organizational support positively predicted nurse faculty's organizational commitment to the academic organization [24]. Another study carried out in Jordan showed that perceived organizational support was significantly related to faculty members' commitment [6]. The supportive argument related to association between perceived organizational support and organizational commitment is that employees who perceive a high level of organizational support may feel confident and hopeful about their desired job goals and are more likely to be committed towards their organization. Therefore, providing more support to nursing faculty by adopting faculty centered strategies such as taking into consideration of their best interests, valuing their work, and providing help when they face difficulties may enhance organizational commitment.

Conclusion

In conclusion, university nursing faculty have moderate level of organizational commitment. Higher education in nursing, position, type of appointment, current organizational tenure and job satisfaction are predictors of organizational commitment. Hence, human service organizations must focus on developing strategies to retain experienced employees by offering permanent appointments and provide professional and academic career development tools. They must do more to offer novel faculty developmental opportunities, provide

organizational support, and improve job satisfaction. These cumulative actions will foster an environment for enhancing organizational commitment amongst nursing faculty. Effectively, such an ecosystem will reduce turnover, improve quality of teaching, lower absenteeism, improve the student's satisfaction level, and enhance organizational effectiveness.

Limitations

The limitations of this study were: the results were derived only from the self-reported techniques based on perceptions of nursing faculty using Likert items. There is a possibility of social desirability and central tendency biases, which may have distorted the true organizational commitment. Moreover, the generalizability of the study's findings is limited because of the study population, which was based on responses from nursing faculty of different nursing colleges within Kathmandu Valley. To obtain more generalizable results, future investigations should include nursing faculty working outside Kathmandu Valley as well. The findings were drawn from cross-sectional data obtained from self-administered questionnaires and this study had not included other variables that may influence organizational commitment i.e., organizational culture, job involvement, job stress, job insecurity, workplace harassment, organizational communication and so on. Therefore, this study was not able to present definitive conclusions about the direction of causality and reveal the factors, which have long-term effects on organizational commitment. Hence, prospective longitudinal research should be conducted to identify the antecedent and consequences factors associated with organizational commitment among nursing faculty in different colleges affiliated to different universities of Nepal.

However, this study has methodological strengths. It was a large survey including major universities in Nepal with a range of nursing faculty using random sampling technique with precise sample size. In addition, a high response rate (94.3% after eliminating the missing data) strengthens the generalizability of the study findings within the nursing faculty of Kathmandu valley.

Abbreviations
JSS: Job Satisfaction Survey; OCQ: Organizational Commitment Questionnaire; POS: Perceived Organizational Support; SPSS: Statistical Package for the Social Sciences

Acknowledgements
We express our thanks to the authors and developers of the JSS, POS and OCQ tools. We would like to express our sincere thanks to authorities of different colleges for granting permission to carry out this study. Finally, we would like to thank all the respondents for their untiring, exceptional effort and cooperation by giving their valuable time to participate in this study.

Funding
This study was funded by University Grant Commission (UGC), Sanothimi, Bhaktapur, Nepal under the Small Research Development and Innovation Grant and research team of UGC supervised our work throughout the research process.

Authors' contributions

RT had worked on this research from the conceptual phase to the dissemination phase. RT, NR and AC collected data, entered in Epidata software, and analyzed the data in SPSS software. RT and NR participated in literature review and report writing. Professor S. K.C. supervised the research process and manuscript writing. RT wrote the manuscript and all the authors read and approved the final manuscript.

Competing interests

The authors declare that they have no competing interests.

Author details

[1]Patan Academy of Health Sciences, School of Nursing and Midwifery, Lalitpur Nursing Campus, Lalitpur, Nepal. [2]Dristi Nepal, Kathmandu, Nepal. [3]Tribhuvan University Teaching Hospital, Maharajgunj, Kathmandu, Nepal.

References

1. Meyer JP, Allen NJ. TCM employee commitment survey: academic users guide 2004. (2004). Available from http://employeecommitment.com/.
2. Allen AJ, Meyer JP. Affective, continuance, and normative commitment to the organization: an examination of construct validity. J Vocat Behav. 1996; 49(3):252–76. Available from https://doi.org/10.1006/jvbe.1996.0043.
3. Bali R, Vaidya D. Study on the organizational commitment in the faculty of an educational institute. Int J Farm Sci. 2012;2(2):167–73. Available from www.inflibnet.ac.in/.
4. Awang Z, Ahmad JH. Modeling job satisfactions and work commitment among lecturers: a case of UITM Kelantan. J Stat Model Anal. 2010;1(2):45–59. Available from http://www.academia.edu/.
5. Warsi S, Fatima N, Sahibzada SA. Study on relationship between organizational commitment and its determinant among private sector employees of Pakistan. Int Rev Bus Res Pap. 2009;5(3):399–410. Available from www.bizresearchpapers.com/.
6. Al-Hussami M, Saleha MYN, Abdalkader RH, Mahadeen AI. Predictors of nursing faculty members' organizational commitment in governmental universities. J Nurs Manag. 2011;19(4):556–66. https://doi.org/10.1111/j.1365-2834.2010. 01148.x.
7. Adenuga RA, Adenuga FT, Ayodele KO. Organizational commitment and turnover intention among private universities' employees in Ogun state, Nigeria. Open J Educ. 2013;1(2):31–6. https://doi.org/10.12966/oje.05.04.2013.
8. Khan Y, Batool S. Comparative study of qualification and organizational commitment among the faculty of private universities. Int J Busi Manage. 2017;5(1):51–61. https://doi.org/10.20472/BM.2017.5.1.004.
9. Timalsina R, Rai L, Gautam S, Panta P. Factors associated with organizational commitment among nurses. J Stud Manag Plan. 2015;1(1):558–71. Available from http://internationaljournalofresearch.org/.
10. Sample size: Simple random sample. (2017). Available from http://stattrek.com/.
11. Sample size: Stratified random samples. (2017). Available from http://stattrek.com/sample-size/stratified-sample.aspx.
12. Random number generator. (2017). Available from http://stattrek.com/statistics/
13. Kothari CR, Garg G. Research methodology: methods and techniques. 3rd ed. New Delhi, India: New Age International (P). Ltd; 2014.
14. Spector P. Job satisfaction survey. 1994. Available from http://shell.cas.usf.edu/.
15. Eisenberger R, Hungtington R, Hutchison S, Sowa D. (1986). Perceived organizational support. J Appl Psychol. 1986;71(3):500–7. Available from http://eisenberger.psych.udel.edu/.
16. Eder P, Eisenberger R. Perceived organizational support: reducing the negative influence of coworker withdrawal behavior. J Manage. 2008;34(1):55–68. https://doi.org/10.1177/0149206307309259.
17. Lee SP, Chitpakdee B, Chontawan R. Factors predicting organizational commitment among nurses in state hospitals, Malaysia. Int Med J Malaysia. 2011;10(2):23–30. Available from http://iiumedic.net/imjm/v1/.
18. Gautam T. Organizational commitment in Nepal. Kathmandu, Nepal: Tribhuvan University; 2003. Available from: http://www.ssrf.org.np/.
19. Elsabahy HE, Sleem WF, El-Sayed NM. Effect of organizational climate on organizational commitment of nurse educator at faculty of nursing Mansoura university. J Educ Pract. 2013;4(27):41–8. Available from http://www.iiste.org/Journals/.
20. BinBakr MB, Ahmed EI. An empirical investigation of faculty members' organizational commitment in the kingdom of Saudi Arabia. Am J Educ Res. 2015;3(8:1020–6. https://doi.org/10.12691/education-3-8-12.
21. Miligi SM, Habib F, ALFozan H. Assessment of work environment and employee's commitment in college of nursing. Int J Adv Res Comput Sci Manag. 2015;3(4):147–56. Available from www.ijarcsms.com.
22. Quiambao DT, Nuqui A. Determinants of organizational commitment among the faculty members of private tertiary institutions. J Soc Sci Humanit Res. 2017;3(1):1–14. Available from http://jsshr.anveshika.org/article/.
23. Khan H, Shah B, ul Hassan FS, Khan S, Khan N. Impact of personal attributes over the commitment level of teachers: a context of higher education institutions of Pakistan. J Bus Stud Q. 2013;5(2):1–14. Available from http://jbsq.org/wp-content/.
24. Gutierrez AP, Candela LL, Carver L. The structural relationships between organizational commitment, job satisfaction, developmental experiences, work values, organizational support, and person-organization fit among nursing faculty. J Adv Nurs. 2012;68(7):1601–14. https://doi.org/10.1111/j.1365-2648.2012. 05990.x.

11

From apprehension to advocacy: a qualitative study of undergraduate nursing student experience in clinical placement in residential aged care

Heather Moquin, Cydnee Seneviratne and Lorraine Venturato* ⓘ

Abstract

Background: Undergraduate nursing placement in aged care is forecast to grow in importance with the increasing aging population, and to help to reverse trends in student lack of interest in gerontology careers. However, there is a need to better understand undergraduate nursing students' experiences on placement with older adults, as well as key features of quality learning within residential aged care. The aim of this study was to explore how nursing students understand learning within residential aged care.

Methods: This qualitative study used a participatory action research approach, and this paper reports on the thematic analysis of data from one cycle of undergraduate nursing placement in a Canadian residential aged care setting, with two groups of 7–8 students and two university instructors. Staff and residents at the research site were also included. Researchers interviewed both groups of students prior to and after placement. Instructors, staff and residents were interviewed post placement.

Results: Students commenced placement full of apprehension, and progressed in their learning by taking initiative and through self-directed learning pathways. Engagement with residents was key to student learning on person-centred care and increased understanding of older adults. Students faced challenges to their learning through limited exposure to professional nursing roles and healthcare aide/student relationship issues. By placement end, students had gained unique insights on resident care and began to step into advocacy roles.

Conclusions: In learning on placement within residential aged care, students moved from feelings of apprehension to taking on advocacy roles for residents. Better formalizing routes for students to feedback their unique understandings on resident care could ensure their contributions are better integrated and not lost when placements end.

Keywords: Nursing students, Nursing education, Action research, Residential aged care facilities

Background

Creating an age friendly workforce – a difficult but necessary endeavour

"Because most patients in almost all settings are older, there is little place for the nurse who does not wish to work with older adults or who lacks the knowledge to provide this care" ([1], p. 24). Nurses must therefore emerge from their preparatory education ready and willing to provide the specific nursing care this population requires [2]. However, there is a general lack of interest among nursing students in gerontology careers [1, 3, 4]. This has been linked to persistent broad-scale ageism within society [1, 4, 5]; occurrences of negative stereotypes towards working with older adults within the nursing profession [6]; drops in students' interests in gerontology careers as they progress through their studies [6, 7]; and a dominance of a cure versus care focus within health care [8]. Nursing schools have also been

* Correspondence: lventura@ucalgary.ca
Faculty of Nursing, University of Calgary, 2500 University Dr NW, Calgary, AB T2N 1N4, Canada

described as providing insufficient education on care of older adults [9].

This is further complicated by challenges in developing quality clinical learning environments for nursing students to learn and work with an older population. A growing shortage of nurses in Canada [10], means that nursing schools are under increased pressure to develop innovative educational programs and augment numbers of nursing professionals prepared for delivering on future healthcare needs [2, 11, 12]. Such interlinked understandings help to clarify why the development of an age-friendly nursing workforce is certainly not a straightforward task.

Despite its limited use thus far, residential aged care (RAC) is forecast to grow in importance as a site for undergraduate nursing education [2]. Placement within RAC settings, though traditionally used early in nursing programs for education on basic nurse competencies, offers potential for advanced knowledge and practice [2]. Cartwright ([13], p. 243) notes that: "Community-based long-term care provides abundant opportunities for transformative learning and practice in areas that are core to 21st century nursing: managing chronic illness and palliative care in ways that are patient-centred and evidence-based, working in interdisciplinary teams, supervising unlicensed caregivers, and developing systems for ongoing quality improvement."

"Therefore, RAC is a key setting to kindle student interest in the care of older adults, while developing essential and advanced proficiencies in contemporary nurse practice."

To ensure placements in aged care settings contribute to the preparation of an age-friendly nursing workforce, the diverse influences on undergraduate student perceptions of practicum learning in aged care and with older adults must be explored. Evidence already suggests that students tend to find these placements "unsatisfactory and/or unsettling" and experience a sense of powerlessness on placement, reinforced by financial constraints, an unaccommodating learning/working environment, and a lack of readiness to encounter and care for ageing bodies ([14], p. 14). A further challenge with gerontological placements is that they are often located within impoverished care environments [7, 8].

Clinical placement is a key contributor to cementing student attitudes [8], and much effort is being made to counter these negative trends by designing placements in aged care that positively shape student perceptions. These efforts range from ensuring placements involve interaction with older adults in diverse settings [4], integrating creative and reflective pedagogies for shifting perceptions [15], and enriching placement environments

[7, 8]. Within this body of work, it is important to maintain distinction between students' perceptions of older adults and their perceptions of gerontological careers [5]. Within the context of a clinical placement with older adults, the aim of this study was to explore how nursing students understand learning within residential aged care.

Methods
Design
This paper reports on one 13-week undergraduate placement cycle that occurred in the summer of 2016. The study followed a participatory action research (PAR) design, involving cyclic, iterative processes for investigation, action, reflection and collaboration in the inquiry [16]. Action research methodologies are established approaches for practitioner research [17] and are particularly useful for nurse researchers in centring the research endeavour within the context being studied and involving research participants as partners in the inquiry [18]. A thematic qualitative approach was used for data analysis, a method often used within action research for uncovering meaning [17].

Development of a positive person-centred placement model
The first stage of this research involved the collaborative and ongoing development of a person-centred placement model aimed at enhancing the interests of undergraduate nursing students in working with older adults. In the spring of 2016, a working group consisting of university educators and researchers, site staff, and residents met in seven 1-h sessions to begin to co-develop the placement model. The working group developed and planned a person-centred placement model for the upcoming student placement, incorporating elements such as the concepts of person-centred care and intergenerational learning; student and resident orientations; communication of student skills and developing capabilities; and roles and expectations of residents, staff, and students.

Setting
Two groups of undergraduate nursing students, with 1 instructor respectively, were placed at two supportive living facilities owned and operated by the same non-profit provider and co-located on the same campus. The 13-week practicum cycle (249 total hours) occurred in the summer of 2016.

Facility 1: positive person-centred placement model
At the intervention site, eight students and residents were matched by the working group and structured time was accommodated in the student schedule. Students

spent 1.5 days per week at the sites and worked with healthcare aides (HCAs), particularly during morning care routines. Students also worked one-to-one with residents on a care plan assignment.

Facility 2: traditional clinical placement model

The second site used a traditional clinical placement model. Here, seven students chose which residents to work with and their time with residents was less structured. Like Facility 1, students spent 1.5 days per week at this site, worked with HCAs, and worked one-to-one with residents on a care plan assignment.

While there were some variances between the placement models at site 1 and 2 in relation to orientation to site, intentionality and focus in the student–resident interactions, in general the placement model at the intervention site was not fully implemented and there were minimal differences between groups. Therefore findings for both groups are presented together to further understanding of student learning within RAC.

Participants

Qualitative data was collected with both groups of students ($n = 15$) and instructors ($n = 2$), and with site staff ($n = 8$) and residents ($n = 5$) involved at the intervention site. Instructors in this study were experienced RNs employed by the university, on a contractual basis, to accompany and facilitate undergraduate student learning during clinical placement. Student participants were second year, first term undergraduate students undertaking their first clinically focused placement. Staff included were HCAs, licensed practice nurses (LPNs) and site management (RNs and allied health personnel).

Data collection

Focus groups were held with students pre- and post-placement, and with residents and staff post placement. Individual interviews were held with instructors and site management post-placement. Data collection was conducted by two members of the research team and sessions took one hour. Interviews and focus groups were conducted in a meeting room at the site or university. Interviews and focus group questions explored

participants' experiences during the placement, and learning facilitators and challenges. Questions were framed temporally (see Table 1 in Appendix for a list of questions by participant group). Focus groups and interviews were all digitally recorded and transcribed verbatim.

Data analysis

Data was analyzed thematically [17]. Transcripts were read and analyzed by two of the authors. Initial readings and analysis resulted in general theming of the data. A series of meetings between the authors allowed for agreement on a set of broad themes under which subcategories were placed. Meetings between the authors on the initial draft prompted a temporal frame as a useful lens for analysis. Subheadings were created to structure and frame the writing so that it flowed temporally from anticipation and beginning placement to completion and final reflection. The authors included further data related to 'process' and redrafted the writing until coming to an agreement on the findings.

Results

This study found that undergraduate nursing students began their placements in RAC with a range of apprehensions and expectations. On placement, encountering challenges in working with HCAs and with a lack of professional nursing roles, students sought out mentorship and learning opportunities. Pairings with residents on placement helped students gain appreciation for older adults and learn person-centred care. Over time and with encouragement, students developed initiative and capacity so that by the end of placement they more actively created their own learning opportunities and stepped into advocacy roles for residents.

Beginning placement: Concerns and expectations

Both groups of students felt hesitant and had concerns prior to placement. One student explained, *"I was just nervous in general...I didn't really know what we would be expected to do"* [N-S-P7]. With this being their first practicum involving care provision, students were acutely aware of their possible limitations: *"I was...concerned about not being ready or not*

Table 1 Interview & Focus Group Questions by Participant Group

Participant Group	Interview/Focus Group Questions	
	pre	post
Students	At end of placement, what do you hope to have learned? How have your courses prepared you for this placement?	Tell us about your experience learning on this placement. (Learning from staff, residents, instructors, highlights, challenges) How has your placement experience shaped your perceptions of older adults/work with older adults?
		post
Staff/Residents/Instructors	Tell us about your experience with this placement. (highlights, challenges)	

knowing my skill set" [P-S-P5]. Students felt uncertain about what they would be doing and on their preparedness for the placement. One student explained, "*I didn't know how I was going to handle peri care...I didn't know how I was going to react to that*" [P-S-P6].

As learners in the environment, students worried they might get in the way, upset routines, or become a bother to staff or residents. Students explained that they did not want to be 'useless' and there was worry about how staff might perceive them: "*We really haven't had a placement with a nurse yet so...you just don't want to be like the annoying student that just annoys the nurses and makes their job difficult*" [P-S-P4].

Students also worried about their abilities in care provision and interacting with residents. One student explained, "*some people really hate their hair being brushed in a certain way and you are not going to figure it until you do it...that was where I was like a little nervous*" [N-S-P2]. Concerns related to care of residents were often associated with limited previous experience with older adults and with dementia. Where students had past experiences with LTC, there was apprehension on whether the care environment would be positive or not, and the emotional and practical implications that might have: "*My great aunt was in a residence so I guess it was more the environment, if it was going to be a happy environment*" [P-S-P6].

It was clear that students wanted to gain skills in care delivery and learn person-centred care from their placements. One group explained that they would like to learn everything "*hands-on*" [N-S-P1] and "*everything that a healthcare aide does basically, [and] a little bit of what an LPN does*" [N-S-P5]. Another student felt that learning in this environment was about getting comfortable with the tasks learnt at the university: "*[It's] a comfort level...just doing certain tasks like the morning care...feeling ... comfortable in doing it by myself*" [N-S-P3]. Learning hands-on skills extended for some to include aspects of person-centred care: "*I don't necessarily mean hands on skills in terms of like starting IVs and... catheters, but ...I have learned about communicating with older adults with dementia*" [N-S-P3]. Many students discussed how they hoped to learn aspects of person-centred care on placement through communication with residents and their families, enriching quality of life, and delivery of care beyond a task focus. Students wanted to learn person-centred care alongside "*how you maintain like the medical side of things...how patient care is delivered...while also keeping it personal and individual and how those two kind of marry*" [P-S-P5].

On placement: Seeking mentorship and learning progression

Students worked with HCAs for morning care on these placements, which allowed them to build their skills in the delivery of personal care of residents. By the end of placement, students explained that working with HCAs allowed them to learn to recognize differences in quality of care that were key to their understandings of person-centred care:

If you have a really good [HCA] you work with, you can see how it really sets [residents] up for a really good day and makes things a lot better so you can really see how that care impacts the residents [P-S-P2].

Role hierarchies and lack of role clarity caused awkwardness and general anxiety, and meant that both students and HCAs were often unsure on the best ways to work together. As one resident put it, "*already the students are more educated than the [HCAs] and the [HCAs] have more experience so I'm sure it was awkward*" [P-R-P1]. HCAs were unsure of the tasks and skills students could do and were reluctant to provide students with learning opportunities. This was frustrating for students: "*It's not like we lack motivation...someone needs to tell us what we are supposed to do...if there is zero instruction there, it can be a little bit uncomfortable because you feel like you are in their way*" [N-S-P3]. One of the instructors explained that this largely had to do with teaching being outside HCA scope:

[HCAs are] not equipped to take students...and you can't fault them either because within their scope it's... task-orientated nursing. So for them to take on a BN student...it can be challenging because they're not sure what level our students are at, what they can do and can't do [N-I-P1].

Even when provided with a list of student skills, HCAs were still reluctant to undertake mentoring. Students felt they were chasing HCAs and felt abandoned when HCAs were busy in their routines and did not have time or skillset to consistently integrate the student into potential learning opportunities. As one student explained, HCAs and students danced around each other: "*We were asking: what would you like us to do? And they are like, what can you do? What have you been doing? They don't have time to like hear that at 7 in the morning*" [N-S-P1].

It was crucial that students developed confidence in their abilities and learned to take initiative in their learning. Confidence and initiative took time to develop, but both groups of students became more confident over the period of the placement and began to have greater autonomy and independence in their own learning and in the delivery of care: "*We just over the time got more comfortable working on our own*" [N-S-P1]. Over time students became more at ease actively seeking out opportunities: *"It will take a few weeks for you to figure out what you want to do and what you haven't learned yet... to ask those specific questions too"* [P-S-P1]. In some cases, students needed to be more direct about gaining opportunities they felt they needed: *"I spent a lot of time...observing at first...it was until the end that I realized like if I want to make something happen...I just have to force my way in there"* [P-S-P2]. Actively instructing students to take initiative helped students with this learning progression: *"[The instructor] prompted us... next day, 'I want you to take control' and we were like 'okay,' so we did"* [N-S-P4]. Where staff-student pairings were consistent, greater time on placement also helped staff become more familiar with student skillsets, which facilitated student learning: *"[We] got to know the staff as well, and they became comfortable working with us and understanding what our abilities were, so I found that helped also"* [N-S-P5]. Not setting up expectations that site staff would seamlessly provide mentorship seemed to also help bolster students to build their own capacity to seek out learning opportunities: *"I feel like it was kind of our job to make the learning opportunities that we wanted"* [N-S-P1]. It was up to the instructors and the students to maintain the educational focus and ensure learning took place. As one student explained, it was necessary for students *"to advocate for yourself [and] find things when you can"* [P-S-P4].

An important aspect to students being able to take initiative on placement was conceptualizing learning as self-directed. Students worked with their instructors to access the learning opportunities they felt they needed for their RN professional development. As one instructor explained, *"because everybody's learning needs are different...their skillsets were theirs to try and identify...I tried to help them find those opportunities"* [P-I-P2]. There was an element of chance with this, where students needed to be ready and willing to grab any learning experiences that came their way: *"In the morning, if something came up we were like 'yes'! I would absolutely jump in there and do it, if they allowed us to. That was the best way in our unit to get those opportunities."* [N-S-P5].

Instructors also encouraged students to create the learning opportunities they required, which sometimes meant resituating repetitive task-based activities for aspects relevant for their education. For example, while serving breakfast to residents many students spent time conversing and getting to know residents, which strengthened their understanding of person-centred care. Instructors took care to build student capacity and agency over the placement period so the process was progressive. For example, students were encouraged to begin working in pairs and not *"break*

off from your pairs until after mid-term and start taking more initiative and more responsibility to your workload" [N-I-P1].

Students felt that RN and LPN job shadowing opportunities would have been a natural learning progression while on placement:

> *I think it would be beneficial to have like a progression. Like start working with the [HCAs], learn what they do, learn their role and then maybe move on to the LPNs and shadow them and see what they do and move up to the RNs and see what they do in this facility* [N-S-P4].

Job shadowing was discussed as a way for students to learn about the more managerial aspects to nursing within residential aged care:

> *I think I could have really benefited from some more like LPN and RN time...we've been learning...how like RNs are like case managers and all these different roles that they could have taken, so I would've benefited from seeing how an LPN organizes their day and leads the team* [P-S-P8].

Though discussed as key opportunities for students, job shadowing of LPNs or RNs occurred very rarely at either placement site. As one student explained jokingly, *"we don't get to hang out with the RNs much. They are like the cool kids"* [N-S-P5].

Limited RNs employed within these settings was an obvious barrier to job shadowing; however, a predominant view of nursing as 'hands-on' seemed to also contribute to this missed opportunity. One RN staff member explained, for example, *"sit[ting] in the office all day and push[ing] paper and call[ing] families on the phone... would not have given that student anything I don't think"* [P-St-P1]. Despite acknowledgements that nursing within RAC has become more managerial, a preference to see, do and learn nursing as 'hands-on' was a predominant theme. These views seemed to block opportunities for understanding the role of the RN in LTC and learning progression beyond basic care.

On placement: Engagement with residents and building relationships

Interactions with residents allowed for positive outcomes in student learning. Students at both sites worked with residents on a one-to-one basis to complete a care plan assignment. Relationship building between students and residents also occurred through more generalized time together during placement, from students assisting with personal care of residents to spending time together in everyday activities such as mealtimes.

Spending time together enabled students and residents to build positive relationships. Residents discussed how they really enjoyed spending time with the students, students felt their time with residents was a consistent highlight of their placements, and site staff were grateful for the extra quality time students could provide to residents. While residents understood that these relationships may not last beyond placement, that the students were *"here for a purpose"* with a *"full schedule"* [P-R-P1], this did not detract from the positive bonds built while the students were there. It was clear that the residents missed the students after the placement ended and were very much looking forward to the next placement and having students on site again.

Lack of experience with older adults prior to placement had contributed to students' early apprehensions: *"My concerns were just like lack of practice, skills and just lack of exposure to older adults"* [P-S-P2]. Reflecting after placement, students confirmed that their perceptions of older adults had changed: *"I didn't think that I would enjoy working with older adults as much and I really did enjoy working with them"* [P-S-P2]. An increased understanding of older adults came from having the chance to spend extended time with a resident and sharing life stories and lessons: *"The person I worked with she...lived her life and it didn't matter what happened; she looked forward, she didn't dwell on what was happening to her...her outlook was amazing and you learn a lot from them I think"* [P-S-P1]. Students gained appreciation both for the residents they paired with and for older adults more generally: *"I would say the one word: underestimate. Do not underestimate them"* [P-S-P6].

Greater understanding of older adults was often linked to recognizing the commonality of human experience students shared with older adults. As one student explained, *"they are just as fragile as us"* [N-S-P7]. Student learning also extended to recognizing unique attributes of older adults:

Of course you treat older adults like you would treat anybody else...but then also seeing like why that can be challenging. Like all these people are dependent on other people and of course they don't like to be...there are just challenges that I never realized [N-S-P1].

Engagement with residents also allowed students to refine and practice their understandings of person-centred care. Students emphasized how greater familiarity with residents through *"trying to get to know the patient...personally and not just...from their charts or records or whatever you see in their reports"* [N-S-P6] allowed the care provider to gain a sense of

personality and behavioural norms for each individual resident. This familiarity was seen by the students as a basis to be able to deliver care that is person-centred: *"Understanding who the client is, and then you can see fluctuations in that and you can do...your care based on that... baseline"* [P-S-P7]. Person-centred care was described by the students both as integration of life histories into care tasks, as well as an extra aspect to care routines: *"just having the time to take that extra two minutes...to sit with them and listen...just that extra...communication piece"* [N-S-P6]. Prioritizing unique engagement with each resident also meant learning to dismiss broad stereotypes: *"Not making assumptions like you are old you can't do this...just ask them like how would you like to do this or what works best for you...because they know their body best and they know what works"* [P-S-P3]. Students recognized that person-centred care can be more of a challenge for staff due to time and budget constraints, but felt it was crucial for sites to deliver care that is person-centred: *"Nurses are busy and it is hard to take the extra time...just taking the time to actually wait and listen...that patient space is really important...to find out the whole story"* [N-S-P4].

Engagement with residents with or without dementia was differentiated, but both opportunities were appreciated. Because learning was self-directed, students worked with their instructors to build in rotations to different units that they felt worked best for their learning. However, placement in supportive living did provide students with less experience with dementia than they would have liked:

It sounds like most of the other [students] were like in [a] long term care home so a higher level of care...that is something that still kind of makes me a little uneasy is I don't feel like I'm that comfortable in dealing with people let's say with really, really high levels of dementia [P-S-P2].

For those who did have those opportunities, working with residents in a memory care unit allowed students to learn specific strategies for working with people with dementia. One student explained that getting to know and observe one resident over time allowed her to recognize changes in eating patterns even when communication was difficult:

One of the really good eaters if they are not eating breakfast...Okay, well that's not how this person normally is. So, even though he can't communicate with me if he is not feeling well, just because I know him as an individual then I am able to assist him better [N-S-P4].

Students were able to build different types of relationships than those staff have with residents. As one student explained, *"there is a different feel for nursing students; like our presence here compared to the people who work here. They kind of treat us differently, well, I would say nicer"* [N-S-P1]. These different types of relationships allowed students to gain insights on residents beyond what staff know:

> *For the care plan [assignment] I got to know like her background and where she was coming from...she loves to be alone on her room but with me I got to know like the reason behind that, which I don't think the [HCAs] had time to know cause they were always busy, or the LPNs...she wouldn't really trust...the workers there but, me like I am the outlier, I am the student so she was more open to me...I got to know the reason why she acts the way she acts. That's something they were missing* [N-S-P6].

This different element to student-resident interactions was attributed to the fact that these exchanges were framed as educational and not carrying the same "real-life" weight as staff-resident interactions: *"[Residents] were open to helping you and answering your questions, doing assessments and like kind of letting you role play with them...because our assessments don't really go into their chart so there's no threat there"* [P-S-P3].

Reflections on placement: Finding a role in RAC

A lack of insight into the RN role, student preference for hands-on nursing, and systemic shifts in the role of the RN away from direct care delivery all contributed to dissuading students from envisioning themselves working in these settings in the future. When asked if they would work in aged care, most students responded that without spending enough time with practice RNs, they were still unsure on the RN role and scope of practice: *"I really want to work on long-term care; I thought it would be great but then having worked or done this placement I don't really know how the RN fits in"* [P-S-P7]. Despite spending very little time with RNs, students recognized the more administrative nature to the RN role and expressed a preference for nursing that was more hands-on with greater resident contact:

> *I don't think I've seen enough of the RN to be like ok this is what I want to do...I'm definitely more hands on so I don't want to like sit in the office and do like documenting and like stuff like that so for that reason I would probably...not do long term care* [P-S-P6].

Students recognized that systemic pressures were shifting the RN role away from hands-on nursing, which also contributed to the predominant choice of not wanting to work in RAC: *"[RNs at the bedside] would be something I would be interested in doing...because [older adults] are definitely like an interesting dynamic and like a great population but it is unfortunate the system doesn't support it"* [P-S-P8].

Despite not envisioning themselves working in RAC, students recognized that knowledge specific to the care of older adults is very much needed beyond this setting and envisioned themselves working with older adults in other settings. As one student summarized, *"no matter which setting you are working in, in health care you will be dealing with older adults and you can learn so much from that experience with them"* [P-S-P1].

Where students learned greater appreciation for older adults and person-centred care within these placements, some felt this would not have been as easily learned in acute settings. It was seen as beneficial to learn these skills here in a *"safe environment where you can constantly be interacting with people, where it is not changing everyday like in an acute setting"* [P-S-P1]. These aptitudes were seen by students as transferable to other settings and applicable to their future provision of care to older adults:

> *Learning how to build the relationships with older adults...I hopefully will end up working in a hospital setting...so you know where they are coming from and then when they leave the hospital where they are going back to...how can I best set them up for success as they go back to the long-term care setting* [P-S-P4].

In the face of systemic pressures impacting aged care settings, students took steps towards placing themselves in advocacy roles for residents. With current restraints on staff time and quality of care, students felt residents needed greater advocacy: *"They just need someone...who could advocate for them...because everyone else is so busy running around just trying to help them with ...daily activities"* [P-S-P3]. In taking initiative, students tried to help provide quality resident care:

> *The lady who had an edema in her leg, and the [HCA] was putting on her pressure socks...she was quite rushing [sic]... 'why don't you just go to the next client while I just take my time with this one?' Because...I [can take] my time to put on her pressure socks. Less pain* [N-S-P6].

Discussion

This study aimed to explore how undergraduate nursing students understand learning on placement in RAC. It was found that students began their placements with various apprehensions and expectations before taking more initiative and seeking out learning and mentorship opportunities. Learning on placement was affected by challenges in students' relationships with HCAs and little exposure to professional nursing roles, impacted by a prevailing view of nursing as hands-on. Students spent extra time with residents and began to step into advocacy roles by placement end. Pairings with residents contributed to students gaining greater appreciation for older adults and learning person-centred care.

Theme 1: Moving on from initial apprehensions by taking initiative

Students began their placements experiencing a mixture of different apprehensions. Anxiety when first undergoing placement is recognized across the literature as students encounter "the culture and ethos of nursing with its complexities and challenges...often for the first time [which]...can be both terrific and terrifying" [15, p. 31]. In this study, along with general anxieties about the newness of the setting and concerns over their own readiness and skillsets, students explained that they worried about how to most usefully interact with staff and residents, while simultaneously learning and gaining tangible skills. Brown et al. [8] developed a temporal model of student placement with a progressive shift of student foci—from self, course, professional care, to patient as person—depending on the support provided by their mentorship and learning environment. The first stage of this model aligns with our findings on student apprehensions, as Brown et al. [8] indicated that students' experience anxiety and insecurity as outsiders within their first placement environment, looking to fit in while also accomplishing their learning outcomes.

As outsiders, students' work with HCAs was consistently awkward and challenging. This was attributed to role hierarchies, uncertainties around student skill-sets, mentoring as beyond HCA scope, and concerns over the best ways to work together. In a comprehensive study investigating capacity of RAC settings to support student placement, students reported encountering similar challenges, including few learning opportunities and being asked to observe rather than engage in care provision [19]. Such challenges are brought into immediate focus with the study by Robinson et al. [19] that detailed how staff working in RAC consistently *live on the edge* in their roles, which provides little-to-no excess capacity for contributing to student learning on placement. Though research on HCA-student interactions in aged care placement is scarce, a study by Annear et al. [20] developed an educational resource – a Carer Assessment and Reporting Guide – to better prepare HCAs and undergraduate nursing students to learn and relate interprofessionally. Our findings confirm the need for further

research in this area to better understand the challenges and to develop further strategies for improving the relationships between HCAs and students within RAC placements.

Students reported an element of *chance* to their learning opportunities, a recognized element of the clinical experience: "education by random opportunity" ([21], p. 170). To move beyond chance, it was up to students to progressively take initiative in their relationships and in the setting to ensure they accessed the learning opportunities they wanted and required. Taking initiative is recognized as a key element contributing to a positive RAC placement experience for students [22] as it complements development of self-reliance [8] and is an important component to active involvement and learner responsibility on clinical placement [23]. In our study, support and encouragement for self-directed learning from instructors was important in allowing students to move beyond their initial anxieties to actively seek out and accomplish their learning goals.

Theme 2: Learning progression through job shadowing

Along with fewer numbers of RNs working in RAC—a decline recognized even a decade ago [19]—a predominant view of nursing as hands-on care seemed to limit the opportunity for students to have exposure to RN/LPN roles. With limited insight into RN and LPN roles, students felt unsure about their future role, and failed to see value in professional practice in this setting. Abbey et al. [14] similarly found that limited exposure to RNs left students with little to no understanding of the complex responsibilities involved with the role and the professional supports available. Students in our study consistently described a lack of RN/LPN exposure as a missed learning opportunity.

Despite having little exposure to RNs, students were aware that the RN role in this setting has shifted away from hands-on care towards a more administrative focus. The literature provides some evidence for why students may hold preferences for hands-on nursing. Ironside et al. ([24], p. 188) explained that students undertaking clinical education tend to be very focused on task completion to the point where "doing more tasks" is equated with "promot[ing] learning and ensur[ing] success in [their] clinical course", despite this potentially being at odds with comprehensive practice learning. Further, Abbey et al. [14] found that students conceptualize 'real nursing' as technical skills – a message reinforced through popular culture – and surmised that a 'normalization movement' in RAC, or purposely enhancing the domesticity of these settings, can mask the clinical content and reinforce student perceptions that these settings are de-medicalized requiring less technical skills. Further, undergraduate nursing students can feel ill-prepared and intimidated by the managerial role of RNs working in nursing homes [25]. These three elements of student focus within clinical education—an overemphasis on task completion, an underappreciation of technical content within aged care and a lack of preparation for administration—helps to provide greater context to a preference for hands-on nursing evident within our study.

Comparisons of hands-on nursing versus 'sitting in the office' within the data highlight how hands-on care is also seen as contact with residents and tied closely to nursing professional identity. With little exposure to RNs working in the setting and with an understanding that RNs work in more managerial positions, students explained that they wanted to work in future positions that involved contact with residents – and felt that the RN role in RAC would not provide them with that. Aged care nurses themselves feel less satisfaction with their roles, due to greater responsibilities and lack of role clarity, and this has been linked to a limited capacity of some RAC sites to support clinical placement [19]. Care must be taken to ensure students have positive experiences in aged care nursing, this ultimately informs their career decisions [19, 26]. With the real challenges facing aged care nursing as a profession, support for student learning requires exposure to professional role models who can highlight and communicate positive aspects of aged care nursing [1, 14].

Greater exposure to positive professional nursing roles could help promote the reality of nursing as a profession involving a broader spectrum of knowledge and services, including administration and case coordination. Abbey et al. ([14], p. 17–18) explain that "exposure to, the decision making, care planning and assessment procedures undertaken by registered nurses in aged care. . . may help to illustrate that the role is more demanding and better supported than the students are easily able to see." Overtly designing placements that go beyond basic competencies could also positively influence student perceptions of working in RAC [14] and could help dispel perceptions that aged care nursing requires lesser skill-sets and know-how than nursing in acute care settings [4].

Theme 3: Gaining appreciation for older adults and moving into advocacy roles

During placement, students engaged one-to-one, spent extra time generally with residents and formed relationships with older adults living in the aged care setting. These opportunities helped students develop their understandings of person-centred care and gain greater appreciation for older adults. Aud et al. [4] indicated that students gain greater respect for older adults and learn to dispel stereotypes through spending time, and having

the chance to interact and build relationships. Students also gained appreciation for older adults through recognizing their shared experiences, as well as the unique aspects of the lives of older adults. Importantly, students come to understand older patients as 'people' when they are able to relate the experiences of older people to their own lives [8]. Further, Elliot et al. [27] identified that residents and family members felt student placement in RAC resulted in a wide array of benefits, including increased social interaction. Indeed, social interaction with students was reported by residents in our study as rewarding and enjoyable.

Spending time with residents facilitated unique insights for students, who used these to step into resident advocacy roles. At both sites, students worked to integrate their unique insights into care delivery through using the extra time they had with residents to build personal relationships, and deliver person-centred care and individually targeted interventions for residents. Feeding back these insights at the organisational level was more problematic. As outsiders, students have little power to enact change in resident care or access formalised processes within the organisation. Elliot et al. [27] discussed student placement in RAC as a unique way to increase capacity in an over-strained sector. That study reported that students on placement improved quality of care and oversight, and offered unique supports to the sector, shifting the focus from managing workforce issues to learning – though the ethical implications to accommodating the student role in care delivery are underscored.

Where students in our study described being able to build different types of relationships with residents than staff, the potential of student presence on placement supporting person-centred care and resident advocacy is highlighted. Intergenerational service learning initiatives align learning objectives with community-identified priorities [28] and have become a "global phenomenon" over the past decade in clinical nursing education, particularly for placement in community settings ([29], p. 378). With their ability to directly incorporate student advocacy for patients into learning (e.g. [30–32]), integrating intergenerational service learning approaches into aged care placement may better support and utilize the extra role of students on placement. Supporting a more active role for students and formalizing ways for student perspectives to be fed back could help to ensure their unique contributions are better integrated into ongoing site operations and not lost when placements end.

Limitations & suggestions for future research

This study focused on two undergraduate student groups from the same university within the supportive living settings of one RAC organization, therefore the generalizability of the findings is limited. However, the study provides insights on student learning trajectories, integration of staff mentorship to support student learning and the benefits of student-resident engagement opportunities within placements in RAC. There is a need for further investigation into the potential benefits of communicating self-directed learning pathways to students, methods for better integrating professional nursing roles into student learning in RAC and formalizing feedback of unique contributions gained through student-resident engagement opportunities.

Conclusion

This study found that taking initiative was important for undergraduate nursing students to move from initial apprehensions to create their own learning opportunities and begin to step into resident advocacy roles while on placement in RAC. Similar student trajectories on placement within RAC are reported in the literature, and methods to enrich mentorship and learning environment are highlighted [8, 20, 22, 26]. Conceptualizing their learning as self-directed was key to students undertaking learning progression within our study. It would be ideal to communicate self-directed learning pathways to students undergoing their first placements in RAC, not to offer prescriptive templates to follow, but to better prepare novice students, set expectations, and optimize learning on placement.

Placements in RAC can better support positive learning progression pathways through including RN and LPN job shadowing experiences for students. However, where there are consistently low numbers of senior staff in RAC to contribute to student learning, there must also be real work accomplished on affirming and communicating the value of care aide competencies to students training to be RNs and easing the working of this key relationship within placement. Shaping learning progression pathways within aged care placements as positive with clear guidelines on how sites can contribute to student mentorship could provide greater opportunity for students to gain a more fulsome understanding of the nursing profession within RAC. This may help set the groundwork for students to better picture themselves working in these settings in the future.

Including student-resident engagement opportunities on placement was found to help students build their understanding of older adults and learn aspects of person-centred care. Where students had extra time to spend with residents and as these interactions were framed educationally, students described building more personal relationships with residents than staff and gaining unique insights into the lives of residents. Better formalizing and supporting this extra time and attention students spend with residents while on placement could facilitate the unique contributions of students into care delivery.

Appendix

Abbreviations
HCA: Healthcare aide; LPN: Licensed practical nurse; LTC: Long-term care; RN: Registered nurse

Acknowledgements
The authors acknowledge and thank the collaborators and participants of the study including the staff and students from the university and the residents and staff from the residential care facilities involved. The authors are also grateful to Jill Norris for reviewing and editing the manuscript.

Funding
This work was supported by a Scholarship of Teaching and Learning (SoTL) grant from the Taylor Institute for Teaching and Learning, University of Calgary [2016–2018]. The funding body approved the study design, including methods for data collection and analysis/interpretation of data. The funding body had no role in the writing of the manuscript.

Authors' contributions
HM- helped develop the study design, undertook data collection and analysis and drafted the manuscript. CS – participated in study design, recruitment of students and instructors, and coordinated faculty involvement through the clinical placement. LV – conceived, designed and coordinated the study and helped draft the manuscript. All authors have read and approved the manuscript.

Competing interests
The authors declare that they have no competing interests.

References
1. Cozort R. Student nurses' attitudes regarding older adults: strategies for fostering improvement through academia. Teach Learn Nurs. 2008;3:21–5.
2. Melillo KD, Abdallah L, Dodge L, Dowling JS, Prendergast N, Rathbone A, Remington R, Shellman J, Thornton C. Developing a dedicated education unit in long-term care: a pilot project. Geriatr Nurs. 2014;35(4):264–71.
3. Burbank PM, Dowling-Castronovo A, Crowther MR, Capezuti EA. Improving knowledge and attitudes toward older adults through innovative educational strategies. J Prof Nurs. 2006;22(2):91–7.
4. Aud MA, Bostick JE, Marek KD, McDaniel RW. Introducing baccalaureate student nurses to gerontological nursing. J Prof Nurs. 2006;22(2):73–8.
5. Gould ON, MacLennan A, Dupuis-Blanchard S. Career preferences of nursing students. Can J Aging. 2012;31(4):471–82.
6. Higgins I, Van Der Riet P, Slater L, Peek C. The negative attitudes of nurses towards older patients in the acute hospital setting: a qualitative descriptive study. Contemp Nurse. 2007;26(2):225–37.

7. Brown J, Nolan M, Davies S, Nolan K, Keady J. Transforming students' views of gerontological nursing: Realising the potential of 'enriched' environments of learning and care: a multi-method longitudinal study. Int J Nurs Stud. 2008;45:1214–32.

8. Brown J, Nolan M, Davies S. Bringing caring and competence into focus in gerontological nursing: a longitudinal, multi-method study. Int J Nurs Stud. 2008;45:654–67.

9. O'Lynn C. Comparison between the Portland model dedicated education unit in acute care and long-term care settings in meeting medical-surgical nursing course outcomes: a pilot study. Geriatr Nurs. 2013;24:187–93.

10. Canadian Nurses Association. Tested solutions for eliminating Canada's registered nurse shortage. 2009. https://cna-aiic.ca/~/media/cna/page-content/pdf-en/rn_highlights_e.pdf. Accessed 23 March 2017.

11. Canadian Nurses Association. Policy Brief #2: Meeting future healthcare needs through innovations in nursing education. 2013. https://www.cna-aiic.ca/~/media/cna/files/en/hhr_policy_brief2_e.pdf?la=en. Accessed 1 April 2016.

12. Barnett T, Cross M, Jacob E, Shahwan-Akl L, Welch A, Caldwell A, Berry R. Building capacity for the clinical placement of nursing students. Collegian. 2008;15(2):55–61.

13. Cartwright JC. Opportunities for practice and educational transformations through unlikely partnerships. J Nurs Educ. 2010;49(5):243–4.

14. Abbey J, Abbey B, Bridges P, Elder R, Lemcke P, Liddle J, Thornton R. Clinical placements in residential aged care facilities: the impact on nursing students' perception of aged care and the effect on career plans. Aus J Adv Nurs. 2006;23(4):14–9.

15. Brand G, McMurray A. Reflection on photographs: exploring first-year nursing students' perceptions of older adults. J Gerontol Nurs. 2009; 35(11):30–7.

16. McIntyre A. Participatory action research. Thousand Oaks: Sage; 2008.

17. McAteer M. Action research in education. Thousand Oaks: Sage; 2013.

18. Streubert HJ. Action research method. In: Streubert HJ, Carpenter DR, editors. Qualitative research in nursing: advancing the humanistic imperative, vol. 2011. New York: Lippincott Williams & Wilkins; 2011. p. 300–18.

19. Robinson AL, Andrews-Hall S, Fassett M. Living on the edge: issues that undermine the capacity of residential aged care providers to support student nurses on clinical placement. Aust Health Rev. 2007; 31(3):368–78.

20. Annear M, Lea E, Robinson A. Are care workers appropriate mentors for nursing students? An action research study in residential aged care. BMC Nurs. 2014;13:44.

21. Leflore JL, Anderson M, Michael JL, Engle WD, Anderson J. Comparison of self-directed learning versus instructor-modeled learning during a simulated clinical experience. Simul Healthc. 2007;2(3):170–7.

22. Lea E, Marlow A, Bramble M, Andrews S, Crisp E, Eccleston C, Mason R, Robinson A. Learning opportunities in a residential aged care facility: the role of supported placements for first-year nursing students. J Nurs Educ. 2014;53(7):410–414.

23. McIntosh A, Gidman J, Smith D. Mentors' perceptions and experiences of supporting student nurses in practice. Int J Nurs Pract. 2013;20:360–5.

24. Ironside PM, McNelis AM, Ebright P. Clinical education in nursing: rethinking learning in practice settings. Nurs Outlook. 2014;62:185–91.

25. King BJ, Roberts TJ, Bowers BJ. Nursing student attitudes toward and preferences for working with older adults. Gerontol Geriatr Educ. 2013; 34(3):272–91.

26. Lea E, Marlow A, Bramble M, Andrews S, Eccleston C, McInerney F, Robinson A. Improving student nurses' aged care understandings through a supported placement. Int Nurs Rev. 2015;62:28–35.

27. Elliot KJ, Annear MJ, Bell EJ, Palmer AJ, Robinson AL. Residents with mild cognitive decline and family members report health students 'enhance capacity of care' and bring 'a new breath of life' in two aged care facilities in Tasmania. Health Expect. 2014;18:1927–40.

28. Karasik RJ, Berke DL. Classroom and community: experiential education in family studies and gerontology. J Teach Marriage Fam. 2001;1(14): 13–38.

29. Knecht JG, Fischer B. Undergraduate nursing students' experience of service-learning: a phenomenological study. J Nurs Educ. 2015;54(7): 378–84.

30. Bell ML, Buelow JR. Teaching students to work with vulnerable populations through a patient advocacy course. Nurse Educ. 2014;39(5):236–40.

31. Hamel PC. Interdisciplinary perspectives, service learning, and advocacy: a nontraditional approach to geriatric rehabilitation. Top Geriatr Rehabil. 2001;17(1):53–70.

32. Hermoso J, Rosen AL, Overly L, Tompkins CJ. Increasing aging and advocacy competency. J Gerontol Soc Work. 2008;48(1–2):179–92.

Design and evaluation of the StartingTogether App for home visits in preventive child health care

Olivier Anne Blanson Henkemans[1]* , Marjolein Keij[2], Marc Grootjen[3], Mascha Kamphuis[4] and Anna Dijkshoorn[1]

Abstract

Background: The StartingTogether program (in Dutch SamenStarten) is a family-centred method for early identification of social-emotional and behavioural problems in young children. Nurses in preventive child health care find it challenging to: determine family issues and need for care; provide education; refer to social services; increase parent empowerment. To mitigate these challenges, we developed and evaluated the StartingTogether App, offering nurses and parents conversational support, tailored education and information on social services.

Methods: A mixed method design, consisting of a qualitative evaluation of the StartingTogether App, with group discussions with nurses ($N = 14$) and a pilot test ($N = 5$), and a randomized controlled trial, evaluating the effectiveness of the app. Nurses ($N = 33$) made home visits to parents ($N = 194$), in teams with or without the app. Nurses were surveyed on the challenges experienced during visits. Parents ($N = 166$) were surveyed on their satisfaction with health care and app. Nurses were interviewed on the benefits and barriers to use the app.

Results: Parents with the StartingTogether App were more satisfied with the visits than parents without ($p = .002$). Parents with a high educational level were more satisfied with the visits than the parents with a low educational level. With the app, their satisfaction level was similar ($p < .001$). Nurses using the app felt more equipped to communicate with parents ($p = .012$) and experienced that parents were more knowledgeable and skilled ($p = .001$). Parents felt that with the app the nurse was more polite ($p = .02$), listened more carefully ($p = .03$), and had more time ($p = .02$). Nurses with the app gave parents more opportunity to ask questions ($p = .001$) and gave clearer answers ($p < .001$). The qualitative evaluation indicated that some nurses needed extra time to develop the habit of using the app.

Conclusions: The StartingTogether App contributes to parents' satisfaction with home visits. An interaction effect between parents' educational level and rating of home visits indicated that the app has an additional value for parents with a lower educational level. Applying mobile applications, such as the StartingTogether App, potentially has a positive effect on communication between nurses and parents about the family situation in relation to parent empowerment and the child's development.

Trial registration: The study is registered with ISRCTN under the number ISRCTN12491485, on August 23, 2018. Retrospectively registered.

Keywords: mHealth intervention, Family-centred care approach, Self-management, Parent empowerment, Randomized controlled trial

* Correspondence: Olivier.Blansonhenkemans@TNO.nl
[1]TNO, Child Health, Schipholweg 77-89, 2316 ZL, Leiden, The Netherlands
Full list of author information is available at the end of the article

Background

Dutch preventive child health care

In the Netherlands, approximately 8% of the children experience behavioural and social-emotional difficulties, such as displaying disruptive behaviour, being socially withdrawn, or lacking concentration [1]. These difficulties can be caused by both personal and environmental factors. Children with learning or developmental difficulties, such as speech and language problems, are more at risk to develop behavioural and social-emotional difficulties. In addition, adverse early childhood experiences, such as parental conflict, separation or neglect, can have a negative impact on development and increase the risk of behavioural and social-emotional difficulties [2]. Early identification of and intervention on social-emotional and behavioural difficulties can prevent problems, by optimizing the environment of the child and promoting his or her development [3].

The Dutch preventive child health care (PCH) takes an holistic approach, focusing on both personal and environmental factors. PCH professionals, including doctors and nurses, monitor children's development during routine assessments at well-child clinics and offer additional interventions at the child and family level [1]. The StartingTogether (ST) program (in Dutch SamenStarten) is a family-centred intervention method for PCH, which aims to contribute to the early identification of social-emotional and behavioural problems in children, aged 0–4 years. The program focuses on building a relationship of trust between the professional and the parent(s), mapping the situation in which the child is growing up, and empowering parents, by expanding their knowledge and improving their skills and self-efficacy [4]. The program is based on the evidence-based Sure Start program in the UK, which offers outreach care (i.e., delivering services in local settings and family environment) to enhance the life chances of young children and their families [5, 6]. Similar to the Sure Start program, ST offers parenting support through home visits and, if necessary, referral to social services in the community. Home visits have been proven to be an effective approach for providing parental support, stimulating children's development and improving their health [7]. In the Netherlands, this family-centred care approach has proven to contribute to better attuning PCH to the parents' preferences [8].

The ST program has many components which are described herein. At the well-child clinic, PCH professionals assess the social-emotional and behavioural development of the child and the family situation. The PCH professional uses an interview protocol, called DMO-p (Dienst Maatschappelijke Ontwikkeling [Social Development Services]) [9]. This protocol is based on a bio-ecological model, which emphasizes the importance of understanding bidirectional influences between individuals' development and their surrounding environmental contexts [10]. The protocol distinguishes five domains: competence of the parent; role of the partner; social support; perceived barriers and life events within the context of the parent (including finance, housing and use of substances); well-being of the child. When parents express a specific need or experience concerns in regard to one or more of the five domains of the DMO-p, the professional provides the parents with educational materials. If more specific support is needed, the professional offers them a home visit by the PHC nurse (in approximately 10% of the cases) [11]. During the home visit, the nurse can personally obtain a clear view of the family situation and has more time for in-depth interviewing with the parent and to build a relationship of trust. The nurse and parents collaboratively re-assess the social-emotional and behavioural development of the child and family situation. Nurses offer parenting support, health advice, and specific support(e.g., post-natal depression). If necessary, the nurse can refer the parents to services in the community, such as a training course on positive parenting.

At the clinic, the nurse adopts a more directive approach, while during the home visits, he or she assumes a more collaborative and/or coaching role. The PCH nurses are trained to apply principles of parent empowerment, as described by Olin and colleagues [12], during these home visits. They strive to recognize, promote and enhance parents' abilities to meet their own needs, solve their own problems, and activate the necessary resources in their community in order to feel in control of their own lives [13]. They take a positive approach, activate parents as change agents in meeting their children's physical and mental health needs, provide structure (e.g., goal, clarity, timeliness), and discuss important relational aspects (i.e., reliability, openness, equality, collaboration and attending to needs and possibilities).

Home visit play a key role in the ST program for outreaching and parent empowering child health care. However, previous evaluations of the program in the Netherlands showed that nurses experience a number of challenges during these visits [9], namely:

1. Identifying the family situation and parents' associated care needs can be arduous. Parents have difficulties verbalizing their needs. Also they are overwhelmed by a multiplicity of family issues and lack knowledge of how to resolve these issues;
2. Nurses lack materials, such as a guide for conversational techniques, to provide information and communication tailored to the family situation and care need;

3. Nurses do not always have the interventions at their disposal to apply during the home visit;

4. Parents are not always referred to relevant social services. An overview of the available services in the community is missing.

These challenges obstruct the identification of personal and environmental factors, influencing the children's social-emotional and behavioural development. Also, they hinder the empowerment of parents and their ability to cope with their family situation independently.

Apps for preventive child health care

Mobile eHealth applications, also called mHealth apps, are increasingly used to supplement health care interventions. Benefits of apps are that they are mobile and can be easily applied during home visits. For instance, professionals can use mobile devices to interact with their clients to access and share online information, or for assessment purposes. Recent meta-analyses have shown that mobile technologies in behavioural interventions lead to better treatment outcomes than interventions without any form of mobile technology [14]. Also, they can contribute to the effectiveness of health care delivery services [15] and enhance the efficacy of health care interventions, for example by increasing adherence to guidelines, enhancing health surveillance, reducing medication errors or decreasing rates of redundant of inappropriate care [16].

Table 1 lists various mHealth apps (Smartphone or Tablet PC) that are developed to support PCH. These apps offer support for monitoring children's development, parent education and empowerment or support for PCH professionals, such as social workers. However, none of these apps cover all steps of a home visit, nor do they offer communication support for the conversation between the nurse and parents. Moreover, none of the apps has been evaluated on its

effectiveness in regard to identifying the family situation, determining care needs and increasing parent empowerment.

To mitigate the challenges experienced during the ST home visits, the StartingTogether App (ST App) was developed. It runs on a Tablet PC, which the nurse uses during the home visits, in collaboration with the parent. It covers: 1) textual and visual conversational support for nurses and parents, 2) education and information on social services in the community, tailored to the care need and the living location, 3) email reports of the home visit for both the parents and the nurse and 4) tools for the nurse to prepare the home visit. See section Intervention for further details.

The aim of this study is twofold: 1) to describe the development process of the ST App and 2) to evaluate its effectiveness in a) facilitating a partnership between professionals and parents b) enhancing the identification of the family's needs c) empowering parents to address these factors themselves and effectively cope with their family situation.

Methods
Evaluation framework
To fulfil our research aim, we used an exploratory sequential mixed method design, in which the qualitative study is combined with the quantitative [17]. The value of this design exists in the fact that results are enhanced to a greater level than the quantitative or qualitative component on their own, and that the approach allows for development and evaluation of the app at the same time (see Fig. 1). The first part of the study consisted of a qualitative, formative evaluation of the ST App, with the aim of improving its design and implementation. The second part of the study consisted of a Randomized Controlled Trial (RCT) to evaluate the effectiveness of the ST App when applied during home visits. Finally, we have integrated the results of the two parts, to come to

Table 1 mHealth apps for preventive child health care

Function	App (country)	Goal
Monitoring child development	*My child's eHealth* record (Australia)	Child's health record with information about the child's development
	Baby Connect, Baby Food Pee Poo, and Total Baby (US)	Graphical reports and charts, weekly averages, medicine, vaccine and growth tracking, and allergies. Also, timers, notifications, reminder alarms, and appointments for doctor visits
Parent education and empowerment	*WhatToExpect* (US)	Day-by-day pregnancy guide, with personalized content, parenting news and health information. Can be connected to a community of expecting moms
	Breastfeeding Management application (US)	Information about breastfeeding, such as guidelines for the use of medications during breastfeeding
Support for child health care professionals, such as social workers	*Child Development 0–6 Years* app (Ireland)	Information on child developmental norms relevant to the 0–6 year's age group

Activity	Qualitative Evaluation	Quantitative Evaluation
Needs assessment	Reviewing research StartingTogether	
	Meeting two groups of nurses (N=14)	
Pilot test	Meeting group of team leaders (N=5)	
	Evaluating prototype with nurses for one month (N=5)	
	Interviewing nurses (N=5)	
Trial and process evaluation		Evaluating StartingTogether App for 1 year
	Periodic meeting representatives intervention group (N=4)	Surveying nurses (N=33)
		Surveying parents (N=166)
		Dossier auditing
	Surveying nurses (N=4)	
Assessment future use	Surveying nurses (N=4)	

Fig. 1 Flow chart of quantitative and qualitative evaluation

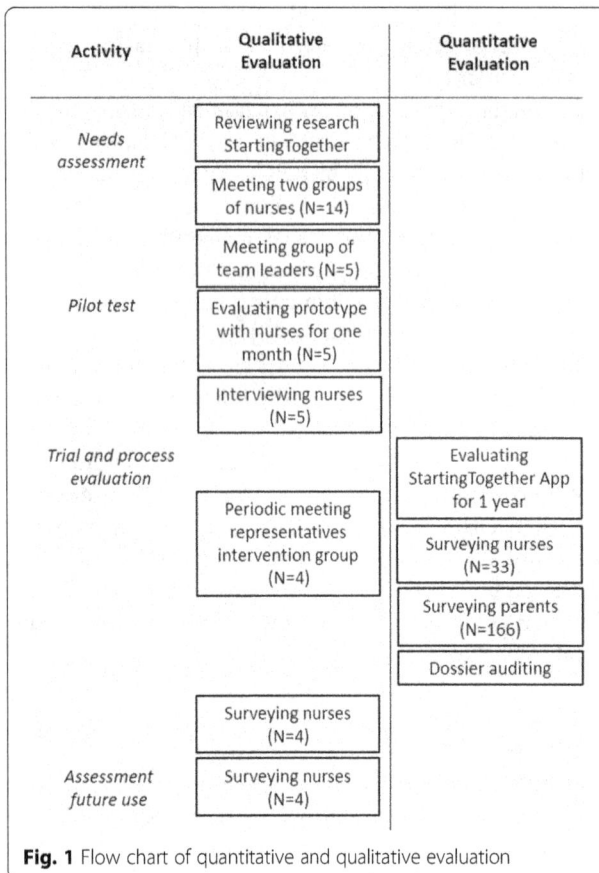

strengths and weaknesses of the app in regard to future use, and strategies for implementation.

Qualitative study design

The main research questions for the qualitative study, that guided the evaluation were: What needs do nurses and parents have, with regard to the home visits? How can the ST App be applied during home visits, so as to contribute to patient-centred quality of care? What issues are important for further implementation? To answer these questions, we conducted: a needs assessment; a pilot test; a process evaluation during the iterative development of the app; and an assessment for future use.

The study design was based on a user centred design (UCD) approach for mobile applications, situated cognitive engineering, and intervention mapping. UCD for mobile applications is a process in which the needs, wants, and limitations of end users of mobile apps are given extensive attention at each stage of the design process [18]. Situated cognitive engineering is an iterative development process with active involvement of users [19]. This process stems from UCD, but has an additional scientific research component. It aims to establish and test theories from the domain for which the

application is developed. Finally, intervention mapping is a development process of health promotion programmes. It aids mapping the path from recognition of a health need or problem to the identification of a solution [20].

Recruitment of participants

The participants were nurses and team leaders working at the PCH Service in Amsterdam. A total of 13 PCH team leaders and approximately 35 nurses were invited to participate in focus groups for the needs assessment, of which five team leaders and fourteen nurses volunteered.

Qualitative data collection

For the needs assessment, two focus groups with the 14 nurses and one focus group with the five team leaders of the PCH service were held in Amsterdam. During these group meetings, they shared their experiences with home visits and expressed how they felt a mobile application could provide them the necessary support. The following topics, as derived from previous research on StartingTogether [9], were used to stimulate the discussion: preparation for the home visits; identifying family needs; strengthening parents skills and motivation; referral to services; offering additional care; other points in regard to StartingTogether. Also during the focus groups, a first mock-up of the app was shown to the nurses for inspiration. It consisted of rough sketches of its interface for navigation and possible functionalities (i.e., media functionality and referral functionality). They were invited to reflect on this first mock-up, provide additional suggestions and to give suggestions for improvement.

Based on the challenges elicited from previous research [9] and the needs assessment, a first version of the ST App was build. It was pre-tested with nurses (n = 5) from the intervention group, divided across different teams. They used the app for one month in a pilot field-test and we evaluated their experience through short interviews. The outcomes of the interviews were used to refine the app. We added more "affordance" to improve the usability of the app, such as buttons for navigations in addition to tabs at the bottom of the screen, redesigned the emoticons as to make them more recognizable, added a direct search option for educational materials (without selecting topics of discussion) and used simpler wording to make the app easier to understand for a layperson. Finally, we resolved some final technical bugs. A process evaluation took place parallel to the RCT (see part Quantitative study design), to ensure that the ST App matched with the PCH work process and needs. Focus groups with representatives of the different intervention group teams (N = 4) were held to investigate the professionals views about the app. They were asked about their experiences with the app and suggestions for possible improvements for the future. After the RCT, we administered a survey among the nurses in the intervention group. We asked them about strengths and weaknesses of the app in regard to future use.

Quantitative study design

The second part of the study consisted of a Randomized Controlled Trial (RCT) to evaluate the effectiveness of the ST App when applied during home visits. The main research questions for the quantitative study to measure the effectiveness were: how satisfied are nurses' and parents' with the home visit; how do they rate the usability of the app; and what is the proportion of valid referrals made after the home visit? Secondary outcome measures included demographics of the nurses, children and parents, to explore potential interaction effects (see Table 2).

Recruitment of participants

The participants were PHC nurses in Amsterdam. They made home visits to parents with children aged 0–4 years in which family issues and/or needs for support were identified with the DMO-p. A total of 17 PCH teams (120 nurses) were invited to participate in the study, of which 9 teams volunteered ($N = 34$ nurses). Reasons not to participate included lack of time or capacity to participate in the study. There were no exclusion criteria. All PCH teams in Amsterdam were invited to participate in the study and all parents and nurses who had agreed to participate were included in the study. One nurse dropped out early in the study and her data were excluded from the analysis.

Intervention

Figure 2 shows the first function of the ST App: textual and visual conversational support for nurses and parents. The parents first select one or more pictograms (e.g., sleeping child or a couple with a heart) that illustrate the topic(s) they want to discuss with the nurse, eliciting a conversation about their family situation (e.g., the babies' sleeping rhythm, or the relationship with their partner). Then, they value these issues with the use of emoticons (i.e., sad/happy, angry/calm, insecure/secure, and shameful/proud). Parents can rate their current emotional state on a scale from 1 through 10 (e.g., 4, somewhat sad), define their goal state (e.g., 5 or 6, somewhat happy) and determine their personal needs. These ratings are meant to promote self-reflection, prioritization of their needs and self-activation. Also, they can determine what they can do themselves, with the help of their social environment, to achieve this goal state.

The concept of selecting and discussing pictograms is derived from *context mapping*. This technique consists of people selecting and discussing artefacts (in this case pictograms) and to make their tacit experiences and feelings explicit [21]. This approach can aid parents and nurses to understand the bidirectional influences between their contexts and their child's development. Also, it can aid them to talk about sensitive topics, which is known to be a barrier for nurse-parent interaction [22]. The valuing of the pictograms stems from both context mapping and solution focused (brief) therapy (SFBT). In SFBT, through precisely constructed questions about the family situation, parents can focus on identifying their goals and generating a detailed description of what life will be like when the goal is accomplished [23]. Thus, the focus lies on constructing situations in which the problem is resolved rather than solving problems.

As illustrated in Fig. 3, the app provides educational materials (i.e. websites, flyers and videos), and lists social services in the community, tailored to the family's situation, need and living location. Examples are an educational video on shaken baby syndrome, pamphlets on upbringing and websites with self-management programs for parents with psychological problems. The educational materials and social services in the community were provided and reviewed by the nurses and team leaders, and added to the app by

Table 2 Overview of primary and secondary outcome measurements per group

Outcome measures	Nurses	Parents
Primary outcome measures		Time of measurement
Evaluation of home visit: challenges experienced during the Starting Together	At the end of the visit	–
Evaluation of home visit: patient-centred health service, quality of care, overall satisfaction	–	At the end of the visit
Usability of StartingTogether App	–	At the end of the visit (intervention group)
Secondary outcome measures		Time of measurement
Demographics nurse	Onset of study	–
Demographics child	At the end of the visit	–
Demographic parents	–	At the end of the visit

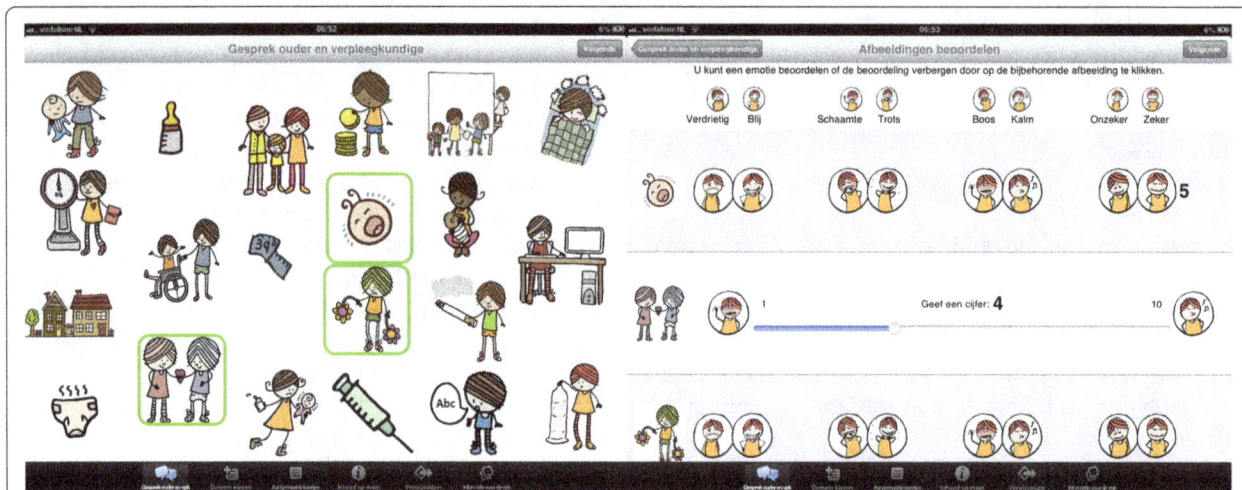

Fig. 2 ST app: Conversational support

the researcher, before and during the study. The DMO-p domains are used to guide the selection of relevant materials, tailored to the social-emotional and behavioural development of the child. The nurse selects one or more domains, based on the parents' selection of topics and evaluation of their family situation. Earlier research has shown that tailoring can enhance the users' participation and engagement in the intervention and, in turn, patient empowerment (i.e., knowledge and skills for self-management) [24]. After choosing one or more domains, the app provides relevant education and social services in the community. The parents and nurse can browse through these services and compare them; who is the target group, what is the service, how much does it cost and is it in the neighbourhood? The locations of the services in the community are displayed on a map, showing the current (home) location and the locations of the selected service. This is meant to facilitate shared decision-making about which care will be provided, which can contribute to parent empowerment, as well as to the parents' satisfaction in regard to the home visit [25].

The app keeps a record of the home visit, which is sent by email to the parent at the end of the visit. The report covers the family's situation and evaluation, the selected educational materials and information about social services (with contact details), notes and follow-up appointments. With the parent's consent, the nurse can send the email to him- or herself, for future reference. For privacy purposes, once the email is sent, the record is removed from the app. Finally, the app offers tools for the nurse, such as official websites for PCH-professionals on youth and upbringing. Here, they can access the relevant care standards for preparation of the home visit.

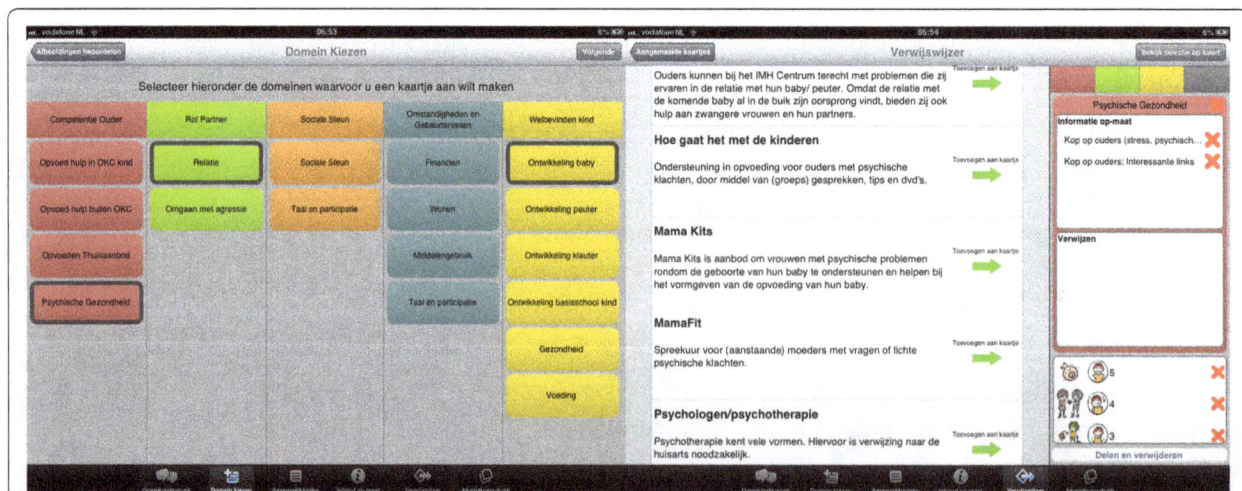

Fig. 3 ST app: Tailored education (websites, flyers, videos) and information on social services

Quantitative data collection

The RCT was conducted over a period of one year (October 2012 through September 2013). As illustrated in Fig. 4, teams of nurses were assigned to the intervention group (STA), which made home visits with the ST App, or the control group, which made home visits as usual (CAU). We applied a stratified randomization method: four teams were allocated to the intervention group ($N = 16$) and five teams were allocated to the control group ($N = 17$). All participating nurses received a two-hour training to complete the survey and administer it to the parents. The STA nurses received a four-hour training to use the ST App, covering a theoretical and practical module.

The nurses in the STA condition made 98 home visits and the nurses in the CAU made 96 home visits. After each home visit, nurses completed a survey about the home visit and invited parents to also complete a survey, after informed consent. The survey for the parents was in four languages: Dutch, English, Arabic and Turkish. The STA group completed the survey on the Tablet PC (a special survey app was developed) and the CAU group completed the survey on paper.

The survey for parents contained questions about their demographics (country of birth, language spoken at home, educational level, age of child). Subsequently, it asked to evaluate the home visit with the use of the validated ($\alpha = .75$) Consumer Quality Index for PHC (CQ-Index JGZ), based on the American Consumer Assessment of Healthcare Providers and System [26]. The CQ-Index JGZ assesses patients' views, which are essential to provide a patient-centred health service and to evaluate the quality of care [27]. Table 3 lists the items proposed to the parents to rate on a 5 point scale (1, not agree at all, through 5, fully agree). Finally, parents were asked to rate their overall satisfaction with the home visit on a scale from 1 (lowest) to 10 (highest). Parents in the intervention group were also asked to rate the app's usability on a scale from 1 (lowest) through 5 (highest).

The survey for the nurses contained questions about their experience with Tablet PCs and apps, at work and at home, the characteristics of the child (gender and aged), and which functions of the app they used. In addition, it asked to evaluate the home visit, in relation to the challenges experienced during the ST home visits. Table 4 lists the items proposed to the nurses to rate on a 5 point scale (1, not agree at all, through 5, fully agree).

As part of their care as usual, nurses in both groups made reports of home visits in the electronic child dossier of the PCH Service in Amsterdam. A dossier audit was conducted to determine the number of valid referrals for each group during the RCT.

Data analysis

For the qualitative study, the data was analysed using a content analysis approach. The conversations during the focus groups and interviews were recorded, and moderators made notes during the meetings. The principles of interpretive description were used to guide the data collection and analysis of the needs assessment, pilot field-test, and the interviews about the process and implementation.

For the quantitative study a power calculation was run. The use of the ST App was used as the dependent variable and the quality of home visits as rated by the parents as the primary independent variable. We applied a formula for statistical superiority design to calculate the a sample size, assuming that our new treatment ST App is more effective than a standard treatment (CAU) from a statistical point of view (Lesaffre, 2008). The main hypothesis was that the use of the app would lead to a higher rating for quality of care perceived by the parent. Other hypotheses were the use of the app would lead to better establishing parents' care need, offering tailored advice and referral, and parent empowerment. Power calculation showed that a sample sizes of 15 nurses in group one and 15 nurses group two (assuming

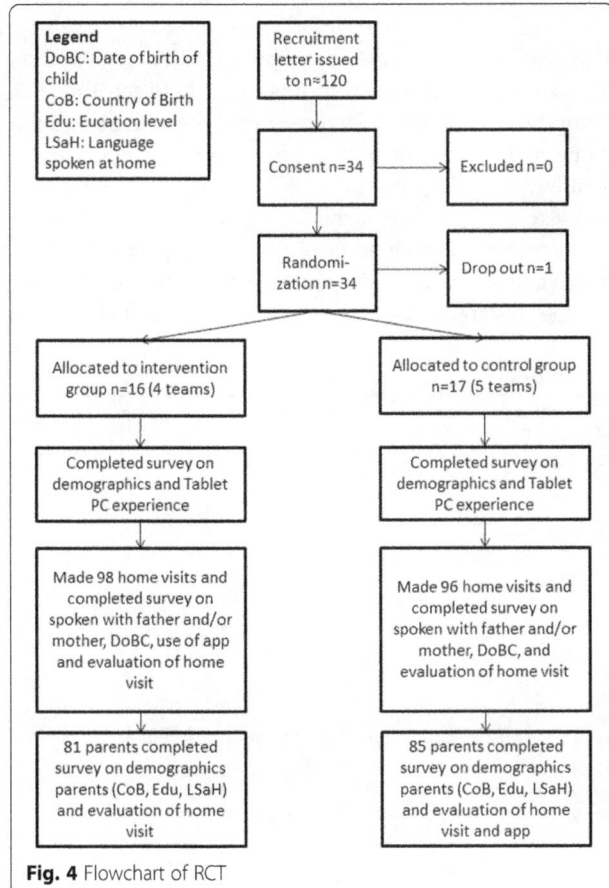

Fig. 4 Flowchart of RCT

Table 3 Parents' evaluation of the home visits, with and without the StartingTogether App, controlled for controlled for the characteristics of the family (covariates) (N = 166)

Covariate	Dependent Variable	df	Mean Square	F	Sig.
Condition (with or without app)	The nurse understood what the parents wanted to talk about	1	1.12	2.23	.14
	The nurse was polite to the parent	1	2.35	5.05	.03
	The nurse listened carefully to the parents	1	2.44	5.45	.02
	The nurse had enough time	1	3.54	5.23	.03
	The parents could ask questions	1	3.66	13.03	.001
	The nurse provided clear answers	1	4.00	9.38	.003
	The advices were usable for the parent	1	.01	.01	.92
	The parents were well referred (if relevant)	1	.08	1.00	.76
	The rating of the parent of the home visit	1	15.02	10.60	.002
Education level parent (high/low)	The nurse understood what the parents wanted to talk about	1	6.32	12.60	.001
	The nurse was polite to the parent	1	4.65	10.00	.002
	The nurse listened carefully to the parents	1	4.57	10.20	.002
	The nurse had enough time	1	3.94	5.82	.02
	The parents could ask questions	1	3.65	12.99	.001
	The nurse provided clear answers	1	.74	1.74	.19
	The advices were usable for the parent	1	.10	.13	.72
	The parents were well referred (if relevant)	1	9.73	11.40	.001
	The rating of the parent of the home visit	1	.82	.58	.45

20% drop-out), each including 10 home visits with parents, would achieve 71% power to detect a difference between the group proportions of 0.100. The group one proportion was assumed to be 0.250 under the null hypothesis and 0.350 under the alternative hypothesis. The test statistic used is the two-sided Z test (pooled). The significance level of the test was 0.05.

Data of the quantitative evaluation were checked for normal distribution using graphical summary of data,

assessment of skewness, descriptive statistics, and tests of normality. A comparison was made between the STA group and CAU group in regard to the evaluation of the home visit by nurse with a non-parametric Two Independent Samples test (Mann Whitney). A comparison was also made between the STA group and CAU group in regard to the evaluation of the PCH by parent with a multivariate analysis. We analysed the effect of the app on the different dependent variables reported by the

Table 4 Nurses' evaluation of the home visits, with and without the StartingTogether App (N = 33)

Item	With StartingTogether App		Without StartingTogether App		P-value
	Mean	SD	Mean	SD	
The care need was clear for the nurse	28	.71	38	.64	.32
The care need was clear for the parent	41	.72	30	.79	.31
The parents and nurse had a shared view of the care need	06	.61	05	.77	.91
The nurse was capable of communicating with the parent(s)	30	.46	01	.79	.002
The nurse was capable of informing the parent(s)	25	.52	15	.79	.32
The parents knew how to cope with their family issues at the end of the home visit	28	.82	3.81	.81	.000
The parents felt competent to cope with their family issues at the end of the home visit	3.97	.98	3.53	.84	.001
The parents were motivated to cope with their family issues at the end of the home visit	24	.69	17	.85	.56
The parents had the intention to follow the referral advice at the end of the home visit (if relevant)	30	.70	39	.70	.56

parents, controlled for characteristics of the family: child's age, child's gender, parent(s) spoken to during the visit, country of birth parent, language spoken at home, and education level parent. Finally, the number of valid and invalid referrals was compared with an Chi square-test.

From the dossier audit reports, we measured the number of referrals per group and validity of the referral. The auditor, a staff nurse at this Service, retrieved reports from the period November 2012 through August 2013. She reviewed if the parent was referred to social services in the community or not. Then, she reviewed if the (non)referral was valid. Validity of referrals was determined through level of adherence to PCH evidence-based protocol [28] The auditor looked at the topic (e.g., sleep), type of issue (e.g., child has difficulty sleeping), the level of complication (e.g., past week or multiple months), and the prescribed intervention or referral (e.g., sleep training or referral to psychologist). Referral was valid or invalid based on how accurate the nurse followed the protocol. For reliability of the audit, at the beginning of the review, a second auditor reviewed 10% of these reports, and the two auditors discussed the reviews which differed to come to a consensus. The goal of the discussion was to increase the main auditor's rating accuracy. By discussing if and when a dossiers was valid or not, based on the PCH protocols and expertise of two auditors, the main auditor could sharpen her rating skills. The inter-rater reliability was 0.79 (Cronbach's alpha).

Ethics, consent and permissions

At the onset of the RCT, parents, nurses and their team coordinators received a letter with information about the study (goal, results, data processing and rights) and an invitation to participate. The nurses, parents and team coordinators, who were willing to participate in the study, gave their informed written consent. The study protocol was approved by the ethics committee of TNO (Nederlandse Organisatie voor Toegepast Natuurwetenschappelijk Onderzoek [Netherlands Organisation for Applied Scientific Research]) registered under the number 05101117.

The digital surveys were directly emailed from the Tablet PC to the TNO main researcher. The paper surveys were put in sealed envelopes by both parents and nurses. Thus, the surveys completed by the parents were collected without the nurses reviewing them. These envelopes were stored in a dedicated locker at the well-child clinic and periodically retrieved by the TNO researcher (time between retrievals was a maximum of 3 weeks). After collecting the data from the surveys, the envelopes were stored in a TNO archive, only accessible by the researchers of TNO involved in the project. The data were saved in a digital safe on the TNO server, only accessible for the involved researchers of TNO. Data and envelopes were stored for a 10 year period, after which they will be destroyed. The audit complied with the privacy law and administration of patient data. Audit data could only be retrieved anonymized and could therefore not be matched with the survey data.

Results
Qualitative findings
Participants

Five team leaders and 14 nurses participated in the needs assessment. The nurses came from different regions in Amsterdam, namely the Centre ($N = 3$), West ($N = 2$), North ($N = 3$), Amstelland ($N = 1$), East ($N = 3$) and New-West ($N = 2$). The residents of these regions vary in ethnicity, Socio-economic status (SES) and family issues.

Outcomes needs assessment

As listed in Table 5, four important topics were addressed in the needs assessments by the nurses, which were: preparation for the home visits; referral to services; identifying family needs; strengthening parents skills and motivation. For these topics, three needs were stated, each with their own rationale. First, nurses indicated that it would be helpful to have a map of social services in

Table 5 Outcomes of the needs assessment

Topic	Needs elicited	Rationale
Preparation for the home visits Referral to services	A map with social services in the community within reach of the family, listing information for the parents, such as registration procedures, waiting lists, costs and location	An overview of available services in the neighbourhood is lacking. Also, these services change frequently. This can make nurses feel unprepared for the home visit, especially if they have to consult the office to discuss the next steps and potential referral to other social services
Identifying family needs	Instruments, in addition to the standard DMO-p, to identify sensitive issues causing the family needs	Time is needed to build a relationship of trust and make the parents feel comfortable to discuss sensitive topics. In some cases, families have multiple problems at the same time, and the nurse has to help ordering and prioritizing these problems to know where to start.
Strengthening parents skills and motivation	The communication should be adaptive and fit the family's profile, in order to achieve shared decision making	There is variation in families' request and need for support, due to differences in intrinsic/extrinsic motivation, level of empowerment and autonomy

the community and that each service listed would present information for the parents, such as registration procedures, waiting lists, costs and location. Second, they asked for additional instruments supporting the conversation with parents to assist in identifying and articulating root causes of sensitive family issues. Third, these instruments should be adaptive, to match the family's profile (e.g., intrinsic/extrinsic motivation, level of empowerment and autonomy), in order to achieve shared decision making.

When asked about suggestions for the ST App, nurses indicated they wanted it to contain documents they generally use. Team coordinators suggested a systematic approach in the app, as it is a requirement for evidenced-based work. That is to say, an approach based on scientific methods and applied similarly by the different nurses. Furthermore, the nurses requested that the functions of and interaction with the app matched their standard work methods in preparation for and during home visits.

The responses to the mock-up varied. First, they were shown a draft of a "media functionality" of the app, which contained information and educational media (fact sheets, video, websites) to aid communication with the parents about their care question(s). Nurses were positive about this component and felt that the app contained media they generally use, and that the form and functions of the app matched their standard work methods. A suggestion for improvement, was tailoring the media more to the parents than to the nurses, so they can walk through the information in the app together, without difficult language or jargon. Another suggestion was to offer the materials to the parents online, so they can look things up themselves after the home visit.

The "referral functionality" in the app contains a map of social services in the community. Nurses positively evaluated this functionality and found it helpful to find relevant information about available services. As suggestions for improvement, they indicated it could be useful to have an email function, so that when parents are being referred, they could send an email to the concerned institution together with the nurse. Also, they suggested a function that allows parents to evaluate the social service. Team coordinators recognized a systematic approach in the app, but provided a number of suggestions for improvement in regard to the interaction (for example, legend for the emoticons).

Outcomes pilot field-test, process evaluation and assessment future use

The outcomes of the needs assessment and suggestions for improvement of the draft version were used to build a first version of the ST App. Subsequently, the app was piloted for one month in a field-test with nurses ($n = 5$)

from the intervention group. We evaluated their experience through short interviews at the end of the pilot. In general, the nurses and coordinators expressed that the app fulfilled their needs and followed their suggestions formulated in the group meetings. Suggestions for improvements, which were mainly at the level of the interface (e.g., navigation through use of buttons at tabs, reposition of items in the screen), were applied in the ST App evaluated in the RCT.

During the process evaluation, nurses mentioned several benefits of the ST App. They felt that the app provided parents insight into their family situation and care needs; they felt more able to relate to the parents (during the home visit, they could literally sit next to the parents with the Tablet PC on their lap or on the table); that the textual and visual conversational support helped parents to express their needs; and they could collaboratively set up a personal plan to address the family situation. The nurses also suggested a number of challenges for the ST App for future use. To implement the app on a broader scale, nurses have to be willing to use the app for the first time. They might need to experience the benefits of the app themselves and need time to adopt the app, in order to develop the habit of using the Tablet PC and the app during home visits. Also, it is important that the management expresses its support for the app throughout the organisation. Finally, nurses missed a tool to easily maintain the educational materials and information on the app themselves (during the study, this was done by the experiment leader). The results of process evaluation are used to further improve the app and develop a training of the app.

Quantitative findings
Participants
PHC nurses from nine teams working in Amsterdam participated in the RCT. In the STA group, nurses from four different teams ($N = 16$) visited 98 families of which 85 parents agreed to complete a survey. In the CAU group, nurses from five teams ($N = 17$) visited 96 families, of which 81 parents agreed to complete a survey. One nurse allocated to the control group dropped-out and her data were excluded. The participating nurses were all women. The average age of the nurses in the intervention group was 43.8 years (SD = 13.1) and in the control group 37.1 years (SD = 10.2) ($p = .11$). All nurses had a Bachelor degree in nursing. More than half of the nurses in the intervention and the control group (respectively 62.5% and 52.9%) had no previous experience with a Tablet PC.

As listed in Table 6, the nurses visited parents with different countries of birth (such as, the Netherlands, Morocco and Turkey) and educational levels (raging from none to Master degree). Parents spoke different

Table 6 Demographics of parents ($N = 166$)

Item	With StartingTogehter App	Without StartingTogehter App	Total
Country of birth			
Netherlands	45	41	86
Morocco	9	16	25
Turkey	7	4	11
Other	25	19	44
Total	86	80	166
Language spoken at home			
Dutch	45	49	94
Turkish	11	6	17
Arabic	8	8	16
Other	22	17	39
Total	86	80	166
Education level			
None	2	2	4
Low (Primary)	8	6	14
Average (General Secondary Education)	21	26	47
High (BA, MA)	55	46	101
Total	86	80	166

languages at home (such as, Dutch, Turkish and Arabic). The average age of the visited children in the control and the intervention group was, respectively, 4 and 6 months. The country of birth, language spoken at home, educational level and age of the child did not differ significantly between the groups.

Parents and nurses discussed the following topics derived from the five domains of the DMO-p. In approximately half of the home visits, the parents and nurses spoke about parenting (59.3%) and the well-being of the child (48.5%). In approximately one in six home visits they spoke about the psychological well-being of the parent (18.0%) and nutrition of the child (including breastfeeding) (15.5%). Other topics discussed less frequently were the relationship between parents, aggression at home, language, finance, housing, use of substances, and disability of the child.

Ratings for the home visits

Table 3 lists how the parents rated the home visit with and without the ST App, along the CQ-Index JGZ items, controlled for the characteristics of the family (covariates): age child, gender child, parent(s) spoken to during the visit, country of birth parent, language spoken at home, education level parent. In addition to the use of the app, education level of the parent affect the evaluation of the home visit, see section below 'Interaction effects: Educational level and satisfaction ratings'. The other covariates did not significantly affect parents' evaluation of the home visits.

Some items received a significantly higher rating with the app than without the app. The CAU group (without app) gave the visits an overall rating of 8.04 (SD = 1.03), on ascale from 1 (lowest) through 10 (highest). The STA group gave an average rating of 8.82 (SD = 1.21) ($F(1)$ = 10.60, $p = .002$). In regard to the nurse being polite, STA parents gave an average rating of 4.58 (SD = .75) and CAU parents an average rating of 4.46 (SD = .60) ($F(1) = 5.45$, $p = .02$). In regard to listening carefully by the nurse, STA parents gave an average rating of 4.68 (SD = .71) and CAU parents an average rating of 4.43 (SD = .61) ($F(1) = 5.05$, $p = .03$). In regard to the nurse having enough time, STA parents gave an average rating of 4.61 (SD = .67) and CAU parents an average rating of 4.41 (SD = .76) ($F(1) = 5.45$, $p = .02$). In regard to the opportunity to asking questions, STA parents gave an average rating of 4.64 (SD = .51) and CAU parents an average rating of 4.28 (SD = .66) ($F(1) = 13.03$, $p = .001$). In regard to the clarity of the answers provided by the nurse, STA parents gave an average rating of 4.56 (SD = .59) and CAU parents an average rating of 4.20 (SD = .66) ($F(1) = 9.38$, $p = .003$). The multivariate analyses also showed that education level explained variance in how parents rated how the nurse's understanding of what the parents wanted to talk about ($F(1) = 12.60$, $p = .001$) and the quality of their referral (if relevant) ($F(1) = 11.40$, $p = .001$), whereas the use of the app did not ($F(1) = 2.23$, $p = .14$; ($F(1) = 1.00$, $p = .76$).

Table 4 lists how the nurses evaluated the home visit with and without the ST App, regarding the challenges experienced during home visits. Also according to the nurses, some items received a significantly different rating with and without the app. In regard to communicating with the parent, STA nurses gave on average a significantly higher rating (M = 4.30, SD = .46) then CAU nurses(M = 4.01,SD = .79) (Z = 2.66, p = .008). In regard to the parent's knowledge how to address the family situation, STA nurses gave on average a significantly higher rating (M = 4.28, SD = .82) than CAU nurses (M = 3.81, SD = .81) (Z = 3.97, p < .001). In regard to the parent's skills to address the family situation, STA nurses gave on average a significantly higher rating (3.97, SD = .98) than CAU nurses (M = 3.53, SD = .84) (Z = 3.35, p = .001).

During the audit, 93 reports from the intervention group and 95 reports from the control group were reviewed. In the intervention group, 33% of parents were referred, while in the control group, 50% of the parents were referred, which is a significantly higher percentage ($X^2(3)$ = 55.26, p < .001). The auditor rated 96% of the (non)referrals in the intervention group as valid and 95% in the control group.

Interaction effects: Educational level and rating of home visits

As listed in Table 7, a linear regression, with age child, gender child, parent(s) spoken to during the visit, country of birth parent, language spoken at home and education level parent as predictors showed that variance in parents' rating of the home visits was explained by educational level (Beta = .16) (R^2 = 03, p < .05). When we divided parents along the median in two educational level groups (high and low), data showed that parents with a high educational level gave the home visits an average rating of 8.58 (SD = .97), while parents with a low educational level gave the home visits an average rating of 8.13 (SD = 1.41) (F(162) = 2.46, p = .015). As illustrated in Fig. 5, parents in the CAU group with a high educational level gave home visits an average rating of 8.37 (SD = .78) and parents with a low educational level gave the home visit an average rating of 7.47 (SD = .99). In the STA group, parents with a high educational level gave home visits an average rating of 8.76 (SD = 1.07)

and parents with a low educational level gave the home visit an average rating of 8.90 (SD = 1.45). The analysis showed an interaction effect (F(57) = 4.91, p < .001).

Usability ratings

On a scale from 1 (lowest) through 5 (highest), parents gave the ST App an average rating of 4.21 (SD = .81). The nurses used different functions of the ST App during the home visits: 58.2% used the textual and visual conversational support for nurses and parents; 80.6% provided education (website, flyer, video) and/or information on social services in the community; all nurses sent an email report of the home visit for the parents and the nurse; 24.5% used the tools for the nurse, such as professional websites on youth and upbringing.

Discussion

The aim of this study was to describe the development process of the ST App and to evaluate its effectiveness in improving the quality of care of PCH home visits. The first part of the study consisted of a qualitative evaluation. Nurses were positive about the app. They felt that it contained media (fact sheets, videos and websites) they generally use; the form and functions of the app matched their standard work methods; it provided parents with insight in their family situation; helped parents to express their needs; and enabled nurses to better connect to the parents and address their situation. Lastly, the referral aid turned out to be helpful in finding information about available services, and team coordinators were positive about the systematic approach in the app.

The second part of the study consisted of a quantitative evaluation of the PHC with and without the ST App. The ST App had additional value for the ST home visits regarding communication and parent empowerment. Overall, parents gave the home visits a positive rating. However, when the ST App was used, their ratings improved. Parents felt that the nurse with the app listened more carefully. Also, they felt the nurse had more time and gave them more opportunities to ask questions and provided clearer answers. Finally, parents

Table 7 Model for variance in parents' rating of the home visits, explained by parent and child characteristics

Coefficients Parents' rating of home visit						
Model	Variable	Unstandar-dized B	Coefficients	Standardized Coefficients Beta	t	Sig.
1	(Constant)	7.76	.33		23.19	.000
	Education level	.14	.07	.16	1.98	.049
Excluded Variables						
Model	Variable	Beta In	Partial Correlation	Collinearity Statistics Tolerance	t	Sig.
1	Age child	−.06	−.06	1.00	−.78	44
	Country of birth	.06	.06	.96	.78	.44
	Language spoken at home	.99	.09	.93	1.07	.29

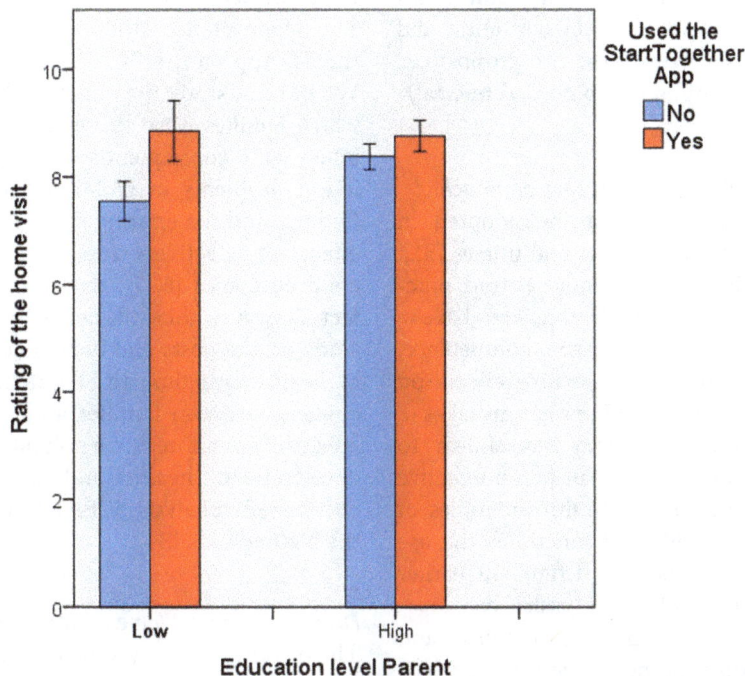

Fig. 5 Evaluation of home visit by parents with high and low educational level with and without StartingTogether App

felt that with the app nurses were more polite. This is notable as previous research found that mobile applications can disconnect us from the surrounding social environment (e.g., nurses have less attention for the parent as they are more focused on the app) [29].

The nurses in the STA group felt that the communication with the parents improved. Also, parents were more knowledgeable and skilled to address their family situation independently, as to contribute to their child's development. These findings are in line with the findings of previous research, that has shown that the use of mobile technology in health care interventions can improve communication between clients and health care professionals [30]. With the ST App, parents were less often referred; however, in both groups most referrals were rated as valid. This is in line with previous research, that has shown that the use of mobile technology in (preventive) health care interventions can decrease rates of potentially redundant or inappropriate care [6]. Finally, parents with a low educational level rated the home visits lower than the parents with a high educational level. However, when the app was applied, the ratings were similar for both groups. A possible explanation for this interaction effect is that parents with a low educational level have more difficulty expressing their needs, and therefore benefit more from the textual and visual support than parents with a high educational level. Another explanation is that parents with a high educational level find it easier to

look up information and ask for help themselves, without the help of the nurse, and benefit less from the information and educational materials provided by the app. Illustratively, we found that education level explained variance in referral. Parents with a higher education level were more likely to be referred accurately to local social services, when relevant. Future research could investigate this effect further.

Our study also showed a number of non-significant effects. First, the use of the ST App did not lead to a clearer or increased shared understanding of parents' need for care. Results show nurses more often than not succeeded in eliciting parents' care need, which is contradicting previous studies findings [9]. Apparently, for the nurses in the current study, obtaining a shared understanding of parents' need for care was less of a challenge. Second, when using the app, the nurses' advice was not more usable for the parents, nor were the nurses better capable of informing the parents. This shows that there is room for improvement when it comes to the content of the app, in regard to fact sheets, videos and websites. During the study, we strived to fill the app with relevant information, but found that this was quite laborious. This may also explain why parents did not have a stronger intention to follow the advice and often opted to cope with their family issue themselves. Third, we did not find a significant effect of the app on the referral of parents. Referral was only relevant in a small number of the parents. We presumably did not have enough power to find significant differences through the surveys. However, the dossier audit did show significant differences between the two groups (i.e., fewer parents in the intervention group needed referral).

Implications

Mitigating challenges in a family centred care approach

Family-centred care is increasingly being adopted in PHC and is positively valued by families and nurses [31]. Previous research has shown that family-centred practices and particularly participatory help giving have a positive influence on parenting confidence, competence, and enjoyment, which in turn have positive effects on parenting behaviour [5]. As the ST program takes a family-centred approach to PHC and has shown to facilitate participatory help giving, it can be an effective way to improve developmental and health outcomes of children [32]. By combining different functions, the use of the app mitigated the challenges defined in earlier research [8, 9]. Through textual and visual conversational support, parents were able to verbalize and prioritize their needs. After the home visit, the parents felt more empowered and better equipped to resolve family issues. These results indicate that mHealth apps can be an effective means to contribute to existing family-centred approaches.

Early identification of parents and their children's' needs

Parents are often faced with a multitude of daily family issues affecting the child's development, such as parenting, relationships, and language. For these parents, it is not always possible to exactly pinpoint what lies at the root of these issues, and more importantly, to focus on a situation in which the problem is resolved by themselves. Once their questions or care needs are identified, simply offering generic information and education is insufficient to help these parents to cope autonomously. Many parents currently go online in search of information, but find it difficult to decide which information is most relevant and reliable for them. Sitting together with the nurse and going through the different functionalities of the app appeared to be helpful. Together they could summarize the family's situation, set goals, and pick relevant educational materials and information to help families to achieve them.

Our expectation is that by simply providing stand-alone apps to the parent or the professional, individually, outside of the context of the home visit, this effect could not have been achieved. Through blended care, risks of crisis and issues in communication (at a distance) are avoided, and social support is facilitated [33]. Therefore, we strongly advise a similar approach for future application of (preventive) child care apps and mHealth in general.

Costs and benefits of the ST app

The scope of this study was establishing the effect of the ST App on the PCH, in the context of home visits. We did not study the effect of the app on the extent to which families were successful in resolving their family issues and consequently social-emotional and behavioural problems in children. Considering the current findings and the existing literature, showing the positive effects of effectiveness of home visiting programs on child outcomes [6, 7], the app may have a positive effect. However, this still needs to be validated through a study on the costs and benefits of the ST App, in terms of health care time (e.g., number of home visits and contacts between families and PCH), costs of the app, effectiveness in resolving family issues and children's development, health and quality of life. Such a cost-benefit analysis (CBA) is currently conducted in the Netherlands [34].

Future use and implementation of the ST app

The results of the study provide important pointers for future adoption and implementation of apps in the context of PCH. One suggestion for improvement is to support nurses to develop the habit of using the Tablet PC and the app during home visits, by experiencing the benefits of the app themselves. Training-on-the-job could be a useful strategy to achieve this [35]. Another remark that the nurses made, is that they would have liked to easily edit and maintain the content of the app themselves. For example, an online tool for nurses to add and update their preferred folders, websites, videos and information on social services, could be added. A final suggestion for improvement was to involve the management, in an early phase of implementation, to create support for the app within the organisation. Therefore, we suggest to organize meetings to introduce the app and ask managers to facilitate their nurses to go on home visits with the app. Later on, management should be informed about the results of the use of the app.

Limitations

First, it was beyond the scope of this study to investigate how the use of the app influenced the parents' action after the home visit. Surveys asked the parents and nurses to evaluate the home visits, and the parent's intention to work at their family issues and follow-up the referral. It was too burdensome for nurses to contact families to collect data on parents' activities undertaken after the visit (in addition to the training, completing and administering surveys, and group meetings). For future studies, we strongly advise to look at the app's effect on the parents' activities in a follow-up.

Second, the study data has a nested structure. In both the STA and CAU group, nurses visited multiple families, completed a survey about this visit and invited parents to do the same. It may be the case that groups of parents visited by one nurse could show more similarity than responses of individual parents between nurses. In case of such as structure, an approach such as hierarchical linear modelling is favoured. However, due to privacy reasons, data were collected anonymously and we do not know which nurse saw which parents which makes such as approach impossible.

Third, the study was conducted in the city of Amsterdam (population approximately 800.000, of which almost half is immigrant). As a result, it is uncertain if our findings are replicable in rural areas. After the current study, the ST App has been piloted in two rural areas in the Netherlands. The first reactions from the nurses in these areas indicate that the app is equally beneficial. However, an important requirement is that the education and information on community services are local.

Finally, it was not possible to connect the survey and audit data. Due to privacy reasons, the audit data could not be allocated to individual families. As a result, our findings only apply to the control and intervention groups as a whole. We can state that the group with nurses using the ST App refers less to social services than the group without the app. We do not know how these findings relate to the individual characteristics of the nurses and how they used the app.

Conclusions

The ST App contributes to the positive experience with the PCH home visits and improves communication between nurses and parents. Also, results suggest that application of the ST App in home visits improves parents' knowledge and skills to cope with their family issues, and reduces rates of potentially redundant care. Especially for home visits to parents with a low educational level, the app has an additional value. Overall, it can be concluded that applying mobile applications, such as the ST App, can contribute to the quality of care within family centred care approaches in PCH and increase parent empowerment.

Abbreviations
CAU: Control group applying Care As Usual; PCH: Preventive child health care; SFBT: Solution focused brief therapy; ST App: StartingTogether App; ST: StartingTogether; STA: Intervention group using StartingTogether App

Acknowledgements
We would like to thank the child health care nurses from the preventive health care service (GGD) in Amsterdam and the families who partook in the study. Also, we would like to thank Anita Cremers from TNO for her contribution in designing the SamenStarten App. Finally, we would like to thank Ferko Öry, who conceived the study and contributed to the acquisition of funding.

Funding
This research was funded by The Netherlands Organisation for Health Research and Development (ZonMw) program 'Vernieuwing Uitvoeringspraktijk Jeugdgezondheidszorg.'

Authors' contributions
OBH has conceived the study, contributed to acquisition of funding, participated in the study's design and coordination, collected the data, performed statistical analysis, and was in the lead to draft the manuscript. MKE participated in the study's design and coordination, collected and interpreted that data and helped to draft the manuscript. MG was in the lead of the iterative development of the ST App, including the group meetings with nurses and team coordinators and piloting. He helped draft the manuscript. MKA and AD participated in the study coordination and helped revising the manuscript critically. All authors read and approved the final manuscript to be published.

Competing interests
The authors declare that they have no competing interests.

Author details
[1]TNO, Child Health, Schipholweg 77-89, 2316 ZL, Leiden, The Netherlands.
[2]Pharos, Arthur van Schendelstraat 620, 3511, MJ, Utrecht, The Netherlands.
[3]Eaglescience B.V. , Naritaweg 12K, 1043, BZ, Amsterdam, The Netherlands.
[4]JGZ Zuid-Holland West, Croesinckplein, 24-26 2722, EA, Zoetermeer, The Netherlands.

References
1. Reijneveld SA, Brugman E, Verhulst FC, Verloove-Vanhorick SP. Identification and management of psychosocial problems among toddlers in Dutch preventive child health care. Arch Pediat Adol Med. 2004;158(8):811-7.
2. Rutherford RB Jr, Quinn MM, Mathur SR. Handbook of research in emotional and behavioral disorders. New York: The Guilford Press; 2004.
3. Beauchaine TP, Neuhaus E, Brenner S, Gatzke-Kopp L. Ten good reasons to consider biological variables in prevention and intervention research. Dev Psychopathol. 2008;20:745-74.
4. Dijkstra N, Detmar S, Schoenmakers A, Öry F. Samen Starten: ondersteuningsbehoefte van ouders bij het opvoeden van jonge kinderen [StartingTogether: needs for parental support in parents with young children]. Leiden: TNO Preventie en Gezondheid; 2004.
5. Dunst CJ, Trivette CM, Hamby DW. Meta-analysis of family-centered help giving practices research. J Ment Retard Dev Disabil Res Rev. 2007;13:370-8.
6. Melhuish E, Belsky J, Leyland AH, Barnes J. Effects of fully-established sure start local Programmes on 3-year-old children and their families living in England: a quasi-experimental observational study. Lancet. 2008;372:1641-7.
7. Peacock S, Konrad S, Watson E, Nickel D, Muhajarine N. Effectiveness of home visiting programs on child outcomes: a systematic review. BMC Public Health. 2013;13:17.
8. Hielkema M, De Winter AF, Feddema E, Stewart RE, Reijneveld SA. Impact of a family-centered approach on attunement of care and Parents' disclosure of concerns: a quasi-experimental study. J Dev Behav Pediatr. 2014;35(4):292-300.
9. Tan N, Bekkema N, Öry F. Toepasbaarheid van opvoedingsondersteuning voor Marokkaanse en Turkse gezinnen in Nederland, in het bijzonder van het programma Samen Starten/DMO-P [applicability of parental support for Moroccan and Turkish families in the Netherlands, specifically the program StartingTogether/DMO-p]. Leiden: TNO Preventie en Gezondheid. p. 2008.

10. Bronfenbrenner U, Ceci SJ. Nature-nurture reconceptualized in developmental perspective: a bioecological model. Psychol Rev. 1994;101(4):568–86.

11. Gemeente Amsterdam. Eerste bestuursrapportage 2014 Amsterdam [First policy report 2014 Amsterdam], Municipality of Amsterdam, 2014.

12. Olin SS, Hoagwood KE, Rodriguez J, Radigan M, Burton G, Cavaleri M, Jensen PS. Impact of empowerment training on the professional work of family peer advocates. Child Youth Serv Rev. 2010;32(10):1426–9.

13. Gibson CH. The process of empowerment in mothers of chronically ill children. J Adv Nurs. 1995;21:1201–10.

14. Lindhiem O, Bennett CB, Rosen D, Silk J. Mobile technology boosts the effectiveness of psychotherapy and behavioral interventions: a meta-analysis. Behav Modif. 2015;39(6):785–804.

15. Free C, Philips G, Watson L, Galli L, Felix L, Edwards P, Patel V, Haines A. The effectiveness of mobile-health technologies to improve health care service delivery processes: a systematic review and meta-analysis. PLoS Med. 2013; 10(1):1–26.

16. Chaudhry B, Wang J, Wu S, Maglione M, Mojica W, Roth E, Morton SC, Shekelle PG. Systematic review: impact of health information technology on quality, efficiency, and costs of medical care. Ann Intern Med. 2006;144:742–52.

17. Creswell JW, Plano Clark VL, Gutmann ML, Hanson WE. Advanced mixed methods research designs. In: Tashakkori A, Teddlie C, editors. Handbook of mixed methods in social and behavioral research. Thousand Oaks: Sage Publications; 2003. p. 209–40.

18. Kangas E, Kinnunen T. Applying user-centered design to mobile application development. Commun ACM. 2005;48(7):55–9.

19. Brinkman WP, Neerincx MA. Applying situated cognitive engineering to mental health computing. CHI. 2012;2012

20. Bartholomew LK, Parcel GS, Kok G, Gottlieb NH, Fernández ME. Planning health promotion programs: an intervention mapping approach. 3rd ed. San Francisco: Jossey-Bass; 2011.

21. Sleeswijk Visser F, Stappers PJ, van der Lugt R, EB-N S. Contextmapping: experiences from practice. CoDesign. 2005;1(2):119–49.

22. Regber S, Mårild S, Johansson Hanse J. Barriers to and facilitators of nurse-parent interaction intended to promote healthy weight gain and prevent childhood obesity at Swedish child health centers. BMC Nurs. 2013;12(1):27.

23. Kim JS. Examining the effectiveness of solution-focused brief therapy: a meta-analysis. Res Social Work Prac. 2008;18(2):107–16.

24. Lustria ML, Cortese J, Noar SM, Glueckauf RL. Computer-tailored health interventions delivered over the web: review and analysis of key components. Patient Educ Couns. 2009;74(2):156–73.

25. Suh WS, Lee CK. Impact of shared-decision making on patient satisfaction. J Prev Med Public Health. 2010;43(1):26–34.

26. Delnoij DM, Ten Asbroek G, Arah OA, De Koning JS, Stam P, Poll A, et al. Made in the USA: the import of American consumer assessment of health plan surveys (CAHPS) into the Dutch social insurance system. Eur J Pub Health. 2006;16:652–9.

27. Bos N, Sturms LM, Schrijvers AJ, van Stel HF. The consumer quality index (CQ-index) in an accident and emergency department: development and first evaluation. BMC Health Serv Res. 2012;12:284.

28. Vermeulen H, Berben S, Heinen M. Evidence based richtlijnen, werken volgens de laatste stand van wetenschap. T JGZ. 2017;49(4):67–8.

29. Romão T. Challenges in designing smarter mobile user experiences. FICT. 2016;7. Accessed 5 Apr 2017 http://journal.frontiersin.org/article/10.3389/fict. 2016.00007/full

30. Lindberg B, Nilsson C, Zotterman D, Söderberg S, Skär L. Using information and communication technology in home care for communication between patients, family members, and healthcare professionals: a systematic review. Int J Telemed Appl. 2013;2013:1–32.

31. Harrison TM. Family-centered pediatric nursing care: state of the science. J Pediatr Nurs. 2010;25(5):335–43.

32. Dunst CJ, Trivette CM. Meta-analytic structural equation modeling of the influences of family-centered care on parent and child psychological health. Int J Pediatr. 2009;2009:1–9.

33. Wentzel J, van der Vaart R, Bohlmeijer E, van Gemert-Pijnen JEWC. Mixing online and face-to-face therapy: how to benefit from blended care in mental health care. JMIR Ment Health. 2016;3(1):1–28.

34. ZonMw, 2017. Costs and effects of the StartingTogehter app for the preventive child health care [Kosten en effecten van de SamenStarten app voor de Jeugdgezondheidszorg]. Accessed 26 Jul 2017, URL: https://www. zonmw.nl/nl/onderzoek-resultaten/jeugd/programmas/project-detail/ versterking-uitvoeringspraktijk-jeugdgezondheidszorg/kosten-en-effecten-van-de-samenstarten-app-voor-de-jeugdgezondheidszorg

35. Fleuren MA, Paulussen TG, Van Dommelen P, Van Buuren S. Towards a measurement instrument for determinants of innovations. Int J Qual Health Care. 2014;26(5):501–10.

Surgical patients' perspectives on nurses' education on post-operative care and follow up in Northern Ghana

Bernard Atinyagrika Adugbire[1] and Lydia Aziato[2*]

Abstract

Background: The purpose of the study was to explore surgical patients' experiences of discharge planning and home care in the Northern part of Ghana.

Methods: The study was conducted at a referral hospital located at the Northern part of Ghana. A qualitative explorative descriptive design was adopted for the study. Purposive sampling technique was used to recruit participants. Data was saturated with 15 participants aged between 23 and 65 years. All the interviews were audio-taped and transcribed verbatim. Data analysis was done using the processes of content analysis.

Results: Nurses educated surgical patients on discharge to avoid smoking, alcohol drinking, chewing cola nuts and strenuous exercise to promote healing and prevent complications. Patients were educated to keep their wound dry and clean. Patients were advised to eat nutritious food, vegetables and fruits and take their medications as prescribed. They were to report drug effects and come to the hospital for follow-up visits. Patients were urged to come for daily wound dressing at the outpatient department. On the contrary, some nurses did not educate patients on signs of wound healing or infection. Some nurses were rude to the patients during wound dressing. Nurses did not visit patients at home when they were discharged from the hospital.

Conclusions: The study showed that although nurses were able to educate discharged patients on how to manage their health at home, there is the need to improve communication and attitude to enhance care.

Keywords: Discharge planning, Home care, Patients' education, Patients' experiences, Personal hygiene, Wound care

Background

Early post-operative recovery depends on educating patients on self-care, wound care and providing clear information to discharged patients [1, 2].Early post-operative recovery also depends largely on good interactions between the hospital nurses and the community health nurse to ensure smooth handing over of patients to continue treatment especially patients' wound care. Bodily care includes looking after oneself, eating well and exercising regularly through proper teaching. In a study conducted in Northern Taiwan,the results indicated that to ensure smoking cessation in post-discharged patients, effective cessation counselling including encouraging patients to modify their lifestyle

through effective education is helpful [3].Ineffective teaching following discharge may lead to the patients' lack of knowledge about how to care for self at home and become ignorant of signs and symptoms of impending infections or complications [4, 5].In clinical practice, it is observed that hospital discharge instructions are given at the moment patients are about to leave the hospital instead of being developed throughout the hospitalization period. As a result the patient leaves the hospital with incomplete information about care including instructions for self-care at home [6].

Post-operative wound care is an important part of self-care after discharge. However, it has been stated that discharged surgical patients lack the required knowledge for wound monitoring. This is attributed to poor discharge teaching, lack of self-efficacy for wound care at home and inaccessible communication with nurses about wound; resulting in wound infection [7].This corroborates

* Correspondence: aziatol@yahoo.com; laziato@ug.edu.gh
[2]Department of Adult Health, School of Nursing, College of Health Sciences, University of Ghana, P.O. Box LG 43, Legon, Accra, Ghana
Full list of author information is available at the end of the article

anecdotal evidence at the Regional Hospital, Bolgatanga, Ghana where many of the surgical patients wounds are often infected due to failure of some nurses to educate patients during discharge planning and to properly hand over discharged patients to community health nurse to continue wound dressing.Also it was reported that more than 85% of surgical patients usually rely on family members or friends for support especially with wound care, household activities, and mobility [8]. This demands inclusion of the family in post-operative wound care education. However, the current study recruited only patients as they were the population target of the researcher and were also readily available, Future researchers could consider researching on family education.

Also, the literature revealed that some nurses fail to explain the purpose and side effect of medications to some patients when they are discharged. Those patients that received information on medications such as drug actions and side effects felt that the information was not clear [9, 10]. However, some patients have adequate discharge instructions on their medications including timing and route of administration. Exercise and nutritious diet were also emphasized on discharge [8]. For instance, some discharged patients received tailored discharge instruction on medications, wound dressing and prevention of infection. In a similar study, the results indicated that 72% of patients receive discharge instruction from other health personnel instead of nurses [11].

In some of the studies, patients whose conditions improved during admission were discharged without any guidelines or instructions from nurses. Patients were not accompanied out of the building neither where their departure needs provided. In addition, there was no time a nurse assessed their learning needs, gave them advice on resources or enquired about their home situation with regard to their home care that could help limit their care burden [12, 13] These studies have shown that some nursing staff never planned for the patient discharged and this may compound patients post-operative complications such as infection.

In a survey conducted on patients with complex care needs in 11 countries (Australia, Canada, France, Germany, the Netherlands, New Zealand, Norway, Sweden, Switzerland, the United Kingdom, and the United States), it was reported that one in four patients did not receive instructions for follow-up nor did they receive clear medication directions [14]. Also, there is untimely, infrequent follow up when patients are discharged making it difficult for patients to manage their conditions at home leading to surgical site infection after being discharged. This puts much burden on patients at home who are not well prepared to manage it resulting in readmission [7, 15, 16]. As a result, surgical patients believed that mobile health monitoring is highly acceptable. Nurses need to

provide more frequent, thorough and convenient follow-up to assess their state of health at home upon discharge.This could reduce post-discharge anxiety and help minimize the risk of wound infection and adverse drug effect after hospitalization [7, 17].In a similar study, it was also reported that patients with long term conditions were referred to community services for ongoing support [18]. Comparatively, some of these literatures go to confirm the practice of nursing care at the regional hospital. In Ghana, the training and regulatory body of nursing (Nursing and Midwifery Council of Ghana) curriculum demands that the training of registered general nursing programme should equip qualified nurses the necessary kills to effectively hand discharge patients over to public health nurse or community health nurse at the community for continuity of care. As a result, during training, student's nurses are mandated to write a project work on individual patient care study. This project allows the students to admit and nurse the patient till he/she is discharged. They visit the homes of these patients to assess the patient home environment whilst the patient is on admission in order to prepare the patient well for discharge. They also visit the patient at home upon discharged to assess and see whether the patient is implementing the education. They finally terminate the care by handing the patient over to the community health nurse for continuity of care. However, anecdotal evidence showed that qualified nurses do not perform these functions despite there are no hospital policy restrictions, hence compounding discharged patients problems. Rather, these discharged patients are often referred to the public health unit even though nurses are expected to make follow up at the community level to assess the patient condition and provide necessary education for speedy recovery.

With perioperative care, patients' perspectives on discharge is important since many outcomes such as health related quality of life which includes the desire to regain health and satisfaction of care can only be reported by the patients [19, 20]. This has been confirmed at Kenyatta National Hospital where 167 participants representing 52.4% admitted their satisfaction with nurses' education on their wound dressing when they were discharged [21]. In addition, surgical patients prefer wound dressing materials that promote quick wound healing, reduce pain and ensure shortest hospitalization time [22]. However, at the surgical unit of the regional hospital, there are no specific wood dressing materials that nurses' use apart from the ordinary cotton wool and gauze provided. Besides, despite the fact that each participant went through different surgical procedure, the nurses use the same dressing materials for wound dressing. However, the frequency of wound dressing and the dressing lotion changes −thus as part of the hospital local practices, non infected wounds are being dressed with methylated spirit using alternate days whilst infected wounds are dressed with povidone iodine. Also, when there is need for wound debridement as part of the hospital policy, the patient is readmitted and sent to theatre for wound toileting. Hence, there is the need to educate discharged patients on the kind of wound dressing materials to use at home that will enhance speedy wound healing.

The curriculum use for training nurses in Ghana demands that student nurses be taught effective therapeutic communication skills to enhance good interpersonal interactions with patients at the wards upon completion of their training. They have also been taught on how to prepare a patient for discharge. However, these acquired skills are abandoned by nurses during their duties. This therefore confirms studies that have observed that basic training of nurses on communication skills; regular in-service training and workshops are recommended as ways that could improve on the quality of nursing care especially with discharge preparation [23, 24].Besides, it is important to ensure effective nurse-patient interaction so that nurses would be able to explain the specific disease of the patient [25, 26]. However, some patients claimed nurses spent little time with them and were always in a hurry and busy and as a result communicated poorly with them. This gave them the impression that they lacked time to talk to, listen or be with them [27, 28].

In summary, the literature has indicated that there are gaps with regard to discharged patients' home management of health conditions. The study therefore explored the experiences that discharged surgical patients from the Northern part of Ghana encounter during management of their health condition at home. It examined the techniques and skills that nurse imparted into them during discharge period to enable them care for themselves at home. The literature also examines the interactions that patients encounter at the community level especially, with the handing over of the patients to the community health nurse to continue treatment. The information gathered through this exploration would inform various stakeholders and hospital management including ward managers about the challenges that these discharged patients go through at home.

Method
Design
The study adopted exploratory and descriptive qualitative approach to establish a comprehensive insight into the patients' experiences of discharge and home care provided by nurses. The design allows an exploration of participants' feelings, behaviour, thoughts, insight and action [29].

Setting
Ghana is located in the Western African region, surrounded by the Gulf of Guinea to the South. The country is formed from the union of the Gold Coast, Ashanti Protectorate, Northern Territories and British Togoland. Ghana is slightly smaller in size compared to Oregon. This tropical sub-Saharan nation encompasses approximately 92,000 mile^2 of territory, ranking as the 82nd largest country in the world. Ghana shares around 1500 miles of its land borders with its nearest neighbours, that is, Burkina Faso to the North, Cote d'Ivoire to the West and Togo to the East.

The Upper East Region is located in the northern part of Ghana and is the second smallest of ten (10) administrative regions in Ghana, occupying a total land surface of 8842 km^2 or 2.7% of the total land area of Ghana. The Upper East regional capital is Bolgatanga where the regional hospital is located. The major towns in the region include Navrongo, Paga, Bawku and Zebilla. Comparatively, the region has varied population comprising all manners of tribes with different spoken languages. However, the commonest languages that are spoken are Grunne (local language) and English language.

The study was conducted at the Regional Hospital located at the Northern part of Ghana. The hospital is located at the North-Eastern part of the regional capital, Bolgatanga. The regional hospital is the largest hospital in the region; as a result, it serves as a referral centre for the district hospitals in the region. The entire nursing population of the hospital is about 160 and the total bed capacity is two hundred and six (206) beds. The surgical department is attached to the theatre and about 50 surgeries are performed in a day. Comparing the setting to other settings cited in the study especially the Europeans countries, it is obvious that the study setting is small and does not have the requested logistics to meet the modern standard of care expected. Even though the nurses are trained to provide standardised care, the nature of the setting restricts the kind of care to be provided. Many at time nurses do improvise certain materials to provide certain nursing care to patients. For instance, making a follow up upon the discharge of a patient is often difficult because of lack of means as compare to other settings where means of transport is not a challenge. Also, the hospital telephone network system is poor hence nurses find it difficult to make a telephone call to patients upon discharge. Nurses can only do this by using their cell phones.

Population and sampling technique
The study population was discharged surgical patients who went through either emergency or planned general surgical procedures within 1 month and stayed within Bolgatanga Municipality. The study involved both males and females general surgical patients who came to the surgical unit as outpatients for their daily wound dressing. The study adopted purposive sampling technique to collect the data. Purposive sampling technique was employed

because of the identifiable nature of participants. That is, the study population was participants who have had general surgeries and had been discharged within 1 month. Hence, 15 participants were recruited based on data saturation. The surgical records of the participants at the hospital were used to identify the participants especially records at the male and female surgical wards and the theatre. The participants were also contacted on phone.

Data collection tool and procedure

A semi-structured interview guide was used to conduct face to face interview with the participants. The lead author conducted all the individual interviews after he had acquired the necessary skills through training to conduct qualitative interviews. The interviews were conducted in English and Grunne (local language). Probes were used to generate detailed understanding of participants' experiences of home care and nurses' follow- ups following participants discharged from the ward. The interviews were conducted at a time and place convenient to the participants and lasted between 30 to 45 min. The same interview guide was used throughout for all the participants that were involved in the study. These interviews were continued till the 15th participant, when the researcher realised that all the15 participants were giving similar responses indicating that there will not be any new information to be provided by the participants even if the researcher wishes to continue with the interviews. Hence, base on this, it was an indication that the data were saturated. The interview was also recorded and transcribed in English. Field notes on observations made during the interviews including non-verbal cues of the participants were written during transcription to reflect participants' true experiences of home management and follow-ups by nurses.

Data analysis

The principles of thematic content analysis according to [30] were used to analyse data. The data were analysed concurrently with data collection to allow for the search of important themes and patterns in the data. The authors coded the data independently and the discrepancies were discussed for a consensus during the analysis. The data were organized into themes and sub-themes after making meaning of the transcripts. The authors discussed the themes and sub-themes to ensure the true reflections of participants home management experiences and nurses' follow-ups. The authors managed the data manually to extract data that supported the findings.

Rigour

Rigour was ensured through member checking where participants confirmed their experiences during data analysis. There was team discussion of emerging themes to facilitate an in-depth understanding of the

participants' experiences of home management and nurses follow ups. Also to ensure that the findings can be applied to other settings, we provided a detailed description of the research processes and findings. The same semi-structured interview guide was used to ensure consistency of the data collection.

Results
Demographic characteristics

A total number of 15 participants were interviewed during the research. Eight (8) participants were females and seven were males. These participants were aged between 23 and 65 years. Three of the participants were in their early twenties, five were in their mid-thirties, four were in their mid-fifties, two participants were in their late fifties and one participant being exactly 60 years. Nine (9) of these participants had some sort of formal education and could therefore speak English fluently. The remaining six (6) participants did not have any form of education and therefore could speak only Grunne. Eleven of the participants comprising five (5) males and six (6) females were married while three males and a female were not married.Three of the participants were Muslims, eight were Christians while four (4) were traditionalist. In terms of occupations, eight of these participants were trained teachers, two were motor fitters and the remaining five participants were peasant farmers. All the fifteen (15) participants were resident within Bolgatanga municipality.

Two major themes were identified in the study. These themes included patients' discharge information and nurses' follow ups/ home visits.The sub-themes of patients' discharge information included information on nutrition and lifestyle practices, medications and wound care and nurse- patient interactions.

Patients' discharge information

Participants' experiences on discharge information centered on the education that participants received from nurses before they were discharged to help them care for themselves at home. Participants received educationthat was beneficial to their healthcare at home on areas such as lifestyle modifications, good nutrition, medication and wound care.

Nutrition and lifestyle modifications

All the participants reported that nurses told them that they should not smoke or drink alcohol such as a locally brewed alcoholic beverage (pito) as it could affect wound healing.

"The nurses told me that I should not drink pito or smoke cigarette otherwise my wound would not heal fast" (MP1).

"The nurses told me that I should not drink alcohol otherwise I would get drunk and fall and probably hit the sore on the ground or sit on the scrotum. I should avoid taking cola nut since it can cause irritation that can make me cough and caused pains" (MP7).

Some participants reported that the nurses told them that they should not lift heavy objects or do any heavy work that could lead to complication:

"The nurse told me I should not lift any heavy object and I should not do difficult work that can cause me problem" (FP4).

Some participants reported that nurses educated them to eat nutritious food when they were discharged.

"The nurses told me I should be eating fruits, vegetables, oranges, fish, meat and others" (MP3).

"The nurses advised me that I should not eat hard food but I should be taking light soup, porridge to enhance easy defecation" (FP6).

However, some participants stated that the nurses did not educate them on what food to eat but told them to come for their wound dressing.

"No nurse discussed anything about nutrition to me, like I should eat this food or that food. It is only the dressing day they told to come back for my wound to be dressed" (MP5).

Education on medications
The nurses educated participants on how to take their medications at home prior to discharge but some did not indicate the time interval for the medication to be taken:

"One nurses showed me that I should take one tablet in the morning, afternoon and in evening. She also told my sister to always remind me to take the medicine at home but she did not state the time interval for the medication to be taken" (FP4).

"The nurses showed me how I should take the medications at home. They told me that I should take the drugs in the morning, afternoon and evening without stating the specific hour I should take the medication" (FP13).

Others were told to take the drugs regularly but not given specific details:

"The nurses said I should be taking the medications regularly but they did not tell me the time I should take the drug" (FP12).

Some participants also followed the inscriptions on the sachet to take their medications at home without prior education from the nurses.

"The medications that they gave me from the hospital, it has been indicated on the sachet how it should be taken so I have been following that inscription to take my medications at home" (FP15).

However, all the participants said the nurses did not educate them on the actions and side effect of their medications:

"No nurse told me about the actions and side effects of the medications that I was taking" (MP5).

"The nurses did not educate me on the actions and the side effects of the medications I was taking at home" (FP13).

Education on wound care
All participants reported that the nurses told them to come to the ward for the daily dressing of their wounds. Participants were given different dates to come for the dressing. A participant stated:

"The nurses told me to come to the ward every three days for the dressing" (MP3). *"The nurse told me to come to the hospital every two days for the dressing"* (MP1).

All the participants reported that they received information from nurses on things that they should do to prevent wound infection.

"The nurses told me that I should not let water get to the wound site to promote infection" (MP3).

"My wife always cleaned my body with sponge, soap and water because the nurses told me that the wound should not be wet" (MP5).

However, some participants said they were not told to keep the wound dry:

"The nurses did not tell me that I should keep my wound dry" (FM14).

Some participants added that nurses advised them to keep the wound clean:

"...She said I should not expose the wound to dirty things like my dress and I should wash my clothing well" (MP1).

Other participants stressed that nurses did not educate them on the early detection of the signs of wound infection for them to report early:

"The nurses did not educate me on the signs of wound infection to enable me detect the infection early and report to the hospital" (FP4).

Some participants reported that some of the nurses would dress their wounds and express the pus whilst others did not do so:

"Some nurses would dress the wound and pressed it for all the pus to come out. But other nurses would dress the wound without pressing and you would not even feel any pain" (MP5).

However, all the participants reported that the nurses did not educate them on the signs of wound infection:

"The nurses did not teach me the signs of wound infection" (FM10). *"The nurses did not tell me any danger signs of wound infection"* (MP8).

Follow up/ hand over patients to community health nurse
The participants reported that no nurse visited them at home or even called them on phone to find out how they were doing at home. A participant stated that some nurses informed her to come for review but if there was a problem, she should report to the hospital immediately:

"Some nurses said I should take note of the day that they told me to come for review but if there is a problem I should come and should not wait for that day. They did not visit me at home" (MP9).

"The nurses never visited me at home following my discharge from the ward but rather, theytold me that I should come back today for them to see how I was doing at home." (FP14).

"I wish nurses had visited me at home to see how I was doing. I believed my wound got infected at home. If a nurse had visited me at home she could have prevented this" (MP3).

All the participants stated that nurses did not hand them over to the community health nurse to continue with treatment.

"Nurses did not visit me at home and they did not hand me over to the community health nurse to continue treatment".

"Hmmm I was thinking that the nurses will tell me to go to the community health nurse for my wound dressing but they did not and I did not also go to her".

Nurse-patient interaction
Some participants added that some nurses were good and polite any time they came for dressing;

"In fact some of the nurses were good. When they come in the morning they would greet me nicely and chat with me. Some were also showing respect to me by speaking politely to me and some would ask me whether I had any problem that I want to share with them" (MP3).

Some participants also stated that the nurses have been taking care of their wound well for them to recover fast.

"I am so happy that I have finally done the operation and dressing is also good. At first I could not work effectively because of my swollen scrotum but now I do the basic work without any problem" (MP7).

"As for the dressing, the nurses in the room are doing well. In fact they dress my wound very well. Look at the wound it is almost healed after two weeks of operation" (MP1).

However, some participants felt that the nurses did not communicate well with them during outpatient wound dressing.

"My wound gaped and I was rushed to the ward and the nurses were shouting at me saying that I was careless" (FP4).

A few of the participants said nurses spoke rudely to them:

"One nurse spoke rudely to me at the dressing room. She said you cannot put medicine down and it poured. I could not talk and my tears were flowing from my eyes." (MP8).

Some participants also stated that some nurses deliberately refused to dress their wounds with the excuse that they (participants) came late.

"The nurses refused to dress my wound saying that I came late even though I was feeling pain at the site of the wound. They only added a plaster to hold the old dressing in place" (MP3).

As a result of these attitudes of some nurses, participants had these pieces of advice.

"Hmm, if they could train nurses to dress wound nicely it would help to reduce infection. The doctors would do the operation nicely and everything would be fine but because nurses do not dress the wounds well, the wounds are always infected" (MP5).

Some participants pleaded that nurses should talk nicely to participants to allay their anxiety:

"It is good that nurses should talk nicely to patients during any procedure they are doing especially those who have never had an operation so that their anxiety and fear will be better" (FP14).

Discussion
The study identified that nurses advised patients to stop certain lifestyle practices such as taking alcohol and smoking cigarette after discharge in order to promote their speedy recovery at home. Besides, nurses educated some patients on the need to keep their wounds dry to prevent infection. These findings support previous studies that indicated that nurses often planned with patients and their family members during discharge and educate them to avoid factors that can negatively affect recovery. They also educate patients on proper personal hygiene and prevention of wound complications [1, 3].

Proper nutrition promotes speedy recovery and enhances wound healing [8]. However, the study indicated that nurses did not stress the importance of nutrition to some patients even though some were encouraged to take fruits, vegetables, fish and meat upon discharge to promote wound healing. It could be inferred from the study that nurses did rush to educate some patients and thereby providing them with incomplete information or information that they could not understand [6].

Educating discharged patients on how to take their prescribed medications at home to enhance speedy recovery is important since failure to do so could lead to patients taking overdose or under dose of such medicines [8]. Besides, it is important to educate patients on the side effects of these medicines [9, 10]. However, the study revealed that some patients were not educated on how to take the medicine at home especially on the prescribed time intervals and this compelled some of them to follow instructions on the label. Besides, patients were not educated on the actions

and the side effects of these medications. It is good nurses and pharmacists take their time to educate discharged patients on their prescription instructions to avoid inappropriate usage of medicine at home.

The study revealed that patients were informed of their scheduled days for wound dressing on the ward without educating them on how to change their wound dressing when necessary. Besides, patients were not educated on some of the signs of wound infection. These findings confirm previous studies that indicate that ineffective teaching of surgical patients upon discharge about wound care could lead to patients lacking the requisite knowledge and skills on how to care for the wound at home leading to complications [4, 5, 7]. It is therefore mandatory that nurses spend much time in educating discharged surgical patients to equip them with the necessary knowledge and skills to enable them handle their wounds properly at home. Besides,the study found that some nurses refused to dress some patients' wounds during follow up visit to the hospital dressing room and such patients perceived nursing care as poor. These practices compounded some the patients' problems contributing to their wound infection.

Nursing is a continuous process and there is the need to visit discharge patients at home to find out how they are doing. However, nurses at the surgical unit did not visit patients at home. Many of the patients stated that some nurses told them their wounds were infected when they reported to the ward for dressing. This confirms previous studies that indicate that due to the untimely and infrequent or lack of follow up visits that nurses do, many patients get wound infection at home. Wound infection puts much burden on family members who lack the requisite knowledge to handle it leading to more complications [7, 15, 16]. To close this gap in the nursing care, it is suggested that nurses should incorporate days in their duty schedule to visit discharged patients to assess their environment and provide education as necessary [13].Also, nurses could liaise with the community health nurses to continue caring for patients at home [18] since failure to do so could affect recovery and cause readmission [31].

In surgery, patients' perspectives about care are relevant as a key outcome in areas such as health related quality of life and satisfaction. Hence, some patients were happy and thankful to some nurses for being polite in their communication and interaction during care confirming previous studies that show that good nurse-patient interaction and communication are the key component of quality care since it establishes a healthy relationship that allows participants to voice their concerns freely [8, 26]. However, the study also found that some nurses were using abusive language for patients and were not ready to listen to their concerns as stated in previous studies [27].

However, some patients were full of praises that some nurses were able to dress their wounds skilfully as supported by a previous study [21]. It was also reported that some patients were happy to have resumed their activities of daily living which is supported by previous studies that show that patients desire to get good outcomes such as regaining their normal activities [19, 20].

Conclusion

In conclusion, the study explored the experiences of discharged surgical patients on their preparation by nurses toward home management and how they manage their condition at home either by themselves or by the community health nurses and as outpatients at the dressing unit at regional hospital, Bolgatanga. Despite the fact that nurses did their best to ensure discharged patients were able to manage their conditions at home, the findings from the study indicated that nurses never visited patients at home and never handed the discharged patients over to the community health nurses to continue management. Nurses also exhibited poor attitude such as poor communication toward patients during outpatient care.

The relevance of the study was to find out the challenges that discharged patients faced following the management of their condition at home and the way forward. From the study findings, it is importance to note that nurses at the surgical unit do not adequately prepare patients towards discharge leading to a serious gap on how they should handle themselves well to prevent infections. It therefore important for the hospital management to organize refresher training on patient discharge preparation, nurse-patient interaction, home visit and the need to hand over patients to community health nurses to continue treatment at home. Even though, the study specifically explored the perspectives of surgical patients on nurses' education following discharge, some discharged patients did indicate that family members play a major role intheir home management. Hence, it is recommended that further studies should be conducted on the impact of family members on discharged patient home management.

Acknowledgements

The authors are so much grateful to the hospital management and all patients who participated in the study.

Limitation of the study

The study had some limitations but the key limitations include; the smaller sample size did not permit for generalisation of the findings. Even though the study was conducted at the referral hospital of the region, the restriction of the languages (English and Grunne) language did not allow many participants to express their views. Besides, the study was limited to persons living within Bolgatanga Municipality.

Authors' contributions

AB collected the data, analysed the data and interpreted the patients' experiences about discharged planning and home care. AL has been revising the manuscript as she read through the entire manuscript to make the necessary corrections and approved the final manuscript for publication. Besides, AL agreed to be responsible to all aspect any part of the work. AL also ensures that are questions related to the accuracy and integrity of the work are appropriately investigated and resolved. Both authors read and approved the final manuscript.

Ethics approval and consent to participate

The Institutional Review Board (IRB) of Noguchi Memorial Institute for Medical Research, University of Ghana, Legon, granted ethical clearance with the code NMIMR-IRB CPN 099/13–14 to conduct the study. Besides, the authorities of the Upper East Regional and Municipal Health Directorate and the Regional hospital, Bolgatanga also gave ethical clearance for the study to be conducted. The participants also signed the consent form after the relevant information was provided to them. The participants were informed that their participation in the study was voluntary and that they could withdraw at anytime they wish to do so. The participants were also informed that there will not be direct benefits from the study but their views would help nursing staff at the unit to know what participants want from them. Pseudonyms like female participant one (FP1) or male participant one (MP1) were used to ensure participants' anonymity and confidentiality.

Competing interests

The authors declare that they have no competing interests.

Author details

[1]Nurses' Training College, Zuarungu, Ghana. [2]Department of Adult Health, School of Nursing, College of Health Sciences, University of Ghana, P.O. Box LG 43, Legon, Accra, Ghana.

References

1. Berg K, Arestedt KF, Kjellgren K. Postoperative recovery from the perspectivesof day surgery patients: a phenomenographic study. Int J Nurs Stud. 2013;50(12):1630–8.
2. Hessenlink G, et al. Quality and safety of hospital discharge: a study on experiences and perceptions of patients, relatives and care providers. Int J Qual Health Care. 2013;25(1):66–74. https://doi.org/10.1093/intqhc/mzs066.
3. Li IC, Lee SY, Chen CY, Jeng YQ, Chen YC. Facilitators and Barriers to Effective Smoking Cessation: Counselling Service for Inpatient from Nurse-Counsellors' Perspectives- A qualitative Study. Int J Environ Res Public Health. 2014;11:4782–98. https://doi.org/10.3390/ijerph110504782. Source: PubMed
4. Pieper B, Sieggreen M, Nordstrom C, Freeland B, Kulwicki P. Discharge knowledge and concerns of patients going home with a wound. J Wound Ostomy Continence Nurs. 2007;34:245–53. https://doi.org/10.1097/01.won.0000270817.06942.00.
5. Tanner J, Padley W, Davey S, Murphy K, Brown B. Patient narratives of surgical site infection: implications for practice. J Hosp Infect. 2013;83(1):41–5. https://doi.org/10.1016/j.jhin.2012.07.025.
6. Hessenlink G, et al. Are patients discharged with care? A qualitative study of perceptions and experiences of patients, family members and care providers. 2012; https://doi.org/10.1136/bmjqs-2012-001165.
7. Sanger PC, Hartzler A, Han SM, Armstrong CAL, Stewart MR, Lordon RJ, Evans HL. Patient Perspectives on Post-Discharge Surgical Site Infections:

Towards a Patient-Centered Mobile Health Solution. 2014;9(12) https://doi.org/10.1371/ PLos one.0114016.

8. Foust, J. B., Vuckovic, N., &Henriquez, E. (2011). Hospital to home health care transition: patient, caregiver, and clinician perspectives: 34(2) 194–212. https://doi.org/10.1177/0193945911400448·Source: PubMed.

9. Hundt AS, Carayon P, Springman S, Smith M, Florek K, Sheth R, Dorshorst M. Advances in Patient Safety Outpatient Surgery and Patient Safety- The Patient's Voice. In: Advances in Patient Safety: From Research to Implementation (Volume 4: Programs, Tools, and Products). edn. Edited by Henriksen K, Battles JB, Marks ES, Lewin DI. Rockville: Agency for Healthcare Research and Quality (US); 2005.

10. Holland DE, Mnistiae P, Kathryn B. Problems and unmet needs of patients discharged "home to self-care". 2011;16(5):240–50. https://doi.org/10.1097/NCM.0b013e31822361d8. Source: PubMed

11. Alcala Pompeo D, Pinto Helena M, Cesarino CB, Ferreira de Araujo RRD, Aparecid Poletti NA. Nurses' Performance on Hospital Discharge. Patient Point of View. 2007;20(3):345–50. https://doi.org/10.1590/S0103-21002007000300017. ISSN 1982-0194

12. McMurray A, Johnson P, Wallis M, Patterson E, Grifiths S. General surgical patients' perspective of the adequacy and appropriateness of discharge planning to facilitate health decision-making at home. J Clin Nurs. 2007;16: 1602–9.

13. Mottram A. "They are marvellous with you whilst you are in but the aftercare is rubbish": a grounded theory study of patients' and their carers' experiences after. discharge following day surgery. J ClinNurs. 2011;20(21–22):3143–51.

14. Schoen C, Osborn R, Squires D, et al. New 2011 survey of patients with complex care needs in eleven countries finds that care is often poorly coordinated. Health Aff. 2011;30:243748. Access 20 Feb 2017

15. Kazaure H, Roman S, Sosa J. Association of post-discharge complications with preoperation and mortality in general surgery. Arch Surg. 2012;147: 1000–7. https://doi.org/10.1001/2013.jamasurg.114.

16. Saunders R, Fernandes-Taylor S, Rathouz P, Saha S, Wiseman J. Outpatient follow-up versus 30-day readmission among general and vascular surgery patients: Acase for redesigning transitional care. Surgery. 2014;156:949–58.

17. Mueller SK, Cunningham S, Kripalani S, Schnipper JL. Hospital-BasedMedication Reconciliation Practices: Asystemic Review. 2012;172(14): 1057–69. https://doi.org/10.1001/archinternmed.2012.2246.

18. Healthwatch Croydon (2016). Experiences of discharge From Croydon University Hospital by patients aged 65 years and over: https://pdfs.semanticscholar.org/22be/2384e7ad51bc4279a015e5fd87ec5bec101c.pdf. Access 11 Oct 2017.

19. Grøndah, V. A. (2012). Patients' perceptions of actual care conditions and patient satisfaction with care quality in hospital: Electronic Publication from Karlstad University https://pdfs.semanticscholar.org/22be/2384e7ad51bc4279a015e5fd87ec5bec101c.pdf. Accessed on 10 Oct 2016.

20. Pusic, & Andrea, L. (2014). Understanding the Patient Perspectives on Surgical Outcome and Experience: Strat-Plastic Surgery Foundation, Artington Height, United State: http://grantome.com/grant/NIH/R13-HS023357-01. Access 20 June 2017.

21. Shawa, E. (2012). Patients' Perceptions regarding Nursing Care in the General Surgical Wards at Kenyatta National Hospital. https://www.academia.edu/2435861/Patients_Perceptions_Regarding_Nursing_Care_in_the_General_Surgical_Wards_atb_Kenyatta_National_Hospital_Nairobi_Kenya. Accessed 10 Oct 2016.

22. Association of Perioperative Registered Nurses. Perioperative standard and recommended practices. Denver: AORN; 2012a. Accessed 23 Apr 2014

23. Lane-Carlson M-L, Kumar J. Engaging patients in managing their health care: patient perceptions of the effect of a total joint replacement presurgical class. Perm J. 2012;16(3):42–7.

24. Mensah, O., Nyarko. (2013). Understanding the Nurse-Patient Interaction at Komfo Anokye Teaching Hospital. The Patients' Perspectives and Experiences. http://hdl.handle.net/123456789/5866. Accessed 10 Oct 2016.

25. Sieger M, Fritz E, Them C. In discourse: Bourdieus theory of practice and habitus in the context of communication-orientated nursing model. Journal of Advanced Nursing. 2012;68(2):480–9.

26. Stephanie N, Zoe J. The patient experience of patient-centered communication with nurses in the hospital setting: a qualitative systematic review protocol. 2015;13(1):76–87. https://doi.org/10.11124/jbisrir-2015-1072.

27. Larsson IE, Sahlsten MJM, Segesten K, Plos KAE. Patient Perception of Nurses Behaviour that Influence Patient Participation in Nursing Care: A critic, an incident study. 2011; https://doi.org/10.1155/2011/534060.

28. Teng KYS, Norazliah S. Surgical patients' satisfaction of nursing Care at the Orthopedic Wards in Hospital UniversitiSains Malaysia (HUSM). Health Environ J. 2012;3(1)36–43.

29. Mayan MJ. Essentials of Qualitative Injury. Walnut Creek: Coast Press; 2009.

30. Miles MB, Huberman AM. Qualitative data analysis: An expanded sourcebook. 2nd ed. Thousand Oaks: Sage; 1994.

31. Wennström B, Stomberg M, Warrén M, Marina S. Patient Symptoms after Colonic Surgery in the Era of Enhanced Recovery–a long-term follow-up. Journal of Clinical Nursing. 2010;19(5–6):666–72.

Caring for late preterm infants: public health nurses' experiences

Genevieve Currie[1*], Aliyah Dosani[1,2], Shahirose S. Premji[2,3], Sandra M. Reilly[2,3], Abhay K. Lodha[4,5] and Marilyn Young[6]

Abstract

Background: Public health nurses (PHNs) care for and support late preterm infants (LPIs) and their families when they go home from the hospital. PHNs require evidence-informed guidelines to ensure appropriate and consistent care. The objective of this research study is to capture the lived experience of PHNs caring for LPIs in the community as a first step to improving the quality of care for LPIs and support for their parents.

Methods: To meet our objectives we chose a descriptive phenomenology approach as a method of inquiry. We conducted semi-structured interviews with PHNs ($n = 10$) to understand PHN perceptions of caring for LPIs and challenges in meeting the needs of families within the community. Interpretative thematic analysis revealed PHN perceptions of caring for LPIs and challenges in meeting the needs of families within the community.

Results: Four themes emerged from the data. First, PHNs expressed challenges with meeting the physiological needs of LPIs and gave voice to the resulting strain this causes for parents. Second, nurses conveyed that parents require more anticipatory guidance about the special demands associated with feeding LPIs. Third, PHNs relayed that parents sometimes receive inconsistent advice from different providers. Lastly, PHNs acknowledged that due to lack of resources, families sometimes did not receive the full scope of evidence informed care required by fragile, immature infants.

Conclusion: The care of LPIs by PHNs would benefit from more research about the needs of these infants and their families. Efforts to improve quality of care should focus on: evidence-informed guidelines, consistent care pathways, coordination of follow up care and financial resources, to provide physical, emotional, informational support that families require once they leave the hospital. More research on meeting the challenges of caring for LPIs and their families would provide direction for the competencies PHNs require to improve the quality of care in the community.

Keywords: Infant, Premature, Community health care, Nurses, Public health, Evidenced-based practice

Background

Canada has a preterm birth rate (2014–2015) of 7.8% [1]. In 2014–2015, Alberta's preterm birth rate averaged 8.7%, and Calgary's rate averaged 9.2% [2]. Infants born between 34 0/7 weeks and 36 6/7 weeks' gestation, referred to as late preterm infants (LPIs), comprise approximately 75% of this population [3]. The Canadian Paediatric Society supports the early discharge of stable LPIs, providing they receive appropriate follow-up within 48 h by a community-based health care provider [4]. While LPIs and term infants are similar in terms of size and mature appearance, there are significant differences. When compared to full term infants, LPIs have an increased risk for several morbidities. Specifically, LPIs experience a higher risk of feeding difficulties [5, 6], excessive weight loss [5], hypoglycemia [5, 7, 8], hyperbilirubinemia [5, 7, 8], hypothermia and temperature instability [7, 8], respiratory distress syndrome [8], and sepsis [8]. These medical issues can persist after discharge from hospital, and result in LPIs having a high rate of emergency room visits and hospital readmission within the first two weeks of life [9–12].

* Correspondence: gcurrie@mtroyal.ca
[1]School of Nursing and Midwifery, Mount Royal University, 4825 Mount Royal Gate SW, Calgary, Alberta T3E 6K6, Canada
Full list of author information is available at the end of the article

In Alberta, once LPIs are discharged from hospital, their home care becomes the immediate responsibility of public health nurses (PHNs). Birth and early postpartum hospital records are provided for continuity of care. In Calgary, PHNs contact all parents often within hours of arriving home to offer nursing support [13]. This support ranges from one home visit or clinic appointment to a series of consultations as required on a need-to- basis. The consultations not only focus on the LPIs but also the parents, who require teaching and guidance to become increasingly self-sufficient. Therefore, PHNs need to have an excellent understanding of how the needs of LPIs differ from those of the term infant. In so doing, PHNs typically rely on their empirical knowledge and the guidelines used with term infants, with some modification [14].

This research study aims to understand the lived experience of PHNs in caring for LPIs and supporting families in the immediate postpartum period. These research findings identify what challenges PHNs experience while providing care for LPIs and their families in the community setting, and what additional resources and competencies PHNs require to improve the quality of care for LPIs and their families.

Methods

As part of a larger study using a mixed methods approach [15], this article reports on one aspect of the research. Descriptive phenomenology was used as the method of inquiry to better understand the lived experience of PHNs and parents in caring for LPIs in the community setting [16, 17]. Descriptive phenomenology explores the structure of experience and consciousness within everyday life [17]. This article presents the results of the PHN experience. Other results considering the parent experience appear elsewhere [18, 19]. The study participants, at three postpartum community service sites, completed a demographic questionnaire. A purposive sampling method [17] was then used to recruit PHNs according to years of experience, location, and role. Ten PHNs with a range of clinical experience from 3 to 30 years participated in the study. Some PHNs, considered experts, functioned in the role of charge nurse, lactation consultant, and/or clinical nurse educator. The PHNs determined where and when to conduct the in-depth, face-to-face semi-structured interviews, which ranged from 60 to 90 min in length.

The research questions were: 1) What is your experience in caring for LPIs as a PHN? And 2) What challenges have you experienced in providing care to LPIs and their families?

Researchers (AD, SR) modified or added questions to explore topics as they emerged during the interviews. The process continued until the researchers determined they had reached informational saturation [20]. Interviews were recorded, transcribed verbatim, and checked for accuracy before analyses. Two researchers (GC, AD) numerically labeled the interviews, to preserve anonymity, before they independently analyzed and categorized the themes. Using interpretive thematic analysis, the researchers (GC, AD, SP) assigned codes to various elements that emerged from the transcribed text, then identified narrative ideas before re-organizing these ideas around central themes [21]. In turn, any patterns found in the codes and central themes and relationships, identified across participants and narratives [22], served to answer the research questions.

Results

Four themes emerged from the data. First, the complexity and intensity of care required by LPIs makes stressful demands on caregivers and providers. Second, LPIs have specific feeding challenges when compared with term infants for which parents lack anticipatory guidance. Third, inconsistencies in care practices between health care providers is difficult for parents and PHNs to navigate. Due to the lack of evidence-informed research, providers come to rely on their empirical knowledge, which sometimes leads to contradictory beliefs that can confuse families or lead to inconsistent care. Finally, as with many health promotion activities, the financial costs of a home visitation program raise questions about its sustainability within a publicly funded system, which can frustrate the best efforts of PHNs. Consequently, health resource management and allocation of care of LPIs also appeared as a major area of concern.

Theme 1: The stress of providing nursing care for LPIs: "they think they're bringing home a term baby...so we're the bearers of bad news"

Meeting the physical demands of LPIs and subsequent emotional needs on the parents represent the most common challenge for PHNs. LPIs have multiple health challenges because of their physiological immaturity. They include: feeding difficulties, hyperbilirubinemia, temperature instability and poor temperature regulation, and risk of sepsis. As PHN #8 stated: *"...first of all they definitely tend to usually have problems with higher levels of jaundice so we have to monitor them more carefully for that."* PHN #5 expressed *"They're not warm enough and they're not feeding well enough and the moms maybe are not feeding them often enough"*. PHN #3 described other health challenges:

... yes [we see them] with weight, with poor weight gain, with poor feeding, jaundice – all of that...
And so they are being admitted day 5, day 6 for phototherapy and we have been faithfully following them.

PHNs described feelings of angst and frustration, exasperated by limited time and resources available to PHNs, trying to address these complex and interrelated needs of LPIs and their parents. For example, PHN #5 explained: *"There is a lot of pressure to do a tremendous amount of teaching in a short period of time. A lot of which goes over their heads 'cause they are tired and they don't hear everything you say."* PHNs question whether hospital staff inform parents of the specific needs of their LPIs or parents simply forget some instructions, as some parents have no recollection that LPIs can experience numerous challenges. This can result in parents not having the information required to address these challenges, which puts PHNs in the difficult position of breaking unwelcome news, often when a problem arises, to the chagrin of the parents. A PHN explained:

Sometimes I feel like we're the bearers of bad news because in hospital everything seems to be going so well. And then you go out to the first visit and the jaundice is going up and the baby's lost weight and output is kind of iffy…Things aren't where they're supposed to be at (PHN #2).

Consequently, some parents leave the hospital with the impression that *"… they're bringing home a 'term' baby"* (PHN #5). Thus parents have no forewarning of the homeostatic and feeding problems associated with LPIs. Accordingly, this difference in perceptions must be addressed by PHNs. PHN #5 expressed her perception of how the baby was progressing which was different than the parents:

The problem that we see a little more often is when the ones come home straight out of hospital that are 36 weeks and they're different, cause they haven't been in the NICU yet and they haven't had that experience so they believe that they're bringing home a 'term' baby and often times they're not feeding, or transferring milks as well but the mom thinks the baby is feeding and the baby is really not feeding so they're missing some of the cues of that baby…

PHNs also conveyed that LPIs frequently resemble term infants in size and appearance and this can lead to confusion as they often require more care. PHN #9 explained:

…[Parents] know their baby's early, but… some of them still go home like the next day with their baby, right. Especially if they have a larger late preterm infant like a 6 to 8 pound late preterm infant, which is not unheard of. I think many of them do not perceive their infant as being any different from a term infant.

Moreover, PHNs have to reduce parental anxiety in such situations:

But sometimes they [parents] don't know [what to do]. …And they feel really bad when they do find out, and they realize… my baby's not feeding and the jaundice is now, you know, up in the red zone (PHN #2).

When things are not going well, mothers: *"have a lot of guilt and you're always trying to reassure them… It's very upsetting for them…"* (PHN #2). Hence, in addition to helping parents of LPI manage a variety of often interrelated challenges and identify and implement appropriate care strategies, PHNs must also be able to identify conflicting feelings among parents and address these also.

Theme 2: Feeding challenges for LPIs: "suck, swallow, breathe is complex for these babies"

PHNs reported how infants tire at the breast, with a poor suck reflex, and inadequate suck swallow coordination. *"Suck, swallow, breathe is complex for these babies. They don't coordinate it very well. And they [parents] need to understand that and that's the problem that we have"* (PHN #5). PHN #3 observed that *"typically what we see [are LPIs] sucking a few times at the breast and then falling asleep"* and mothers have difficulties *"recognizing [these] cues"* (PHN #2). These difficulties become problematic because, *"the parents often think that 'oh, they're done. They're full, and in fact, they're not; they're just kind of exhausted"* (PHN #2). To ensure adequate milk intake, PHNs described the significant amount of time they spend with parents: *"…we can provide a tremendous amount of teaching, education, a lot of feeding support one on one, [with]hours of time"* (PHN #5). PHN #9 articulated: *"I will sometimes spend upwards of an hour just working on breastfeeding in the community or in the clinic."* According to PHN #2 *"Well certainly often there's feeding issues so that, that certainly often takes extra time… getting these babies to the breast and feeding effectively at the breast."* The inability of the parents to assess these satiety cues could of course, lead to inadequate feeding and becomes a significant nursing practice issue.

In addition, most parents aspire to breastfeed their LPIs exclusively but this presents more of a challenge with LPIs due to immaturity.

A lot of times these moms want to go to full breast feeding so the challenge is being able to stay with the family long enough to get this baby fully breast fed, you know, to where the mother actually has a good relationship with you and you want to keep that going so that she can meet these goals (PHN #5).

However, it can prove difficult because the infants quickly become physically exhausted and can only breast-feed for less than several minutes before they tire *"...many late preterm babies really tire at the breast quite easily so they're using up almost as much calories working to get the milk and then the calories they are getting"* (PHN #9). In addition, parents are not always aware that feeding is ineffective and this becomes the priority for the PHN despite lack of understanding from parents:

Parents sometimes think everything is going well and the baby's feeding well. And [then] you observe a feed, and you realize, you know, that it's not really going well. I'm not hearing adequate milk transfer. [Consequently] the weights gain's not great (PHN #2).

PHNs relayed specific challenges associated with assisting parents with a range of feeding strategies (breastfeeding, bottle feeding and mixed feedings) and they felt very responsible for promoting correct information. PHN #7 described her experience with bottle feeding:

So I find that it can be a little bit stressful in that they're [parents] not picking up those cues and so I'll teach them...you know the baby is grimacing or the baby's hand goes up, the baby's turning away it means they don't want any more.... So that can be frustrating for me ...Why hasn't anybody told you this...Your baby's at risk of, you know, aspiration...

PHN #4 recalled that parents appear unaware of the developmental challenges associated with being a LPI: *"When the baby's too tired at the breast, you need to give her more of a break."* With bottle-feeding, PHNs noted gaps in parents' understanding of infant cues. It seems that parents sometimes used a *"bottle that's too fast and [the infant was] choking and flooding on the bottle and shutting down and not wanting to eat"* (PHN #5). In these circumstances, parents and infants appeared to work at cross-purposes. PHNs recognized that because of these feeding challenges, weight gain appeared sporadic and not as linear and progressive as with term infants. PHN #6 noted the growth was slow:

...you have to be sort of patient with these, with these families, and that there's little gains and little successes and that they, you know, as long as there's a step forward up then, that, you know, that's good but it's just that they need to take a little bit more time which, you know, and the reassurance to families that they'll look at it as a journey, and that, um the days are long....

Such observations generally prompted *"a lot of follow-up"* (PHN #2) from PHNs and typically for a long period of time to ensure consistent weight gain, and exclusive breastfeeding. In this regard, PHNs evidently provide significant critical analysis of feeding and outcomes for these infants when providing follow up care. *"...I think they have in their mind that they need to catch their baby up, right? It's always a race to catch up and that's a shame. Just let the baby grow at its speed and enjoy the baby..."* (PHN #7).

Theme 3: Inconsistencies between health care providers: "...there needs to be more consistent information"

PHNs report a lack of consistency in the advice that providers give parents. PHN #7 indicated *"...that's a big concern for parents. That the information given in the hospital is different from the information we're giving. So definitely there needs to be more consistent information."* PHNs conveyed experiencing frustration when helping parents make the transition from the hospital to the home. Parents seemed to apply everything that the NICU nurses told them. *"It was really hard to get through to him [the father] the importance [of feeding] 'cause he figured that we couldn't do anything else for him cause the NICU nurses taught him everything they needed to know"* (PHN #4). Parents of LPIs cared for in the NICU *"typically find it quite difficult to go from that rigid, every 3-hour feeding schedule, to knowing when and how to transition or move, um, onto demand feeding"* (PHN #8). Some PHNs expressed that these inconsistencies in messages result from the lack of anticipatory guidance parents received from other health care professionals while in the hospital. *"They [parents] feel very overwhelmed"* (PHN #2) especially if uninformed about the likelihood of multi-faceted health challenges. *"They don't always absorb everything that you're saying cause it's a lot for them"* (PHN #2). The parents of LPIs *"really do struggle... [The] mother is exhausted by the time morning rolls around...then she's got the rest of the family to look after"* (PHN #5).

From PHNs' perception, what parents perceive as inconsistent care is in fact PHNs modifying care strategies relative to the LPIs' inconsistent growth and development patterns. For example, feeding behavior and growth patterns can vary as shared by PHN #7:

...oh the nurse [in the hospital] said the latch looked good. ...Well does it feel good? No it doesn't? Well, it's not supposed to hurt....Well if she told you it was relevant two days ago, ... but now on day six it's no longer the case [because] of what I'm seeing in front of me with the baby's numbers and how you're doing and how you're presenting. So based on my assessment, we're going [to need] to have a new plan.

These differences can prove difficult for parents *"it makes them upset, it makes them feel undermined"* (PHN #3) when their infants' needs change over time, and the care strategies of hospital or community nurses differ. Additionally, the lack of evidence informed practice guidelines or protocols developed for LPIs in the community added to the variability in the care that is provided. PHN #10 described the dilemma succinctly,

> "...there's not much out there [referring to guidelines] ...so what do you compare them to? Do you compare them to the extreme premies or do you compare them to the term babies?"

Since they are closer in age to term infants, *"I think they [PHNs] tend to compare [LPIs]more to term children"* (PHN #10). Consequently, some PHNs treat LPIs like term babies while others rely on their own experiential knowledge. This practice contributes to various PHNs having different ideas about the direction of care for LPIs. PHN #4 indicated that she *"...would have done [things] differently than what the other nurse had done. Like she had just said that we would call her, but I would have seen that baby again."* PHNs also discussed the need for a consistent caregiver to follow the family and follow through on care suggestions: *"...I think it [having the same PHN follow up] would help"* (PHN #2). The reason for this is because *"sometimes we only see them that one time and then someone else will follow up so you don't really get to...see [the] whole thing"* (PHN #2). This lack of continuity of care can be detrimental to the LPI and families since *"you make this promise and then the next day they [another PHN] phone and they don't fulfill that promise with the mother. They change it [the care plan] and that is a downward spiral"* (PHN #1).

Whereas care practices between RNs practicing in the hospital and home do vary, other health care professionals also contributed to the lack of consistency. PHN #5 shared her perspective:

> Unfortunately, sometimes, what happens is they go to the family doctor, and the family doctor tells them everything is okay – see you in two months – and then we don't get a chance to see them again. Because...the baby may not be feeding well, and we may have concerns, but sometimes it's hard to get those families to buy in [to what we can offer].

PHNs also struggle with parental perception of hierarchy with health care professionals. *"...A lot of times the doctor's word is the end word"* (PHN #5). This causes difficulties between the PHN and the parent if they have received conflicting advice from the PHN.

Theme 4: Financial constraints on health promotion: "She had nobody. No vehicle...we might be bringing them into clinic, two, three days in a row and that's pretty punishing for them"

The PHNs expressed concern about the financial constraints on public health funding and the implications for providing postpartum care to an increasing number of families. PHN #1 explained her dilemma as follows: *"if we bring them to clinic [it is more efficient because] more people [can be] seen in the day..."*. However, PHNs understand the limitations of a clinic visit, since the clinic setting does not offer the best setting in which to observe feeding practices. For this reason, they prefer to assess and counsel mothers in their homes. PHN #3 stated:

> as a lactation consultant, I feel strongly that if I can see a mother in her own chair, with her own pillow, to look at her own comfort, in her own home, it is a very different experience from bringing them in to the clinic. And that helps enormously.

PHNs described a preference for delivering care in the home since it provides the opportunity to understand the family's physical environment and social support network first hand: *"...when we are in the home we can see exactly what's in the environment. We probably get a better idea of the social situation probably in their home..."* (PHN #8). Given their fragility, LPIs remain susceptible to environmental influences, and PHNs prefer a home visit to conduct a proper assessment and intervene more effectively. PHN #5 explained, *"The advantage of home visit is you're not bringing out a new baby ...putting her in a car or bringing her for a half-hour drive to see you... They're sore, they're tired, they don't feel great, and they want to be at home."* Furthermore, home visits are preferable *"...if it's especially warm or really cool or really windy or really rainy day, [home visits] help prevent [any associated risks of] these changes in temperature for the babies"* (PHN #9). Finally, home visits are preferable since *"...they're[parents] comfortable in their setting. They're more relaxed in their [home] setting and they can speak freely"* (PHN #5).

PHN #1 stated her rationale for home visits quite convincingly:

> ...When you go to their home, it's easier to see if their living conditions are very poor. If you get to the front door and the screen is all ripped out and there are cigarette butts everywhere outside the front door and beer bottles, it's a different situation than as if they have been asked to come to the clinic and so you need that 2 h to get into even[assess] the finances and start resources for the mother that have not been really worked on enough in the hospital.

Some PHNs voiced concern for families with serious transportation problems. For them, access became an obstacle. In the case of one family: *"She [the mother] didn't have any other family in Calgary... She had nobody. No vehicle, no access to a vehicle"* (PHN #2). The demands could become even more difficult if *"...we are seeing them the next day and we might be bringing them into clinic, two, three days in a row and that's pretty punishing for them..."* (PHN #3). For many vulnerable families, home visitation would more likely ensure that parents and LPIs receive the quality of care required.

Discussion

This study represents the first in-depth exploration of PHNs' lived experience of caring for LPIs in the community. The research findings describe how the lack of evidence informed guidelines, consistent care pathways, coordination of care, and general resources affected nursing care.

PHNs shared their experiences surrounding the care of LPIs in the community and how the vulnerability and fragility of LPIs requires special attention. Multifaceted health challenges include: temperature instability and jaundice, as well as feeding difficulties. These physical challenges relate to the developmental and neurological immaturity of the infant [8, 10]. This becomes problematic for health care providers when there are not specific care guidelines tailored to LPIs experiencing such challenges. Narratives from PHNs told how in the absence of such guidelines, providers and caregivers often treat LPIs as term infants. This thinking reinforces misunderstandings about differences in growth parameters, and how feeding problems related to choking and aspiration, as well as jaundice and temperature instability are sometimes under assessed for LPIs. Our findings suggest PHNs require evidence informed care and feeding guidelines when caring for LPIs. Such an approach has worked successfully in the hospital setting [22].

Home care guidelines would particularly benefit those families of LPIs discharged early [14]. Reyna, Pickler, and Thompson [23] in their study of early preterm infants transitioning home from the NICU environment, suggest focusing on common feeding issues, such as suck swallow breath coordination as well as hunger and satiety cues. Since LPIs face similar challenges, guidelines would apply to them as well. Other researchers have proposed strategies and resources for health care providers working with premature infants. The researchers recommend that providers address the psychological strain parents can experience when caring for LPIs, including anxiety and apprehension relating to feeding difficulties, and the lack of personal confidence to provide the appropriate level of care at home [24–29].

The lack of evidence informed guidelines for LPIs may lead to inconsistent care by health care professionals. These inconsistencies can distress and confuse parents. Boykova [30], Russell and colleagues [31], and Boykova and Kenner [32] found similar results highlighting that parents require nurses with specialized knowledge of the preterm infant and discrepancies in care amongst nurses may not only affect care outcomes, but ultimately results in a lack of confidence and trust in the health care provider.

Our findings suggest that acute care providers in the hospital need to prepare parents for the unique challenges of caring for a LPI. The need for meticulous attention to discharge planning is congruent with a synthesis of literature. Adama, Ayes and Sundin [29], Boykova [30], Griffin and Pickler [26], and Jefferies [33] collectively recommend that preterm infants require early intervention in discharge planning well before the date of discharge. It is important for discharge planning to include assessing parental knowledge barriers surrounding care of the preterm infant. Griffin and Pickler [26] go further to recommend that prior to discharge, nurses should provide a structured and individualized discharge plan, including assessment of suitability for discharge, based on the infant's needs, parental competencies, resources, and risk factors. Furthermore, Boykova [30] suggests conducting an assessment of parents' emotional state as well as the availability and quality of social supports available prior to discharge. Boykova [30] emphasizes that parental learning needs change over time. During the initial period following discharge, parents require information about care giving and medical conditions. Over time, these learning needs change and parents need information regarding growth and development. Hence, it is necessary for PHNs to consider how learning needs evolve and adapt their parental support measures accordingly.

Finally, financial constraints continue to restrict the allocation of resources for PHNs to care and coordinate interventions for LPIs and their families. Time constraints and limitations on the number of visits requires communication and continuity of care with all providers that care for LPIs. An interdisciplinary approach to care, from hospital to home, involving PHNs, physicians, and other health care professionals can be organized into a model of care specifically for LPIs. Follow up care using such care teams for seamless transition into the community is well supported in the literature to address vulnerable populations, including early and very early preterm infants transitioning from NICU [34–36] and medically fragile infants [37, 38].

Our study focused on postpartum community services in Calgary. We interviewed PHNs once during the study and did not return our analyses to them for member checking. We did, however, present our findings to PHNs who agreed with our findings. We did not triangulate the PHNs' perspectives about parents of LPIs with parents' experience of caring for LPIs.

Conclusion

This study contributes to our understanding of how PHNs perceive the challenges of caring for LPIs within the community setting. Given these findings, we believe more research needs to be done to identify the complex health care needs of LPIs and their parents in the community setting. More studies would lead to the development of research-informed practice guidelines; and encourage a more integrated approach of health care delivery from hospital to home, in order to improve the quality of care for families of LPIs.

Abbreviations

LPI: Late preterm infants; PHN: Public health nurse

Acknowledgements

We would like to acknowledge Postpartum Community Services, Calgary, Alberta, public health nurses, and parents who participated in our study. We would also like to thank our research team for their contributions to our study.

Funding

This study was funded by the Alberta Centre for Child, Family & Community Research Centre, and the integrated knowledge translation activities were supported by the University of Calgary Seed Grant. The funding bodies were not involved in the design, collection, analysis and interpretation of data, or the writing of this manuscript. The funds provided were used for operational costs of the project.

Authors' contributions

GC, AD, SSP, SR, AL and MY made substantial contributions to the study design, acquisition, analysis and interpretation of data. GC, AD, SSP, SR, and AL made substantial contribution to the analysis and interpretation of data. GC and AD drafted the manuscript. All authors revised the manuscript critically for important intellectual content; gave final approval of the version to be published; and agreed to be accountable for all aspects of the work.

Competing interests

The authors declare that they have no competing interests.

Author details

[1]School of Nursing and Midwifery, Mount Royal University, 4825 Mount Royal Gate SW, Calgary, Alberta T3E 6K6, Canada. [2]O'Brien Institute of Public Health, University of Calgary, Calgary, Alberta, Canada. [3]Faculty of Nursing, University of Calgary, 2500 University Drive NW, Calgary, Alberta T2N 1N4, Canada. [4]Department of Paediatrics, Section of Neonatology, Alberta Health Services, Foothills Medical Centre, 1403 29th Street NW, Calgary, Alberta T2N 2T9, Canada. [5]Alberta Children's Hospital Research Institute, Calgary, Alberta, Canada. [6]Prenatal & Postpartum Services, Public Health Calgary Zone, Alberta Health Services, 1430, 10101 Southport Road SW, Calgary, Alberta T2W 3N2, Canada.

References

1. Canadian Institute for Health Information. Inpatient hospitalizations, surgeries and childbirth indicators in 2014–2015. https://secure.cihi.ca/free_products/CAD_Hospitalization_and_Childbirth_Snapshot_EN.PDF. Accessed 15 Mar 2016).
2. Canadian Institute for Health Information. Childbirth indicators by place of residents, 2014–2015. https://apps.cihi.ca/mstrapp/asp/Main.aspx?Server=apmstrextprd_i&project=Quick%20Stats&uid=pce_pub_en&pwd=&evt=2048001&visualizationMode=0&documentID=029DB170438205AEBCC75B8673CCE822. Accessed 29 Aug 2016.
3. Kugleman A, Colin AA. Late preterm infants: near term but still in a critical developmental time period. Pediatrics. 2013;132(4):741–51.
4. Whyte RK. Safe discharge of the late preterm infant [position statement FN 2010-01]. Paediatr Child Health. 2010;15(10):665–0.
5. Cleaveland K. Feeding challenges in the late preterm infant. Neonatal Netw. 2010;29(1):37–41.
6. Nagulesapillai T, McDonald S, Fenton T, Mercader H, Tough S. Breastfeeding Difficulties and exclusivity among late preterm and term infants: results from the all our babies study. Can J Public Health. 2013;104(4):e351–6.
7. Laptook A, Jackson GL. Cold stress and hypoglycemia in the late preterm ("near-term") infant: impact on nursery of admission. Semin Perinatol. 2006;30(1):24–7.
8. Wang ML, Dorer DJ, Fleming MP, Catlin EA. Clinical outcomes of near-term infants. Pediatrics. 2004;114(2):372–6.
9. Jain S, Cheng J. Emergency department visits and rehospitalizations in late preterm infants. Clin Perinatol. 2006;33(4):935–45.
10. Escobar GJ, Greene JD, Hulac P, Kincannon E, Bischoff K, Gardner MN, et al. Rehospitalization after birth hospitalization: patterns among infants of all gestations. Arch Dis Child. 2005;90:125–31.
11. Ray KN, Lorch SA. Hospitalization of early preterm, late preterm, and term infants during the first year of life by gestational age. Hosp Pediatr. 2013;3(3):194–203.
12. Goyal NK, Folger AT, Hall ES, Ammerman RT, Ginkel JB, Pickler RS. Effects of home visiting and maternal mental health on use of the emergency department among late preterm infants. J Obstet Gynecol Neonatal Nurs. 2015;44(1):135–44.
13. Berreth K. Public health nurses provide preventative programs, promote health, mobilize communities. Alta RN. 2013;68(4):20–2.
14. Premji SS, Young M, Rogers C, Reilly S. Transitions in the early-life of late preterm infants: vulnerabilities and implications for postpartum care. J Perinat Neonatal Nurs. 2012;26(1):57–68.
15. Hanson WE, Creswell JW, Clark VLP, Petska SK, Creswell JD. Mixed methods research designs in counseling psychology. J Couns Psychol. 2005;52(2):224–35.
16. Starks H, Trinidad SB. Choose your method: a comparison of phenomenology, discourse analysis, and grounded theory. Qual Health Res. 2007;17(10):1372–80.
17. Giorgi A. The theory, practice, and evaluation of the phenomenological method as a qualitative research procedure. Phenomenological Psychology. 1997;28(2):235–60.
18. Premji S, Currie G, Reilly S, Dosani A, Oliver LM, Lodha AK, Young M. A qualitative study: mothers of late preterm infants relate their experiences of community-based care. PLoS One. 2017 Mar 23;12(3):e0174419.
19. Premji SS, Pana G, Currie G, Dosani A, Reilly S, Young M, Hall M, Williamson T, Lodha AK. Mother'S level of confidence in caring for her late preterm infant: a mixed methods study. J Clin Nurs. 2017. Dec 1;27(5-6):e1120–33.
20. Cleary MC, Horsfall JH, Hayter MH. Data collection and sampling in qualitative research: does size matter? J Adv Nurs. 2014;70(3):473–5.
21. Colaizzi PF. Psychological research as the phenomenologist views it. In: Valle R, King M, editors. Existential phenomenological alternatives for psychology. New York: Oxford University Press; 1978. p. 48–71.
22. Baker B. Evidence-based practice to improve outcomes for late preterm infants. J Obstet Gynecol Neonatal Nurs. 2015;44:127–34.
23. Reyna BA, Pickler RH, Thompson A. A descriptive study of mothers' experiences feeding their preterm infants after discharge. Advanced Neonatal Care. 2006;6(6):333–40.

24. McDonald SW, Benzies KM, Gallant JE, McNeil DA, Dolan SM, Tough SCA. Comparison between late preterm and term infants on breastfeeding and maternal mental health. Matern Child Health J. 2013;17(8):1468–77.

25. Hill A. Mothers' Perceptions of child vulnerability in previous preterm infants. ABNF Journal. 2015;26(1):11–6.

26. Griffin J, Pickler R. Hospital to home transition of mothers of preterm infants. MCN Am J Matern Child Nurs. 2011;36(4):252–7.

27. Phillips-Pula L, Pickler R, McGrath J, Brown L, Dusing S. Caring for a preterm infant at home. a mother's perspective J Perinat Neonatal Nurs. 2013;40(6):335–44.

28. Murdoch MR, Franck LS. Gaining confidence and perspective: a phenomenological study of mothers' lived experience caring for infants at home after neonatal unit discharge. J Adv Nurs. 2011;68(9):2008–20.

29. Adama EA, Bayes S, Sundin D. Parents' experiences of caring for preterm infants after discharge from neonatal intensive care unit: a meta-synthesis of the literature. J Neonatal Nurs. 2016;22(1):27–51.

30. Boykova M. Transition from hospital to home in parents of preterm infants. J Perinat Neonatal Nurs. 2016;30(4):327–248.

31. Russell G, Sawyer A, Rabe H, Abbott J, Gyte G, Duley L, et al. Parents' views on care of their very premature babies in neonatal intensive care units: a qualitative study. BMC Pediatr. 2014;14:230.

32. Boykova M, Kenner C. Transition from hospital to home for parents of preterm infants. J Perinat Neonatal Nurs. 2012;26(1):81–7.

33. Jefferies AL. Going home: facilitating the discharge of the preterm infant. Pediatr Child Health. 2014;19(1):31–6.

34. Browne JV. Developmental care for high-risk newborns: emerging science, clinical application, and continuity of from newborn intensive care unit to community. Clin Perinatol. 2011;38:719–29.

35. Ritchie SK. Primary care of the premature infant discharged from the neonatal intensive care unit. MCN Am J Matern Child Nurs. 2002;27(2):76–86.

36. Lasby K, Newton S, Platen A. A New frontier: neonatal transitional care. Can Nurse. 2004;100(8):19–23.

37. Cherouny PH, Federico FA, Haraden C, Leavitt GS, Resar R. Idealized design of perinatal care: IHI innovation series white paper. Cambridge, Massachusetts: Institute for Healthcare Improvement; 2005.

38. Robinson M, Pirak C, Morrell C. Multidisciplinary discharge assessment of the medically and socially high-risk infant. J Perinat Neonatal Nurs. 2000;13(4):67–86.

15

What relatives of older medical patients want us to know - a mixed-methods study

Ditte Maria Sivertsen[1*] ⓘ, Louise Lawson-Smith[2] and Tove Lindhardt[3]

Abstract

Background: Relatives of acutely hospitalised older medical patients often act as case managers during a hospital trajectory. Therefore, relatives' experiences of collaboration with staff and their involvement in care and treatment are highly important. However, it is a field facing many challenges. Greater knowledge of the values and areas that are most important to relatives is needed to facilitate the health care staff to better understand and prepare themselves for collaboration with relatives and to guide family care.

Methods: The aims were to 1) describe the aspects of collaboration with staff during the hospital care trajectory emphasised by relatives of older medical patients 2) compare the characteristics of relatives who wrote free-text notes and those who did not. Relatives of acutely hospitalised older medical patients responded to a structured questionnaire ($n = 180$), and nearly half wrote free-text comments ($n = 79$). Free text was analysed with qualitative content analysis. Differences between (+) free text/ (−) free text groups were analysed with χ^2 test and Kruskal-Wallis test.

Results: Analysis disclosed three categories I) *The evasive white flock*, concerning the experienced evasiveness in staff attitudes and availability, II) *The absence of care* as perceived by the relatives and III) *Invisible & unrecognised* describing relatives' experience of staff's lack of communication, involvement and interactions with relatives especially regarding discharge.
Significant differences were found between relatives who wrote free-text and those who did not regarding satisfaction, trust and having a health care education.

Conclusions: This study provides knowledge of aspects relatives of older medical patients find particularly problematic and, further, of characteristics of relatives using the free-text field. Overall, these relatives were met with evasiveness from staff, an absence of care and felt invisible and unrecognised in the lacking collaboration with staff. Hence, strategies to ensure quality care and systematic involvement of relatives are needed, and the findings in this study may contribute to, and guide, quality improvement of family centered care in acute hospital wards.

Keywords: Acute hospitalisation, Collaboration, Free text, Older medical patient, Relatives

Background

During a hospital stay older medical patients are often accompanied by relatives. These relatives have important knowledge about their older relative, since they are involved in managing their daily life activities [1, 2], and they often feel responsible for the older person's wellbeing, monitor their professional care and advocate for quality care aimed at increasing the older person's chances of staying independent [3, 4].

Health-care utilization, mainly inpatient care, increases with age, especially in high-income countries [5]. In Danish medical wards, patients above 65 years old constitute 53% of all admissions [6]. Both national and international policy strategies focus on increasing the involvement of patients and relatives in care and in care decisions to ensure an individualised care trajectory that meets both patients' and relatives' expectations [7, 8]. However, there seems to be a gap between policy and practice, since a national survey shows that patients and their relatives in the Capital Region of Denmark feel less involved in their care trajectory than in other regions [9].

* Correspondence: ditte.maria.sivertsen@regionh.dk
[1]Optimed, Clinical Research Centre (Section 056), Copenhagen University Hospital Hvidovre, Kettegård Allé 30, DK-2650 Hvidovre, Denmark
Full list of author information is available at the end of the article

Many relatives take on the role as case manager of the hospital trajectory to pursue continuity and high-quality care for the older patient, and their satisfaction with care and treatment is tied to the degree of collaboration with the hospital staff as well as to their reported feelings of guilt and powerlessness [1]. This indicates that relatives have emotional issues related to the hospital context that affect their experience and perceptions. An Australian study explored the immediate needs of relatives of acutely ill older patients through interviews (*n* = 10) and found that *being informed* and *being there* were essential for relatives. However, participants were included at both medical and surgical wards and therefore differs from our patient group of older medical patients [10]. A systematic review from England examining both patients' and relatives' perspectives in acute care settings found that relational approaches to care led to more positive experiences during acute hospitalization [11]. As noted, collaboration between relatives and staff is highly relevant when caring for older patients, but several studies show that this can be hard to achieve [4, 12, 13]. As an example, a review of staff-family relationships found that while families of older people value collaboration in care, staff members acknowledge its importance, but have difficulty translating theory into practice [12]. Relatives report that they have to stand up for themselves and for the patients in order to overcome these conflicts in values and the discrepancies in defining the patient's situation [3, 14]. Greater knowledge of the values and areas that are most important to relatives would help the healthcare staff better understand and prepare themselves for collaboration with relatives.

Asking respondents to add free-text comments in questionnaires is common practice; However, it is less common to use them for analysis. Yet, they may increase our understanding of respondents' responses and experiences and identify areas that are particularly important to the target group. This may guide development of clinical practice as well as future research [15]. An unexpected large amount of questionnaires were returned with free-text notes, and that raised our interest in what they wanted to tell us, as well as in what characterises the respondent, who puts time and effort into making free-text notes in an already comprehensive and demanding questionnaire. Out of respect for this effort, we further found that we had an obligation to use these data. The data material is part of a bigger study, and the quantitative questionnaire results are presented elsewhere [16]. To our knowledge, no studies have, until now, analysed free-text comments from relatives of older acutely admitted medical patients.

Methods
Aim
The aim of this study was to explore the use and content of a free text possibility in a structured survey by:

- Describing the aspects of collaboration with staff during the hospital trajectory emphasised by relatives of older medical patients.
- Comparing characteristics of relatives who wrote free-text notes and those who did not.

Design
A cross-sectional, descriptive and comparative mixed-method design was applied analysing free text data from a structured survey study.

Setting and data collection
The study was conducted at the Medical Department of a Copenhagen University Hospital covering seven wards. Patients matching inclusion criteria were approached consecutively after admission, informed about the project and asked for permission to contact the relative that helped them the most. If patients gave written consent, the relative was contacted by phone to obtain verbal permission to send the questionnaire to them. An envelope containing the questionnaire, written information about the project and a prepaid return envelope was then sent to the relative. Returning the questionnaire was considered as written consent according to Danish law practice. Questionnaires were completed after the patients' discharge. Data collection took place from November 2010–November 2011.

Participants
Relatives of older medical patients (≥65 years, acutely admitted, living at home, able to cooperate, and having comorbidities or receiving home care) were eligible for inclusion. *Relatives* were the persons appointed by the patient as the one providing the most help; this could be a family member, friend or acquaintance.

The family collaboration scale
The Family Collaboration Scale (FCS) is a validated structured questionnaire measuring collaboration with health care professionals as experienced by relatives of older patients [17]. FCS covers four dimensions: 1) Attributes of collaboration; 2) Prerequisites of collaboration; 3) Outcomes of collaboration; and 4) Promoters of and barriers to collaboration. A free-text field on the last page encourages subjective descriptions of experiences and reflections: *"If you have any additions regarding the collaboration with staff that you think the questionnaire did not deal with sufficiently, feel free to write them here"*.

Data analysis
Quantitative data
Respondents who provided written comments were compared with those who did not in terms of age, gender, kinship, education, helping frequency, duration of caregiving

and scores of trust and satisfaction with the hospital trajectory in the structured part of the FCS. To give an overall picture of the comments a frequency count was performed to identify the ratio of positive (i.e. praise) and critical comments. This was done by counting the predominance of sentences with positive respectively critical content. Categorical data were analysed with χ^2 test, and Kruskal-Wallis test was used to analyse numerical data. SAS 9.3 software was used for statistical analysis.

Qualitative data

The handwritten comments were transcribed and merged into one document while keeping the ID number of each comment for identification. Qualitative content analysis was performed [18]. The data set was read several times to achieve a general understanding. Hereafter the text was divided into *meaning units*, which were further reduced into *condensed meaning units*. A *code* was derived representing the core of each meaning unit. Codes were sorted into categories, which were labelled in accordance with the meaning content (see Table 1). Two of the authors (DMS, TL) performed this analysis and discussed the findings until reaching consensus. The authors' pre-understandings will influence the analysis and interpretation of data; hence the two authors strived to be aware of their pre-understandings and challenge each other in the analysis process.

Ethical considerations

Written and oral information was given to both patients and relatives, emphasizing that participation was voluntary, that withdrawal from the project could be done at any time and that participants' identities would be kept confidential. None of the researchers were employed in the participating wards.

Results
Participants

We received 180 of the 279 questionnaires that were sent out (response rate, 64.5%). Of these, 79 (44%) had free-text comments. The comments ranged in length from 5 to 1298 words, with a total of 7662 words and a mean of 97 words per comment. Sixty-eight percent of the comments were written by women (see Table 2). There were significant differences between relatives who wrote comments and those who did not. Of those who provided free-text only 38.4% reported high satisfaction at admission, whereas the no-comment group reported 57.6% ($p = 0.008$). The results were similar for the two groups' satisfaction during hospital stay (41.1% vs. 56.1%, $p = 0.001$) and at discharge (32.9% vs. 43.9%, $p = 0.030$). Also, more respondents who scored low on trust in the structured part of the FCS made notes in the free-text field (39% vs. 54.6%, p = 0.008) and finally those who had a health education elaborated more in free-text (26% vs. 13.3%, $p = 0.033$). There were no significant differences in other background variables between the two groups. However, although not significant, more respondents with high school or university education made free-text comments than did those with public school education.

Five comments were entirely positive expressing praise and satisfaction with the hospital trajectory, 40 comments were entirely critical and 34 comments were mixed. Overall, the positive statements tended to be more general in nature, while the critical ones tended to provide more detailed descriptions.

Findings

The encounter with the hospital system was the overarching theme, and communication seemed to be central in all categories. Three categories emerged: *The evasive white*

Table 1 Example of the analytical process used for qualitative content analysis

Meaning unit	Condensed meaning unit	Code	Category
Most of them [staff] were stressed and had very little time to inform relatives when asked (Daughter, age 43)	Staff was stressed and gave little information	Workload is a barrier for communication	The evasive white flock
I find it very difficult to tell the difference between nurses, doctors, porters etc. it makes it very difficult to approach the right one – in my case a nurse (Son, age 36)	Difficult to distinguish between staff groups	Approachability	The evasive white flock
Even though I made staff aware that my father lived on nutritional protein drinks after surgery for throat cancer, they kept serving him brown bread and stuff like that. For a whole day he got nothing to eat or drink... (Daughter, age 65)	Staff not considerate of eating issues and did not provide appropriate food	Basic care need: Eat and drink adequately	Absence of care
Came home in rainy weather in a taxi wearing nothing but slippers, white long underpants and an undershirt. It was cold. (Son, age 66)	Patient was sent home in his underwear in cold weather	Basic care need: maintaining body temperature and dignity	Absence of care
We had to seek all information ourselves, and a discharge meeting was held only after I put my foot down (Son, age 59)	Information and involvement only happened upon relative's own initiative	Lack of communication and involvement	Invisible & unrecognised
My father was for a while treated as a diabetic patient with insulin injections, although he is not diabetic. I made staff aware of this, but I was rejected. 3 days went by, before they stopped the injections. (Daughter, age 56)	Staff did not pay attention to the relative, and treated the patient incorrectly	Lack of communication and involvement	Invisible & unrecognised

Table 2 Characteristics of relatives who did or did not add free-text comments to the Family Collaboration Scale questionnaire

	Added comments (n = 79)	n	No comments (n = 101)	n	P-value*
Age, years, mean	60.3	78	60.8	98	0.998
Sex, Female, %	67.5	77	66.0	100	0.830
Relationship with patient, %					
Spouse	22.8	79	27.7	101	0.749
Offspring	62.0	79	58.4	101	
Other	15.2	79	13.9	101	
Education, %					
Public school	64.1	78	74.3	101	0.143
High school/ University	35.9	78	25.7	101	
Health education, %	26.0	77	13.3	98	**0.033**
High degree of satisfaction with hospital care**, %					
At admission	38.4	73	57.6	99	**0.008**
During the hospital stay	41.1	73	56.1	98	**0.001**
At discharge	32.9	73	43.9	98	**0.030**
High degree of trust in the provided care**, %					
I trusted that my relative got the care s/he needed	39.0	77	54.6	99	**0.008**

*SAS 9.3 was used for the statistical analysis. The χ^2 test was used to analyze categorical data, and the Kruskal-Wallis test was used to analyze numerical data. P-values < 0.05 were considered significant and are highlighted in bold font
**Response categories in the questionnaire were: high degree, some degree, less degree, not at all

flock describing perceptions of staff attitudes and availability; *The absence of care* describing relatives' perceptions of hospital care; *Invisible & unrecognised* concerning the lack of involvement and collaboration experienced by relatives. The categories were closely interrelated and had in common a predominant sense of 'something' that was missing. We found all of the following categories covered in the questionnaire, hence, these aspects were seemingly either particularly central to relatives, or they were aspects of the trajectory that were particularly poorly handled by the staff, leading to a need in relatives to elaborate further in writing.

The evasive white flock
Staff attitudes and availability was a central issue for relatives in their encounter with the hospital system. Staff approachability was also an issue, and relatives described observing the staff and trying to find an appropriate moment to approach them. Several comments included descriptions of a futile search for someone to talk to among the staff. The staff did not appear to be visible and available, creating an unwelcoming atmosphere for the relatives. The search for a relevant person to contact was like a game of hide and seek and several comments described unfriendly behaviour from the staff. Although some were accessible and helpful, others had dismissive attitudes when relatives approached them with questions.

It was quite impossible to speak to a nurse; they were just simply not there, no matter where we searched.

When we found one, they did not have the time – "ask someone else" or "he belongs to some other nurse" (...) In some cases the nurses were quite rude when we tried to get information (Daughter, age 64).

The nurses' unavailability seemed to be a barrier to interaction. Moreover, relatives found it difficult to identify which staff to approach for information. The uniforms all looked the same to the relatives, and the staff was seen as one big group of people, all dressed in white. The text indicated that relatives experienced the ward as a busy environment in which the staff was always short of time and where it was hard for relatives to identify the right person to approach for information about the care of their hospitalized relative. Many relatives reported that the staff seemed busy and stressed. At times this created barriers in the communication process and made relatives hesitate to approach the staff.

The interaction between staff and relatives could be improved if you did not feel like you were interrupting the staff's routines (...) It is difficult to find the right time to discuss your relative's situation with the staff without feeling a bit "in the way" (Daughter, age 55).

The relatives felt that they disturbed the staff and interrupted their routines when they wished to talk about the patient's situation. The working conditions and time pressure were in some comments used as explaining factors for missing interaction, information and staff being dismissive.

> The staff in the ward was very busy, but in spite of that, as a relative, it was frustrating that there was no proper communication, one could only feel sorry for the staff having the burden they clearly experienced. However, I am sad that I never felt that I could get a satisfactory answer when I approached them (Granddaughter, age 34).

The comments expressed ambivalent feelings about the staff. Although relatives described being frustrated over poor communication and the lack of satisfactory answers, they also expressed understanding for the staff's working conditions and used these conditions as explanations for unfortunate events, praising their efforts in a high-pressure working environment.

The absence of care

This category describes experiences connected to nursing care. Descriptions of basic care needs that were not met were plenty and regardless of their sympathy for the staff's workload and time pressure, the relatives expressed strong concerns over patient needs that were neglected. The comments included descriptions such as lack of sufficient nutrition, insufficient personal hygiene, dirty linen and clothing and a general lack of professional and compassionate care.

One relative considered the absence of care to be a contributing factor to the death of his mother and generalized the experience by expressing concern for other patients as well.

> My mother was sent home without proper clothing, in just underwear and a thin dressing gown in a transport car without assistance. She had to climb up the stairs to the 1st floor. She was hospitalised again the following day, and she died three days later. I hope that other elderly people are not treated in this manner (Son, age 68).

Comments about drug administration raised issues such as patients not receiving sufficient analgesics, medicine given in the wrong dose, adverse drug events and missing medication reconciliation. Medicine-related errors related to lack of communication were described by relatives who had provided the staff with important information about the medication; however, the staff did not seem to be responsive or to take the information into consideration.

> As a daughter, I know all about my mother and her medication, and yet they would not listen, so it

> [medication] was given incorrectly - disgraceful (Daughter, age 59).

The physical environment and especially the lack of a calm, health-promoting environment, seemed to affect the relatives' perceptions of hospital care. Several relatives complained about insufficient cleaning of the wards, which gave them a bad impression of the hospital as a whole. Privacy and dignity issues were also a concern. Some perceived sharing a room to reduce dignity and to affect tranquillity and sleep. Loss of dignity was also described when patients were moved, like pieces of furniture, from one room to another several times during their stay.

Invisible & unrecognised

Analysis indicated that relatives felt invisible and unrecognised in situations where they actually tried to obtain some kind of collaboration with staff. Their expertise was seemingly not requested, and they were not involved at moments where they considered their participation to be crucial, for instance when getting closer to a date of discharge. Information, coordination and involvement were, in the eyes of the relatives, important for a satisfactory discharge process. Extra home care, medicine or rehabilitation were mentioned as interventions relatives needed to collaborate with staff about. Not being informed or involved in planning or decision processes frustrated the relatives, who described how they had to be proactive and persistent in order to get involved and to obtain adequate information. In some cases, missing information even affected the relationship between the patient and his or her relative, and clear and direct information about the patient's status was wanted.

> My mother died during hospitalisation, and I would like to have had specific information about how serious the situation was. Instead, doctors and nursing staff used general terms and hints (Son, age 55).

Lack of information had consequences for the relatives' possibility for providing support and planning of the future care. Several relatives reported that information about discharge was not given until a few hours before discharge. This prevented relatives in preparing the patient's homecoming. Some were not informed of the discharge at all.

> Were never informed of the discharge. Were never involved in the process (...) Very poor communication (Daughter, age 45).

Information about how to care for the patient at home was also called for; some relatives expressed uncertainty about which symptoms they should be aware of or how to react if symptoms worsened.

In some cases, patients seemed to be sent home too soon and were, in the relative's opinion, not ready for discharge. Different kinds of barriers to continuity in the care trajectory were described, e.g. insufficient transition of information through the system and to municipal care agencies, and lack of communication between in-hospital units and other hospitals, as well as between staff and relatives.

The relatives expressed frustration over hospital staff's lack of interest and sense of responsibility for patient after discharge. Sometimes the relatives contacted the discharging hospital unit for some piece of information or follow-up on the discharge arrangements and were met with indifference.

...Then I called the hospital unit the day after discharge, and I was told that the case was filed now that my mother-in-law was discharged (Daughter-in-law, age 59).

In contrast, The Supported Discharge Team was highlighted as a positive and successful initiative that involved relatives in the discharge process. This team was perceived as being empathic and taking the time to understand the patient in his/her daily context.

Discussion

The main aim of this study was to explore aspects of the hospital trajectory, relatives needed to emphasize. The three categories that emerged were: the evasive white flock, absence of care and invisible & unrecognised. Relatives needed guidance and, at the same time, felt that they were in the way and a disturbance to the staff. The first category concerning evasiveness of the nurses seemed central to this paradox. Studies of how nurses view collaborations with relatives have found that although relatives are considered an important resource, in practice nurses try to avoid relatives, particularly if they are perceived to be demanding [13, 19]. Lindhardt et al. [13] found a pattern of 'escape-avoidance' conduct, which, from the relative's point of view, may be perceived as unavailability as described in our study. The nurses' non-verbal communication of time pressure further inhibited communication by making relatives hesitate to approach them to avoid disturbing their work activities. The inaccessibility of nurses and relatives' reluctance to disturb staff are well-known problems in the collaboration between relatives and nurses. Literature has described these problems in different contexts, e.g. in medical wards [4], nursing home [20] and in complaints from both patients and relatives regarding encounters and communication at a large Swedish hospital [21] indicating its persistence and widespread occurrence. Our results indicated that what researchers have found to be culturally embedded behaviour

of nurses is perceived by relatives as inaccessibility and as a barrier to contact and communication.

Absense of care was identified as the second category. Care is the essence of nursing [22]. However, the relatives in our study reported that in their experience, care was not always prioritised in everyday nursing practice, and they described in detail examples of this. There seemed to be a discrepancy between their expectations and the practice they encountered in the acute hospital context. Other studies have shown that relatives of older patients in acute hospital wards provide informal care [23]. Given the inclusion criteria (i.e. comorbidities and receiving home care) it may well be that the relatives in our study were informal caregivers. If so, they may have had special knowledge of the care needed by their hospitalised older relative, and when they observed that these needs were not met by the formal caregivers, it led to frustration. Relatives with a health education more often made comments. Taverner et al. [24] analysed the experiences of registered nurses who were also family caregivers of hospitalised older people, and found that these subjects experienced a culture of care where neglect were normalised, and therefore had to act *"vigil by the bedside"*, causing feelings of distress and disjuncture between their own identity as a nurse and the care they witnessed. Similarly, this vigilant monitoring has been described elsewhere, when caregivers' unmet expectations were replaced by uncertainty and suspiciousness [4]. Theories of informal caregiving has identified *worry* and *the protective dimension* as central aspects [25, 26]. Studies have shown that some relatives in acute medical wards 'stand guard' to protect the patient from flaws and poor care and that they feel responsible for the patient's wellbeing [14]. The perceived absence of care, in our study, may create such worries and awareness, and this may explain the frustrations and the emphasis on the lack of care and collaboration expressed in the study.

In our study the relatives' inclination to write free-text comments was highest among those with negative experiences. This tendency is also seen in a large study of patient satisfaction surveys ($n = 75.769$) where the least satisfied patients were most keen to elaborate in free-text [27]. The same applies to Garcia et al. [15] who has examined the use of free-text comments, and concludes that those who comment are either the articulate ones or those who have something negative to elaborate. However, this did not apply for a survey conducted among relatives of hospice patients, which showed that positive comments accounted for 75% of the free text comments [28]; hence, context seemingly is an influential factor. In the characteristics of the participants, we found that relatives scoring low on trust in our study more often elaborated in free-text writing. We cannot tell if these relatives lacked trust from the beginning and therefore were more observant and critical, or if trust disappeared due to the flaws in the care they experienced. However, trust is a value that lies within the concept of caring [29] and has been found to be central in a relative's collaboration with health care professionals [17]. Relatives hand over their loved ones to the care of hospital professionals, and for informal caregivers, this requires trust. Relatives monitor how this responsibility is handled by the professionals, and whether care is provided with engagement and empathy is likely to form the basis for trust or distrust. In the psychometric testing of the FCS, trust was found to be a special factor dimension, indicating its significance in the nurse-relative collaboration [17]. The trust dimension was shown to be particularly important in the admission phase and to correlate with the quality of contact with nurses, indicating that relational and communicative aspects are related to trust. Further, the physical environment was correlated with trust [17]. The physical environment was mentioned in our study and in conjunction with the evasive nurses, it impaired contact and communication and therefore possibly also trust. Further, the relatives in our study expressed frustration when their need for information was not acknowledged by the staff. Also, if a relative's knowledge about a patient's situation is not taken into account, insecurity may develop and trust may be threatened. Studies have pointed out that a lack of care and information creates worries, doubt and distrust [10, 21], and other studies suggest that an accessible, listening and empathic nurse is a prerequisite for successful collaboration with relatives [12, 30].

Closely connected to the experienced evasiveness from the staff was the feeling of being "invisible and unrecognised" in the third category. The lack of exchange of information between relatives and staff stood out in the comments. Relatives, particularly informal caregivers, are important sources of information, with a special need for information, as they often take over the patient's care after discharge. Communication is a prerequisite for collaboration which again is a prerequisite for sufficient exchange of information between staff and relatives [31]. A Danish study found that poor collaboration was significantly associated with relatives' low satisfaction with the care trajectory [1]. In accordance with this finding, the majority of the respondents in our study were dissatisfied with the care trajectory, and a central complaint was the lack of collaboration and communication between relatives and nurses. Communication seemed negatively affected by several factors. The relatives described how communication with staff happened when they initiated it, which is in accordance with other studies [32]. This means that seemingly even resourceful relatives, such as our respondents, were unable to obtain the communication and information they needed. Further, our study indicated that discharge was an important time at which the need for coordination and communication was crucial. However, the relatives felt ignored and that their knowledge was not granted. Studies of strategies to improve discharge planning and increase satisfaction, emphasizes an individualised approach where involvement, support and communication are important factors [33, 34].

Seemingly, relatives call for nursing delivered in accordance with nursing values, but nurses seem reluctant to provide it. However, nurses report feelings of guilt and frustration because of their inability to provide good patient care in accordance with their own professional ideals [35]. It is noticeable, that although frustrated and worried by the absence of care and evasive nurses, the relatives in our study saw nurses as victims and sympathised with them due to their stressful working conditions. This, in accordance with the study of Lindhardt et al. [14], in which relatives blamed the system rather than the people working in it. Several studies have described the dilemma of today's nurses working conditions, where nursing values compete with more powerful, organisational, value systems [31, 36]. New Public Management (NPM) and its value system governs the public sector and eldercare in Nordic countries including Denmark [37]. It represents an administrative-economic rationale and stands in contrast to nurses' professional medical rationale [36]. Effectiveness and productivity are central values in NPM and form the fundamental conditions for clinical practice in which nurses are supposed to provide care, and the nursing values may therefore be challenged within this context.

Strengths and limitations

Our results disclose aspects seemingly of particular importance to the participants in the survey, since the questionnaire had already dealt with these issues, and yet the respondents felt the need to elaborate further after completing the structured questionnaire. This provides us with information that may be used in quality improvement efforts and when planning collaborative interventions targeted relatives.

There is, however, a risk of a biased sample for several reasons. Firstly, it takes a certain amount of mental strength and energy to add notes to an already extensive structured questionnaire. Potentially, those who did not add free text were the ones under most strain. Secondly, more dissatisfied relatives added free text notes, and the notes were more often critical, a tendency described elsewhere [15, 27]. Thirdly, relatives with a health education more often wrote comments. They may have professionally-based expectations to the care trajectory, be more likely to notice flaws and may possibly be more willing to return the questionnaire. Hence, the sample was not representative, and this limits the generalizability of the conclusion.

This study demonstrated the value of combining qualitative and quantitative elements, since analysis of the survey data offered information both about the issues relatives found especially important and therefore needed to emphasize and the characteristics of respondents with particular need to elaborate in free text.

Implications for clinical practice

The free-text comments analysed in this study indicated that quality of care for older patient varies and that active strategies to ensure quality care and involvement of relatives are needed. Nursing managers should provide a framework and conditions for structured involvement in clinical practice at the cultural-, educational- and organisational levels. The perceived unavailability of nurses should be addressed by nursing leaders and clinical managers, who should encourage and facilitate constructive interactions and collaborations with relatives. There is a need to analyse nursing workloads and to prioritise nursing care. Working systematically with feedback meetings and user panels to analyse individual cases and organisational in-ward developments will ensure that valuable observations and knowledge of patients and relatives are considered. Relatives are clearly allies for nurses: they are motivated to provide good care while having sympathy and understanding for the staff's high-pressure environment. Including relatives in the planning and providing of care may promote nursing core values in clinical settings, increase the quality of care for the patient and the satisfaction among relatives.

Conclusions

In line with other studies investigating the experiences of relatives at hospitals, relatives in our study reported feeling uninvolved and 'in the way', which was a barrier for contact and communication with staff. Furthermore, collaboration was inhibited by the nurses' evasiveness. Experiences with low-quality care seemingly sparked the inclination to write free-text comments, as we identified significant differences regarding the satisfaction and trust scored by relatives who wrote free-text comments versus those who did not. Factors such as lack of contact with staff, absence of information and care and not being involved were frustrating to relatives, who seemed to be keen observers of the busy atmosphere of acute wards and to have a clear vision of good quality care. Further studies are needed to investigate characteristics of relatives who want to collaborate with staff and to test interventions in acute care settings aimed at systematically involving relatives.

Abbreviations
FCS: The Family Collaboration Scale; NPM: New Public Management

Acknowledgements
The authors would like to show our gratitude to the relatives contributing to this study and to the patients for accepting us to contact their relatives. We would also like to thank the participating hospital units and members of the Optimed research programme, especially Janne Petersen for statistics.

Funding
The study received no specific grants from any funding agency in the public, commercial or not-for-profit sectors. The authors were all employed in the hospital's Clinical Research Centre at the time of the data collection period.

Authors' contributions
Study design and idea (TL), data collection (DMS, LLS), analysis (DMS, TL), drafting of original manuscript (DMS), critical revisions & final approval (DMS, LLS, TL).

Authors' information
DMS had 2 years of clinical experience as Registered Nurse (RN) in medical wards and 5 years in research and has not previously worked theoretically with relatives. LLS had 10 years of clinical experience as RN and 5 years in research of older medical patients. TL has 40 years of experience as RN and almost 20 years of experience with research regarding relatives of older patients.

Competing interests
The authors declare that they have no competing interests.

Author details
[1]Optimed, Clinical Research Centre (Section 056), Copenhagen University Hospital Hvidovre, Kettegård Allé 30, DK-2650 Hvidovre, Denmark. [2]Novo Nordisk A/S, Vandtårnsvej 114, 2860 Søborg, Denmark. [3]Department of Internal Medicine, Copenhagen University Hospital Herlev, Herlev Ringvej 75, 2730 Herlev, Denmark.

References
1. Lindhardt T, Nyberg P, Hallberg IR. Collaboration between relatives of elderly patients and nurses and its relation to satisfaction with the hospital care trajectory. Scand J Caring Sci. 2008;22:507–19.
2. Li H. Family caregivers' preferences in caring for their hospitalized elderly relatives. Geriatr Nurs N Y N. 2002;23:204–7.
3. Popejoy LL. Complexity of family caregiving and discharge planning. J Fam Nurs. 2011;17:61–81.
4. Jurgens FJ, Clissett P, Gladman JRF, Harwood RH. Why are family carers of people with dementia dissatisfied with general hospital care? A qualitative study. BMC Geriatr. 2012;12:57.
5. World Health Organization, editor. World report on ageing and health. Geneva: World Health Organization; 2015.
6. Plan for Den ældre medicinske patient (Plan for the older medical patient). Capital Region of Denmark; 2009. https://www.regionh.dk/Sundhed/Politikker-Planer-Strategier/PublishingImages/Sider/Den-%C3%A6ldre-medicinske-patient/PlanforDen%C3%A6ldremedicinskepatientgodkendtafRR173200.pdf. Accessed 24 Apr 2013.
7. Recognised, valued and supported: Next step for the Carers Strategy. HM Government, UK; 2011. https://assets.publishing.service.gov.uk/government/uploads/system/uploads/attachment_data/file/213804/dh_122393.pdf. Accessed 23 Nov 2012.

8. Bruger-, patient- og pårørendepolitik (Policy for Users-, patients- and Relatives). Capital Region of Denmark; 2008. https://www.regionh.dk/Sundhed/Politikker-Planer-Strategier/PublishingImages/Sider/politik/Brugerpatientpolitik.pdf. Accessed 22 Nov 2012.

9. Den Landsdækkende Undersøgelse af Patientoplevelser, LUP 2015 (The National Danish Survey of Patient Experiences 2015). Enheden for brugerundersøgelser (Unit of Patient-perceived experiences), Capital Region of Denmark. 2015. http://patientoplevelser.dk. Accessed 14 Jun 2016.

10. Higgins I, Joyce T, Parker V, Fitzgerald M, McMillan M. The immediate needs of relatives during the hospitalisation of acutely ill older relatives. Contemp Nurse. 2007;26:208–20.

11. Bridges J, Flatley M, Meyer J. Older people's and relatives' experiences in acute care settings: systematic review and synthesis of qualitative studies. Int J Nurs Stud. 2010;47:89–107.

12. Haesler E, Bauer M, Nay R. Staff–family relationships in the care of older people: a report on a systematic review. Res Nurs Health. 2007;30:385–98.

13. Lindhardt T, Hallberg IR, Poulsen I. Nurses' experience of collaboration with relatives of frail elderly patients in acute hospital wards: a qualitative study. Int J Nurs Stud. 2008;45:668–81.

14. Lindhardt T, Bolmsjö IA, Hallberg IR. Standing guard—being a relative to a hospitalised, elderly person. J Aging Stud. 2006;20:133–49.

15. Garcia J, Evans J, Reshaw M. "Is there anything Else you would like to tell us"–methodological issues in the use of free-text comments from postal surveys. Qual Quant. 2004;38:113–25.

16. Lindhardt, T. et al. Collaboration between relatives of older patients and nurses in acute medical wards: confirmatory factor analysis of the revised family collaboration scale. J Nurs Meas. 2018;2:26.

17. Lindhardt T, Nyberg P, Hallberg IR. Relatives' view on collaboration with nurses in acute wards: development and testing of a new measure. Int J Nurs Stud. 2008;45:1329–43.

18. Graneheim U, Lundman B. Qualitative content analysis in nursing research: concepts, procedures and measures to achieve trustworthiness. Nurse Educ Today. 2004;24:105–12.

19. Hertzberg A, Ekman S-L, Axelsson K. 'Relatives are a resource, but…': registered nurses' views and experiences of relatives of residents in nursing homes. J Clin Nurs. 2003;12:431–41.

20. Holmgren J, Emami A, Eriksson LE, Eriksson H. Being perceived as a 'visitor' in the nursing staff's working arena – the involvement of relatives in daily caring activities in nursing homes in an urban community in Sweden. Scand J Caring Sci. 2013;27:677–85.

21. Jangland E, Gunningberg L, Carlsson M. Patients' and relatives' complaints about encounters and communication in health care: evidence for quality improvement. Patient Educ Couns. 2009;75:199–204.

22. Leininger M. Culture care theory: a major contribution to advance transcultural nursing knowledge and practices. J Transcult Nurs. 2002;13:189–92.

23. Ambrosi E, Biavati C, Guarnier A, Barelli P, Zambiasi P, Allegrini E, et al. Factors affecting in-hospital informal caregiving as decided by families: findings from a longitudinal study conducted in acute medical units. Scand J Caring Sci. 2016. doi:https://doi.org/10.1111/scs.12321.

24. Taverner T, Baumbusch J, Taipale P. Normalization of neglect: a grounded theory of RNs' experiences as family caregivers of hospitalized seniors. Can J Aging Rev Can Vieil. 2016;35:215–28.

25. van Manen M. Care-as-Worry, or "Don't Worry, be Happy.". Qual Health Res. 2002;12:262–78.

26. Bowers BJ. Intergenerational caregiving: adult caregivers and their aging parents. Adv Nurs Sci. 1987;9:20–31.

27. Riiskjaer E, Ammentorp J, Kofoed P-E. The value of open-ended questions in surveys on patient experience: number of comments and perceived usefulness from a hospital perspective. Int J Qual Health Care. 2012;24:509–16.

28. York GS, Churchman R, Woodard B, Wainright C, Rau-Foster M. Free-text comments: understanding the value in family member descriptions of hospice caregiver relationships. Am J Hosp Palliat Med. 2012;29:98–105.

29. Martinsen K. Omsorg i sykepleien - en moralsk utfordring. In: Fokus på sygeplejen, udvalgte artikler fra 1979 til 1992 (Caring in nursing - a moral challenge. In: Focus on nursing, selected articles from 1979 to 1992). Copenhagen: Munksgaard; 1995.

30. Jonasson L-L, Liss P-E, Westerlind B, Berterö C. Ethical values in caring encounters on a geriatric ward from the next of kin's perspective: an interview study. Int J Nurs Pract. 2010;16:20–6.

31. Lindhardt T. Collaboration between relatives of frail elderly patients and nurses in acute hospital wards. Doctoral Thesis. University of Lund; 2007.

32. Robben S, van Kempen J, Heinen M, Zuidema S, Olde Rikkert M, Schers H, et al. Preferences for receiving information among frail older adults and their informal caregivers: a qualitative study. Fam Pract. 2012;29:742–7.

33. Bauer M, Fitzgerald L, Haesler E, Manfrin M. Hospital discharge planning for frail older people and their family. Are we delivering best practice? A review of the evidence. J Clin Nurs. 2009;18:2539–46.

34. Shepperd S, McClaran J, Phillips CO, Lannin NA, Clemson LM, McCluskey A, et al. Discharge planning from hospital to home. The Cochrane Collaboration. Chichester: Wiley; 2010.

35. Maben J, Adams M, Peccei R, Murrells T, Robert G. 'Poppets and parcels': the links between staff experience of work and acutely ill older peoples' experience of hospital care. Int J Older People Nursing. 2012;7:83–94.

36. Kjerholt M, Wagner L, Delmar C, Clemensen J, Lindhardt T. Continuity in care trajectories of older chronically ill patients in a battlefield of competing rationales. Int J Older People Nursing. 2014;9(4):277–88. https://doi.org/10.1111/opn.12031. Epub 2013 Apr 30.

37. Trydegård G-B. Care work in changing welfare states: Nordic care workers' experiences. Eur J Ageing. 2012;9:119–29.

38. Danish Law 593. Act on Research Ethics Review of Health Research Projects. 2011. https://www.retsinformation.dk/forms/r0710.aspx?id=137674.

16

Heart health whispering: A randomized, controlled pilot study to promote nursing student perspective-taking on carers' health risk behaviors

Michelle Lobchuk[1]*⬤, Lisa Hoplock[1], Gayle Halas[2], Christina West[1], Cheryl Dika[1], Wilma Schroeder[3], Terri Ashcroft[1], Kathleen Chambers Clouston[4] and Jocelyne Lemoine[1]

Abstract

Background: Lifestyle counseling is described as a "major breakthrough" in the control of chronic diseases. Counseling can be challenging to nurses due their lack of motivation to counsel, hesitancy to appear non-judgmental, lack of empathy, and lack of time. Nurses voice their need for more training in counseling communication skills. Our main objective was to engage in ongoing development and testing of a promising *Heart Health Whispering* perspective-taking intervention on nursing students' clinical empathy, perceptual understanding, and client readiness to alter health risk behaviors.

Methods: In this randomized controlled pilot study, the full intervention (perspective-taking instructions, practice, and video-feedback) and partial intervention (video-feedback only) comprised 24 and 18 nursing students, respectively. Quantitative data were collected with a 10-item pre- and post-intervention clinical empathy tool, a one-item 'readiness to change' health risk behavior tool plus similarity ratings on students' empathic accuracy were calculated. Data were analyzed using Independent Samples t Tests and mixed model ANCOVA models. Students' and actors' evaluative responses toward the intervention phases were collected by handwritten notes, and analyzed using content analysis and constant comparison techniques.

Results: The main finding was that students in the full intervention group reported greater clinical empathy in the post versus baseline condition. Students underestimated their clinical empathy in comparison to carers' reports in the post-condition. In both intervention groups, carers reported more readiness to change in the post-condition. Carers identified favorable and unfavorable *perceptions and outcomes of approaches taken by students*. Students desired immediate and direct feedback after the video-dialogue and -tagging exercise.

Conclusions: *Heart Health Whispering* is a promising intervention to help educators in basic and continuing education to bolster nurse confidence in empathic conversations on health risk behaviors. This intervention incorporates commonly used strategies to teach empathic communication along with a novel video-analysis application of a perspective-taking task. Student and carer actor comments highlighted the value in opportunities for students to engage in self-evaluation and practicing the empathic process of taking the client's perspective on health risk behaviors.

Keywords: Education, Empathy, Video-feedback, Health risk behavior, Carers, Nursing students

* Correspondence: Michelle.Lobchuk@umanitoba.ca
[1]Rady Faculty of Health Sciences, College of Nursing, University of Manitoba, Room 315 – 89 Curry Place, Winnipeg, MB R3T 2N2, Canada
Full list of author information is available at the end of the article

Background

Through the wondrous advancement of medical procedures, treatments and therapies, individuals worldwide are living longer but often with chronic illness [1]. Chronic illness can be costly to affected individuals and to health care systems (i.e., trillions of dollars, globally) [1]. To avert this cost and sub-optimal quality of life often associated with chronic illness, health promotion and disease prevention are "major breakthroughs" in the control of chronic diseases [2]. Evidence demonstrates support for upstream approaches that alter determinants of health by promoting wellness and preventing illness through health behavior choices (e.g., smoking cessation, increased physical activity, and healthy dietary choices) [3–5]. While it remains easier to prescribe medications to avert risk for chronic illness (e.g., aspirin for "cardio-protection"), clinicians' efforts to promote changes in health risk behaviors are associated with improved mortality rates [6]. However, multiple challenges exist in altering health risk behavior choices.

Health risk behaviors are often longstanding, comforting, and tied to stressful situations, psychosocial variables, work and home environments, limited education, or economic factors [6]. For instance, family carers (aka carers) are a segment of our population that tends to engage in health risk behaviors (e.g., smoking, poor diet, or lack of exercise). This may be due to expectations and stressors associated with the dual demands of caregiving and employment [7, 8]. Consequently, carers may develop mental health issues (e.g., anxiety) and exhibit exaggerated cardiovascular responses to stressful conditions that put them at greater risk than non-carers for the development of high blood pressure or heart disease [9–12].

Despite nurses' health promotion and illness prevention education, carers consistently report that interpersonal connection and concern for their wellbeing are absent [13, 14]. Nurses have described a lack of motivation to counsel due to the resistance of clients, hesitancy to appear judgmental, lack of empathy due to a poor understanding of individual challenges with behavior change, and struggles in being patient and listening carefully due to the lack of time [15]. However, person-centered approaches require that health care providers endeavor to understand carers and include them as partners in decision-making about behavior change [16]. Our recent pilot work indicated that carer readiness to take ownership for their health risk behaviors is bolstered when nursing students make it a priority to perspective-take, empathically listen, and discern the carer's unique circumstances, skills, abilities, beliefs, and preferences [17].

Perspective-taking is a teachable component for nurturing clinical empathy. It holds promise in promoting a non-threatening dialogue where individuals can describe their unique contexts and the conditions that underlie unhealthy behaviors or pose barriers to changing unhealthy behaviors [17]. Perspective-taking sensitizes clinicians to: (a) be cognizant of their own thoughts and feelings about health risk behaviors, (b) control their thoughts and feelings to imagine the client's viewpoint of the health risk behavior and barriers for change, and (c) seek validation of his or her inferences of the client's viewpoint. Perspective-taking can enhance empathic accuracy (i.e., the ability to accurately infer another person's thoughts and feelings) [18]. Clients entrust clinicians to take a more person-centered approach and to understand them by identifying obstacles that thwart their readiness to change a health risk behavior [17].

Training opportunities to foster confidence and skills in empathic counseling are needed. This will help nursing students to better understand the underlying influences of health risk behaviors, as well as the stigma and negative attitudes that may implicitly undermine empathic approaches. Our main study objective was to engage in ongoing development and testing of a promising *Heart Health Whispering* intervention as a novel person-centered approach for counseling and health promotion. We posed the following research question: *When nursing students receive perspective-taking instructions and engage in video-feedback (aka Heart Health Whispering) versus video-feedback alone, does this result in increased competence in clinical empathy, student-carer perceptual agreement on carer thoughts and feelings about the health risk behavior, and carer readiness to alter health risk behaviors for protection against detrimental cardiovascular conditions?* We also examined evaluative interview responses of students and carers on the impact, appropriateness, and acceptability of the intervention to aid with further refinement.

Methods
Study design

We conducted a two-center, randomized, controlled pilot study with a full intervention group (Group I) and a partial intervention group (Group PI). Approvals from the Ethics Boards at the University of Manitoba (aka the university) and Red River College (aka the college) were obtained before executing study protocols. Within the present study, we addressed recommendations from our first one-arm pilot study by: launching a randomized controlled study, incorporating a refined recruitment protocol with nursing students, using carer actors, employing a modified video-tagging session, and obtaining data to calculate effect size differences in students' clinical empathy [17].

Participants

Between March 2016 and December 2016, we recruited a convenience sample of undergraduate student nurses and nurse practitioner students. According to our inclusion criteria, the undergraduate sample was comprised of students at: (a) the end of the second year or in the third year of a three-year accelerated baccalaureate program at the college ($n = 5$) or (b) the end of the second year or in the third or fourth year of a four-year baccalaureate program at the university ($n = 15$). All students had completed respective clinical practice, health promotion, relational nursing, family nursing, and adult health courses. Participating undergraduate students received a $20 cash honorarium and a thank you card for their time and effort.

The nurse practitioner sample was comprised of master-level students in a two-year nurse practitioner program at the university who were enrolled in the first term of a clinical practice course ($n = 22$). Students received a pass or fail credit for participating in the study or alternate course assignment. See Additional file 1 for more details on participant recruitment.

No power analysis was performed as this was pilot work addressing participant responses to the recruitment strategy, group assignment, and intervention phases, and the determination of effect size based on the study outcome of clinical empathy for a larger future study.

Intervention Protocol

A fulsome description and schematic of the theory-based *Heart Health Whispering* intervention that was influenced by work in social psychology [19–21] has been published elsewhere [17] and is also located in Additional file 2. The full intervention involved four phases. The Research Assistant (RA) conducted a computerized randomization process to assign students to Group I ($n = 24$) or Group PI ($n = 18$) (Fig. 1). Due to practical reasons, students, the interventionist (JL), and interviewers (ML and LH) were not blinded; only the actor was blinded to group assignment. We employed two female actors (hereafter called the 'carer') from the College of Medicine, Standardized Patient Program. Actors received a script and training to play the role of a stressed middle-aged family carer who is concerned about her health risk behavior.

Phase 1 occurred roughly 2 weeks prior to the in-lab session. In this phase, the interventionist taught individual Group I students about perspective-taking and then the students practiced the technique for 2 weeks. Phases 2 to 4 occurred in the lab 2 weeks after Phase 1. At the lab, individual Group I and Group PI students completed demographic and empathy questionnaires. In a separate room from the student, a carer actor used a tool to identify a health risk behavior to discuss with the student and how ready they were to change that health risk behavior. In *Phase 2*, students had a video-recorded dialogue with a carer actor for 10 min about the carer's health risk behavior. In *Phase 3*, the carer actor was separated from the student. While sitting with the interventionist, the carer

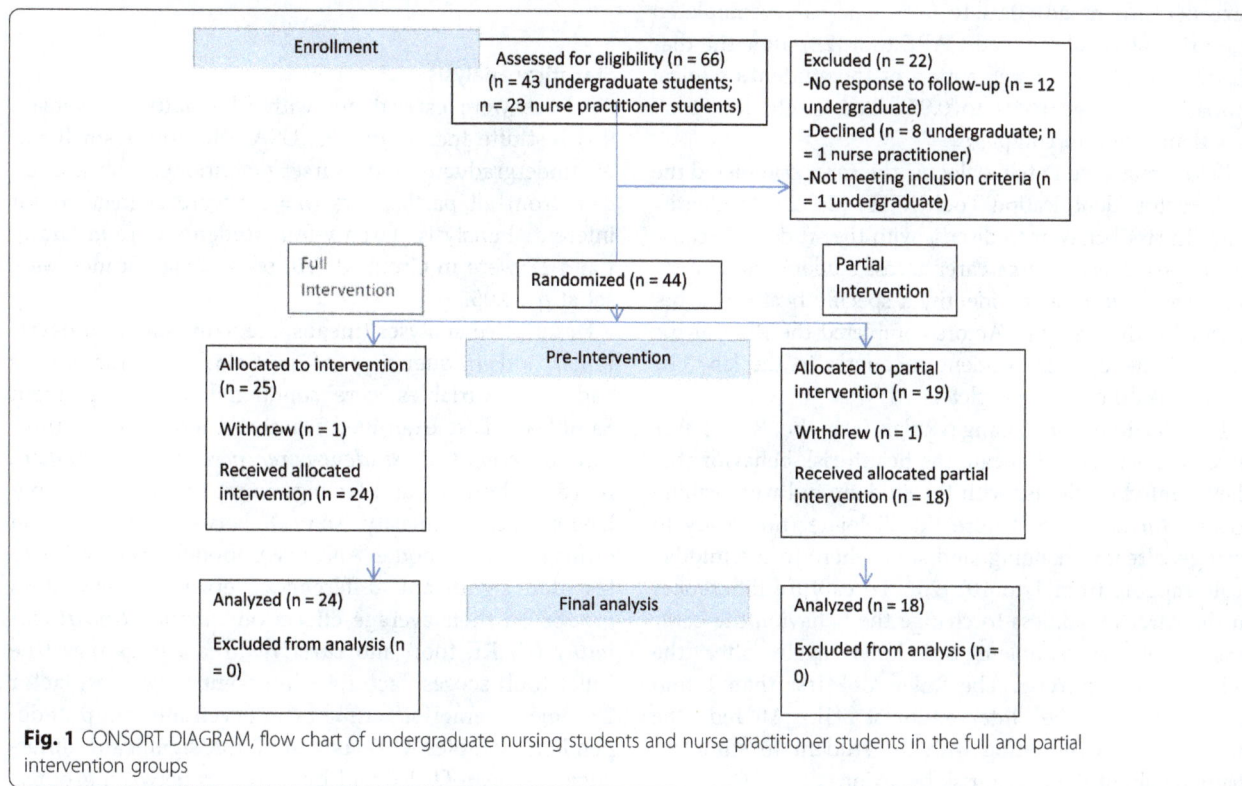

Fig. 1 CONSORT DIAGRAM, flow chart of undergraduate nursing students and nurse practitioner students in the full and partial intervention groups

watched the dialogue video and paused it each time the carer experienced a thought or feeling. The carer indicated: a) whether it was a thought or feeling, b) whether the thought or feeling was positive or negative in tone, and then c) wrote out in sentence-form the context of the thought or feeling. Later, while the carer was completing Phase 4, the student watched the video with the interventionist. The interventionist paused the video each time the carer had indicated experiencing a thought or feeling. The student then inferred what the carer was experiencing at that time. In *Phase 4*, student and the actor (separately) engaged in exit interviews.

Data collection and measurement

Students completed the investigator-developed demographic tool to capture student age, gender, extent of communication training with clients, extent of communication training on health risk behaviors, the student's own experience being a family carer, and the student's own engagement in health risk behaviors and desire to change said behaviors. The demographic tool took less than 5 min to complete.

We employed an adapted version of the Consultation and Relational Empathy (CARE) [22] tool to capture the student's inference of the carer's response to his or her clinical empathy: *Please rate how you feel the carer actor will perceive (perceived) you to be at*, e.g., *"really listening to him or her"*. Students completed this scale before and after the dialogue which included 10 items; 1 (poor), 5 (excellent); α range = 0.91 to 0.95. The carer completed the original version of the CARE tool [23] after the dialogue to capture her perception of the student's clinical empathy (α range = 0.94 to 0.95). The CARE tool took less than 5 min to complete.

Before engaging in the dialogue, the carer completed the Risk Factor Identification Tool (RFIT) [24, 25] to identify a health risk behavior to discuss with the student. Because actors posed as the same carer across student encounters, they were able to easily identify a specific health risk behavior for the dialogue. Actors completed the RFIT at the first, middle, and last student encounter in the lab. The RFIT took 10 min to complete.

The Readiness to Change Ruler (aka the Ruler) was used with carers to indicate the health risk behavior that they wanted to discuss with the student and were willing to rate on the Ruler before the dialogue (not ready to change, already changing, and somewhere in the middle; scale ranging from 1 to 10) [26]. To capture differences in the carer's readiness to change the behavior, the carer was asked to complete the Ruler again after the video-tagging exercise. The Ruler took less than 1 min to complete. The interventionist (JL) shared the pre-dialogue Ruler rating with the student to stimulate dialogue about the health risk behavior.

To measure student perceptual understanding of carers' thoughts and feelings experienced during the dialogue, we were guided by Ickes' [21] empathic accuracy approach. We employed scores of "0" (essentially different content), "1" (similar, but not the same), and "2" (essentially the same content) to determine the similarity between student and carer tags involving three evaluative factors of: a) whether the carer experienced a 'thought or feeling', b) whether the 'tone' of the tagged instance was positive or negative, and c) the 'situation' being referenced in the instance [17]. For each tagged instance, rater scores were averaged. The total similarity score was calculated by adding average rater scores for each instance. We then divided the total similarity score by the maximum points that the student could have obtained to obtain an overall percent similarity score. Fleiss Kappa coefficients for agreement among six investigative team raters across ten students' tagged instances were 0.49 ($p < 0.0001$) indicating moderate rater agreement; for "0" was 0.65 ($p < 0.0001$) indicating substantial agreement; "1" was 0.38 ($p < 0.0001$) or fair agreement; and, "2" was 0.54 ($p < 0.0001$) or moderate agreement [27].

Open-ended exit interviews, as guided by investigator-developed scripts (Tables 1 and 2), were conducted (ML, LH, JL) respectively with each student and carer. Handwritten notes on participant responses about the impact, appropriateness, and acceptability of each phase of the intervention protocol were captured. The exit interviews took 30 min to complete.

Statistical analysis

Analyses were carried out with SAS Software (version 9.4) Institute Inc., Cary, NC, USA. Due to the small size of undergraduate and nurse practitioner sub-groups, data from all participants ($n = 42$) were aggregated for inferential analysis. Twenty-four students were in Group I and 18 were in Group PI. All tests of significance were set at $p < 0.05$.

Descriptive analyses (means, medians, standard deviations, and frequencies) of participant characteristics and study variables were conducted. An Independent Samples t Test examined whether there was a significant difference in *student-carer perceptual agreement* on carer thoughts and feelings about the health risk behavior (i.e., similarity scores) between intervention groups. Mixed model ANCOVA models were used to test for significant differences between intervention groups on their average effects on *student clinical empathy* (CARE tool) and *carer readiness to change* (the Ruler tool) scores: factor 1 = intervention groups; factor 2 = time; interaction = time by intervention group. Independent Samples t Tests tested for significant differences in mean CARE and Ruler scores between groups.

Table 1 Interview questions for nursing students

Question #1

Full intervention group	Can you describe your thoughts and feelings about the empathic technique when you applied it with the carer to help you understand his or her thoughts and feelings about health-risk behaviour?
Partial intervention group	Can you describe the approach that you took with the carer to help you understanding his or her thoughts and feelings about the health-risk behavior? Can you describe your thoughts and feelings about the approach you took with the carer to help you understand his or her thoughts and feelings about health-risk behavior?

Question #2

Full intervention and Partial intervention groups	Can you tell me whether you think that the empathic technique (or approach you took) helped you to better understand the carer's thoughts and feelings about health-risk behavior? Prompt: If yes, I would be interested in knowing 'how' the intervention (or approach you took) helped you? Prompt: Did the intervention (or the approach you took) affect how you felt about the carer? Prompt: Did the intervention (or approach you took) affect your behavior toward the carer? How did the intervention (or approach you took) affect your behavior toward the carer? Can you describe whether your approach in trying to understand health-risk behaviors is different now since you learned this new technique (full intervention group only)? Prompt: Can you tell me whether you plan to continue using this technique (or your approach) to help you understand health-risk behaviors of patients and carers better? If no, why not? If yes, why? Prompt: I am also interested in knowing if the technique (or approach you took) caused you to learn something different about yourself and how you view health-risk behaviors?

Question #3

Full intervention and Partial intervention groups	As a last question, is there anything else you would like to add to help the researchers of this study develop this intervention to help student nurses talk with carers about health- risk behaviors? Example: Were there any comments or concerns about the appropriateness and clarity of demographic data questions and the video-tagging exercise?

Two authors (ML and LH) independently examined hand-written notes of exit interview responses by integrating field notes and using content analysis and constant comparison techniques to identify, code, categorize, and label the primary patterns in the data [28, 29]. When disagreements occurred in the coded data, discussions occurred between ML and LH until consensus was achieved. Supporting quotes from the data were selected for identified themes and sub-themes.

Results

A total of 42 nursing students provided voluntary consent to participate. The undergraduate nursing students ($n = 20$) were between 19 and 35 years of age; nurse practitioner students ($n = 22$) were between 25 to 51 years of age. Across all students, the majority (88%) were female who reported having received communication training to engage with clients in undergraduate coursework, continuing education, or job training. Fifty-two percent of students reported having previously received communication training to dialogue with clients on health risk behaviors in courses at the undergraduate and/or graduate levels of study. Seventeen per cent ($n = 7$) of the participants stated that they were a family carer and 57% ($n = 4$ of 7) had care recipients who engaged in health risk behaviors (e.g., poor dietary intake, misuse of alcohol, and lack of exercise). Regarding student participants' own health risk behaviors, 48% indicated that they had behaviors (often multiple) that they wished they could change (e.g., poor diet, smoking cigarettes or marijuana, lack of exercise, inadequate sleep, and poor coping with stress) (Table 3).

Quantitative findings

Regarding differences in mean *clinical empathy* (CARE tool) (Table 4), a mixed-model ANCOVA analysis revealed no main effects of intervention group, $F(1,40) = 0.75$, $p = 0.391$. Time was significant, $F(1,40) = 7.94$, $p = 0.008$ as well as the interaction between intervention group and time, $F(1,40) = 9.98$, $p = 0.003$. Within-group analysis revealed that students in Group I reported having more clinical empathy at post-measurement than they did at baseline, $t(40) = 4.56$, $p < 0.0001$; 95% CI [2.16, 5.59]; $d = 0.43$. There was no statistically significant difference between baseline and post-intervention clinical empathy in Group PI; $t(40) = -0.23$, $p = 0.822$; 95% CI [-2.20, 1.76]; $d = 0.04$. Between-group analysis revealed no significant difference in clinical empathy between Group I and Group PI at baseline; $t(40) = -0.23$, $p = 0.822$; 95% CI [-4.41, 3.52]; $d = 0.07$. There was also no significant difference in clinical empathy between Group I and Group PI, post-intervention; $t(40) = 1.86$, $p = 0.07$; 95% CI [-0.31, 7.62]; $d = 0.62$. Thus, while Group I and Group PI students scored similarly on clinical empathy, Group I students perceived themselves to increase in empathy, whereas Group PI students did not.

Supplemental analysis revealed a significant difference between Group I students and carers, $t(39.14) = 2.24$, $p = 0.03$; 95% CI [0.52, 10.23]; $d = 0.65$, on student clinical empathy, post-intervention. Similarly, there was a significant

Table 2 Interview questions for carer actor

Question #1	Can you describe your thoughts and feelings about the approach the student nurse took to help him or her understand your thoughts and feelings about the health-risk behavior?
Question #2	Can you tell me whether you think that the approach the student nurse took helped him or her to better understand your thoughts and feelings about the health-risk behavior? Prompt: If yes, I would be interested in knowing 'how' the student's approach helped you to describe your thoughts and feelings about the health-risk behavior? Prompt: Did the student nurse's approach affect how you felt about the student nurse? Prompt: Did the student nurse's approach affect your behavior toward the student nurse?
Question #3	Can you describe whether your 'personal' approach (s) will be different when you talk about your own wellness and health-risk behaviors with other health care providers (e.g., your physician, other nurses)? Prompt: Can you tell me whether you plan to continue using this approach to help your own health care providers better understand your health-risk behaviors? If no, why not? If yes, why?
Question #4	I am also interested in knowing if the student's approach caused you to learn something different about yourself and how you view health risk behaviors?
Question #5	As a last question, is there anything else you would like to add to help the researchers of this study develop this intervention to help student nurses talk with carers about health- risk behaviors? Example: Were there any comments or concerns about the appropriateness and clarity of study questionnaires (i.e., the computer risk identification tool, the 'readiness to change' ruler, and the CARE tool) and the video-tagging exercise?

difference between Group PI students and carers, $t(34) = 8.13$, $p < 0.0001$; 95% CI [10.75, 17.92]; $d = 2.71$, post-intervention. Thus, both groups of students underestimated their clinical empathy in comparison to carers' reports. Of interest, carers' perceptions of student clinical empathy was lower for Group I than for Group PI students; $t(36.49) = -2.24$, $p = 0.031$; 95% CI [-10.11, -0.50]; $d = 0.67$ (Table 4).

With regard to *student-carer perceptual agreement* (i.e., similarity ratings), the overall percent similarity score was higher in Group I (mean 68.41, SD 10.33; range 41.67 to 85%) across 236 instances compared to Group PI (mean 65.24; SD 16.95; range 30.68 to 90%) across 189 instances. However, this difference between the two groups was not statistically significant, $t(26.28) = 0.70$, $p = 0.489$; 95% CI [-6.11, 12.46]; $d = 0.23$. Overall, there was tendency for students in Group I to achieve greater perceptual agreement on carers' thoughts and feelings about health risk behaviors than students in Group PI.

On *carer readiness to change* (the Ruler tool), a mixed-model ANCOVA revealed no main effects of intervention group ($F(1,40) = 0.00$, $p = 0.974$) or interaction effects ($F(1,40) = 0.00$, $p = 0.998$). Time was significant, $F(1,40) = 82.10$, $p < 0.0001$. Within-group analysis revealed that carers in Group I reported more readiness to change at post-measurement (mean 8.22, SD 1.50) than they did at baseline (mean 5.91, SD 1.84), $t(40) = 6.92$, $p < 0.0001$; 95% CI [1.64, 2.99]; $d = 1.38$. Similarly, Group PI carers reported more readiness to change at post-measurement (mean 8.21, SD 1.65) than they did at baseline (mean 5.89, SD 1.96); $t(40) = 6.00$, $p < 0.0001$; 95% CI [1.53, 3.09]; $d = 1.28$. Thus, carers reported a similar readiness to change post measurement regardless of whether they interacted with students in Group I or Group PI.

Evaluative interview responses

Evaluative responses by carers toward students' approach (Additional file 3) and students' responses toward intervention phases (Additional file 4) are displayed along with descriptive response counts and illustrative quotations for each sub-theme. A cursory examination revealed a similar count across most sub-themes by carers and students in both intervention groups. The following summary focuses on the most frequent comments in both groups, except when noted.

Carers

Carers identified varied favorable and unfavorable *perceptions and outcomes of behavior or approaches* taken by students in the dialogue. Favorable comments included 'good communication and listening skills' that were congruent with 'nonverbal communication skills' and evaluated by carers as exhibitions of 'empathy' and caring or intuitive 'responsiveness'. Carers appreciated students who employed a 'gentle, educational approach' about managing the behavior. Although carers felt that Group I students provided more 'summarization' of the dialogue, carers in both intervention groups 'felt understood' and 'felt safe and comfortable in not being judged'. When interacting with Group I students, carers 'felt new resolve to change' their health risk behaviors. They described that they 'learned to take the initiative' in the future to openly share authentic information with their own health care providers. Carers in both intervention groups said that they 'learned more about [their] own feelings' of resentment and guilt relating to their caregiving situation. When carers described 'liking the student or their approach', they felt a connection with the student, which occurred particularly when students' asked the right question and focused on the carer's self-care.

Table 3 Descriptive statistics of nursing students ($n = 42$)

Variable	N (%)
Gender	
Female	37 (88%)
Male	5 (12%)
Age, years (mean; range)	
Undergraduates	25.3 (19 to 35)
Nurse Practitioner	33.0 (25 to 51)
Year in nursing program	
Undergraduates	
2nd year (end)	2 (5%)
3rd year	7 (17%)
4th year	11 (26%)
Nurse Practitioners	
1st year	22 (52%)
Nursing school	
Undergraduates	
College	5 (12%)
University	15 (36%)
Nurse Practitioners	
University	22 (52%)
Received communication training with carers?	
Yes	22 (52%)
No	19 (45%)
Missing	1 (3%)
If yes, what type of communicating training?	Specific courses in undergraduate program ($n = 11$) Non-specific courses in undergraduate program ($n = 7$) Home care companion / Health care Aide orientation training ($n = 1$) Continuing education ($n = 2$)
Received communication training about health risk behaviours?	
Yes	19 (45%)
No	22 (52%)
Missing	1 (3%)
If yes, what type of health risk communication training?	Specific courses in undergraduate/graduate program ($n = 9$) Non-specific courses in undergraduate/graduate program ($n = 6$)
Are you currently a family carer?	
Yes	7 (17%)
No	35 (83%)
Does your care recipient engage in health risk behaviors?	
Yes	4 (57%)
No	3 (43%)
If yes, what type of health risk behaviors?[a]	Poor dietary intake ($n = 2$) Alcohol, smoking, drug, illicit and prescription drug abuse, sexual exposure, lack of exercise, poor diet ($n = 1$)

Table 3 Descriptive statistics of nursing students ($n = 42$) (Continued)

Variable	N (%)
	Self-harm, illicit drugs, and manic behaviours ($n = 1$)
Do you have any health risk behaviors you wish you could change?	
Yes	20 (48%)
No	19 (45%)
Missing	3 (7%)
If yes, what type of health risk behaviors?[a]	Poor diet ($n = 4$) Smoking ($n = 1$) Poor stress coping and lack of exercise ($n = 1$) Poor diet, secluding self when sad or overwhelmed, cigar and marijuana smoking ($n = 1$) Poor diet, lack of exercise, inadequate sleep, poor stress coping ($n = 1$) Poor diet, lack of exercise, inadequate sleep ($n = 1$) Poor diet, lack of exercise, poor diet, poor stress coping, and smoking ($n = 1$) Not identified ($n = 6$)

[a]Participants identified multiple health-risk behaviors either for their care recipient or themselves

Unfavorable comments by carers included descriptions of when 'students needed guidance' from the carer who had to take the lead in the dialogue. For example, during one session, the carer liked that the student allowed the carer to take the lead in the dialogue, however the carer also felt compelled to start the conversation due to student reticence: "She had a very caring, validating, non-judgmental approach. But she didn't explore in any great depth [my] motives for binge-eating. I felt that she was reticent to explore further or didn't feel comfortable delving deeper" (D3 UG Group PI). Of note, carers described 'not feeling heard' by some students in Group I. A number of Group I students tended to take 'paternalistic' stances by offering inappropriate advice or making assumptions about the carer. Carers described 'no delving and/or jumping to intervene' for some Group I students who seemed eager to intervene before fully understanding the carer's triggers for engaging in the health risk behavior. There were additional carer comments about some Group

Table 4 Differences in CARE scores of student nurses and carers

	Baseline Condition		Post-Intervention Condition	
	Intervention Group (I) (Mean, SD)	Partial Intervention Group (PI) (Mean, SD)	Intervention Group (I) (Mean, SD)	Partial Intervention Group (PI) (Mean, SD)
Students	31.67 (6.88)[a]	32.11 (6.27)	35.54 (6.35)[a,d]	31.89 (5.33)[c]
Caregiver	–	–	40.92 (9.91)[b,d]	46.22 (5.24)[b,c]

Common superscripts indicate the same column or row mean scores were significantly different from each other; [a]identifies within-group differences; [b-d]identifies between-group differences. CARE tool range of scores 0 to 50 units (higher ratings indicate greater clinical empathy)

I students who were described as 'inauthentic' in their approach based on behavioral signals (limited eye contact) or robotic verbal responses. Overall, carer actors described a range of mixed emotions and experiences with students in both groups.

Students

In Phase One, students practiced perspective-taking with close others (e.g., their parents and friends) who engaged in health risk behaviors such as smoking and poor diet. Most comments reflected how the practice session helped students to attain a 'better comprehension of others in terms of triggers for engaging in the health risk behavior. A number of students indicated that engagement in perspective-taking was 'not easy to do'. Perspective-taking required a different approach by students. In particular, it required more conscious effort and students reported that they needed to practice taking the other person's viewpoint rather than resorting to a familiar self-oriented way of thinking or making assumptions about another person's risk-taking behavior.

For Phase Two, students revealed three goals for the dialogue: build trust and respect, seek understanding, and provide support. To fulfill these goals, students identified helpful verbal and non-verbal 'communication techniques', such as paraphrasing and maintaining an open body posture. As a result of these techniques, which included perspective-taking (mentioned more frequently by students in Group I), both groups 'gained an appreciation of the carer's perspective' on their health risk behavior as a coping technique. One Group I student stated that the intervention helped her to see that there was more to the carer's situation than just smoking. She thought the dialogue would have been unsuccessful if she had tried to intervene instead of listening to the carer. Despite our instructions to not intervene and seek understanding, students mentioned that they had 'wanted to intervene' and provide the carer with suggestions for improving their situation. Group PI students commented more frequently about their 'self-reflection on improvement' of communication techniques that would come with more practice. Students in both intervention groups perceived Phase Two to be 'a positive experience' with greater 'self-awareness' (of non-verbal cues). They recommended that video-recorded dialogue be incorporated into the curriculum. One student exclaimed, "We need to practice these skills, like today!" (D8 UG Group PI).

Students in both intervention groups commented on their 'appreciation' for Phase Three as an opportunity to see themselves in a new light and think about different approaches they might adopt in similar situations in practice. Reviewing the dialogue video and engaging in video-tagging appeared to be particularly helpful for students to engage in 'self-reflection on improvement'. One

student reported, "I think the video-tagging process is a really great way to pick up on nuances of therapeutic communication, especially non-verbal communication. I think it is a really great way for students to fine tune communication skills in a non-threatening environment so that they may be applied in clinical practice" (D13 UG Group I).

The field notes revealed recommendations for improvement in student video-feedback. Students desired immediate and direct feedback from the carer after the dialogue and/or after completing the tagging: e.g., how accurate they were in the tagging. Although students received this feedback after data analysis, they preferred to receive it more immediately. Taken together, results indicate that students perceived their participation to be worthwhile and the protocol to be effective, appropriate, and acceptable.

Discussion

Family carers need to take care of their wellbeing, but this often does not happen. The ability of nurses to counsel carers on their health risk behaviors in order to maintain or achieve wellness relies on an empathic, therapeutic approach and building relationships with them [30]. Developing the capacity of nurses to demonstrate clinical empathy is "best achieved at the student level" while their attitudes and skills are being formed [31, 32]. In the present study, we followed up on our one-arm pilot study [17] by conducting a two-arm randomized control trial. We sought to obtain preliminary data on the immediate impact of the *Heart Health Whispering* intervention on: student competence in clinical empathy, student-carer perceptual agreement on carer thoughts and feelings about their health risk behaviors, and carer readiness to change the health risk behavior.

The main finding in this study is that students in the full intervention group (Group I) reported greater clinical empathy after engaging in perspective-taking training (post versus baseline condition). Students in the partial intervention group (Group PI; who did not receive perspective-taking instructions or the opportunity to practice perspective-taking) reported no difference in their clinical empathy. These findings support recommendations to include theoretical, didactic, and experiential learning to bolster student knowledge of empathy and the underlying process of perspective-taking [33–35]. Students' qualitative comments demonstrated that their customary responses toward health risk behaviors are driven by erroneous assumptions of individual choice rather than seeking to understand individual circumstances and perspectives regarding the difficulties in changing problematic behaviors. Their comments corroborated previous findings on the value of perspective-taking in allowing them to enhance their 'exploring skills' [36] and encouraging carers to gain trust in exploring sensitive triggers for health risk behaviors. The present study provides promising evidence that the 20–30 min instructional session and a 2-week practice session had a distinct contribution in enhancing students' empathic approach. However, larger studies on the 'dose' of instructional and practice sessions are required before educators incorporate the perspective-taking exercise into educational curricula.

On a promising note, our cursory analysis indicated that post-intervention clinical empathy and similarity scores were greater for Group I students whose qualitative comments indicated a greater appreciation for the carer's viewpoint on health risk behaviors than Group PI students. The lack of significant between-group differences in the post-condition in student self-reports on clinical empathy, carer readiness to change, and student-carer similarity ratings can be attributed to: possible contamination (i.e., Group I students came in contact with Group PI students and may have disseminated perspective-taking information shared by the RA), the small sample size, or the research design (i.e., both groups of students received similar benefits of video-feedback such as the opportunity for self-reflection on their communication styles). Exit interview findings, combined with actors' CARE and readiness to change responses, suggest that students in both groups demonstrated empathy, even if Group PI students did not receive the full intervention. We speculate, as have other researchers [16, 37–40], that having the undivided attention of students who focused on carer self-care helped the carer to take ownership, feel empowered, become positive about personal strengths, and have confidence to change a challenging behavior; this is also supported in a review on the positive impact of self-affirmation on health behavior change [41]. Thus, nursing students were receiving good communication training and acquiring fundamental communication skills. There is potential to enhance this further through the *Heart Health Whispering* intervention introduced in this study.

The second interesting finding is that carers rated student clinical empathy as higher than students' self-assessment. This finding is consistent with a meta-analysis that revealed a limited linkage between objective measures and self-reports on perceptual accuracy [42]. Clinicians are poor judges of their consultation performance in the context of health risk behavior conversations [43]. Similarly, early researchers in social psychology found that 'observer-target' similarity ratings do not associate well with observer self-reports on empathic accuracy [44]. Kalish et al. [45] speculated that their findings of higher preceptor ratings than students' ratings on student compassion were due to different expectations. Students may have also been unduly critical in their approach [45]. Together, these findings indicate that our continued use of objective measures of individuals' attempts to engage in empathy-related behaviors

and empathy-related outcomes is needed to establish the validity of self-reports.

A third interesting, but unexpected finding is that carers rated clinical empathy as significantly greater for Group PI students versus Group I students, post-condition. A differential count of qualitative responses showed that carers reported they felt 'less heard' in Group I compared to Group PI. Carers also commented on students in Group I 'not delving enough', and seeming 'inauthentic', and 'paternalistic' in their responses to the carer. Plausible reasons for this could be that Group I students may have become impatient based on their comments on the difficulties they experienced when engaging in perspective-taking. Jansink et al. [15] described that nurses tend to leap "ahead of the patient" and hold "false or too high expectations" for motivation to change. Perspective-taking requires careful listening skills that are different from customary quick provision of health risk behavior information and advice. On the other hand, Group PI students had less cognitive demands and likely were less distracted in their dialogue allowing them to draw on previously acquired knowledge and skills that was detected by the carer. This is supported by the qualitative responses of Group PI students where they indicated more frequent use of communication techniques than did Group I students. Additionally, Group I students were struggling with practicing their new skills resulting in poorer performance than students in Group PI. Miller and Mount [46] described that learning and practicing new skills takes time and can lead the trainee to experience ill ease and the lack of genuineness. This is consistent with what carers detected in the present study. Carers added that some students required more practice; this is supported by growing evidence on the benefits of repetitive practice and feedback sessions [47, 48] with standardized actors and peers or fellow trainees [37, 49] in tailored clinical contexts where skills will be applied.

The present study has several limitations that pose as potential threats to internal validity (e.g., small scale study, cross-sectional measurement, and contamination). A main concern that requires ongoing attention is the challenge that raters encountered in not achieving substantive agreement on similarity ratings, particularly on the "1" rating (i.e., similar, but not the same content). A key recommendation by the raters, was to develop clearer qualitative decision rules; for each tagged instance, raters should first evaluate 'the situation' followed by 'the tone', and then the 'thought' or 'feeling'. We also did not conduct observational evaluations of students' perspective-taking behaviors that are often incorporated in communication training. However, our main aim was to continue to develop and test our empathy-based video-analysis intervention, and determine its impact on students' perceptual understanding of carers' thoughts and feelings about health risk behaviors.

Notable strengths to this research include our ongoing systematic development of our theory-derived intervention. We addressed key recommendations from our previous pilot work to improve study protocols, including improved recruitment strategies and enhanced instructions for the video-tagging exercise. We employed a highly reliable clinical empathy tool that demonstrated sensitivity to detect differences in pre- and post-conditions. Although *Heart Health Whispering* is comprised of a combination of new and previously developed strategies, our innovative approach integrated them to enhance the way students learn the perspective-taking approach. Our approach encouraged self-awareness of one's beliefs on health risk behaviors, provided perspective-taking instructions with practice sessions, provided the opportunity to hear stories about the impact of the carer role and potential linkages with carers' health risk behaviors, and engaged students in a novel video-analysis application of a perspective-taking task designed to help them infer carers' thoughts and feelings [33, 50–53]. Evaluative feedback obtained from carers and nursing students allow us to make continued improvements to the intervention (i.e., provide more direct and immediate sharing of tagged video-data with students) and develop a reliable similarity rating tool that captures students' perceptual understanding.

Conclusions

While developing and studying the impact of *Heart Health Whispering*, outcomes for students and carers appeared promising and warrant further testing. The video-analysis (tagging video instances) and -feedback (i.e., sharing similarity scores) components of the *Heart Health Whispering* intervention are novel. Nurse educators in basic and continuing education are offered preliminary evidence on how to bolster nurse confidence in having empathic conversations about health risk behaviors. Carers said that empathic conversations help them to take ownership, feel trust that they are understood without judgment, and gives them a voice in exploring solutions as revealed through their stories. Nursing students and practicing nurses who learn these techniques could be encouraged to engage in self-evaluation plus annual re-training or reassessment as part of self-competencies in communication skills. This study has implications for ongoing empirical work to further refine a promising intervention on how to bolster clinician clinical empathy so as to avoid "jumping ahead of the patient" [15] when engaging in therapeutic conversations on carer self-care.

Additional files

Additional file 1: Recruitment Protocol for Undergraduate and Nurse Practitioner Students. (DOCX 14 kb)

Additional file 2: Intervention Protocol. (DOCX 19 kb)

Additional file 3: Family Carer Actor qualitative table. (DOCX 25 kb)

Additional file 4: Student qualitative table. (DOCX 25 kb)

Abbreviations

ANCOVA: Analysis of covariance; CARE: Consultation and relational empathy measure; carers: Family carer actors; Group I: Intervention group; Group PI: Partial intervention group; RA: Research assistant; RFIT: Risk factor identification tool; Ruler: Readiness to change ruler

Acknowledgments

The authors thank Yinghong (Amy) Wu for recruiting and collecting data from undergraduate nursing student participants and Dr. Rasheda Rabbani for statistical advice.

Funding

This work was supported by a Research Manitoba Chair held by Dr. Lobchuk and the Manitoba Centre for Nursing and Health Research College of Nursing Endowment Fund Research Grant in Professional Foundations. The funding bodies had no role in the design of the study and collection, analysis, and interpretation of data and in writing the manuscript.

Authors' contributions

All authors were involved with the conceptualization and production of this manuscript. ML, GL, CW, KCC, and WS were involved in the design of the research project. ML, LH, and JL collected data. JL participated in study coordination, made key observations, and had input in executing study protocols in the Lab. ML, LH, and JL analyzed data. All authors read and approved the final manuscript.

Competing interests

The authors declare that they have no competing interests.

Author details

[1]Rady Faculty of Health Sciences, College of Nursing, University of Manitoba, Room 315 – 89 Curry Place, Winnipeg, MB R3T 2N2, Canada. [2]Max Rady Faculty of Health Sciences, College of Medicine, University of Manitoba, P228-770, Bannatyne Avenue, Winnipeg, MB R3E 0W3, Canada. [3]Red River College, Nursing, 2055 Notre Dame Avenue, Winnipeg, MB R3H 0J9, Canada. [4]Department of Surgery, Section of General Surgery, University of Manitoba, 770 Bannatyne Avenue, Winnipeg, MB R3E 0W3, Canada.

References

1. World Health Organization. World Report on Aging and Health. Geneva: World Health Organization; 2015.
2. Carrera PM. The difficulty of making healthy choices and "health in all policies". Bull World Health Organ. 2014;92(3) https://doi.org/10.2471/BLT.13.121673. Accessed 06 Sept 2017

3. Keleher H, Parker R, Abdulwadud O, Francis K. Systematic review of the effectiveness of primary care nursing. Int J Nurs Pract. 2009;15:16–24.

4. Lin JS, O'Connor E, Whitlock EP, Beil TL. Behavioral counseling to promote physical activity and a healthful diet to prevent cardiovascular disease in adults: a systematic review for the U.S. preventive services task force. Ann Intern Med. 2010;153(11):736–50.

5. Schellenberg ES, Dryden DM, Vandermeer B, Ha C, Korownyk C. Lifestyle interventions for patients with and at risk for type 2 diabetes: a systematic review and meta-analysis. Ann Intern Med. 2013;159(8):543–51.

6. Franklin BA, Vanhecke TE. Counseling patients to make cardiovascular lifestyle changes: strategies for success. Prev Cardiol. 2008;11(1):50–5.

7. Hoffman GJ, Lee J, Mendez-Luck CA. Health behaviors among baby boomer informal caregivers. Gerontologist. 2012;52(2):219–30.

8. Mochari-Greenberger H, Mosca L. Caregiver burden and nonachievement of healthy lifestyle behaviors among family caregivers of cardiovascular disease patients. Am J Health Promot. 2012;27(2):84–9.

9. Haley WE, Roth DL, Howard G, Safford MM. Caregiving strain and estimated risk for stroke and coronary heart disease among spouse caregivers differential effects by race and sex. Stroke. 2010;41:331–6.

10. Lee SL, Colditz GA, Berkman LF, Kawachi I. Caregiving and risk of coronary heart disease in U.S. women: A prospective study. Am J Prev Med. 2003;24(2):113–9.

11. Schulz R, Newsom J, Mittelmark M, Burton L, Hirsch C, Jackson S. Health effects of caregiving - the caregiver health effects study: an ancillary study of the cardiovascular health study. Ann Behav Med. 1997;19:110–6.

12. Shaw WS, Patterson TL, Ziegler MG, Dimsdale JE, Semple SJ, Grant I. Accelerated risk of hypertensive blood pressure recordings among Alzheimer's caregivers. J Psychosom Res. 1999;46:215–27.

13. Ward J, Cody J, Schaal M, Hojat M. The empathy enigma: an empirical study of decline in empathy among undergraduate nursing students. J Prof Nurs. 2012;28(1):34–40.

14. Williams J, Stickley T. Empathy and nurse education. Nurse Educ Today. 2010;30:752–5.

15. Jansink R, Braspenning J, van der Weijden T, Elwyn G, Grol R. Primary care nurses struggle with lifestyle counseling in diabetes care: a qualitative analysis. BMC Fam Pract. 2010; https://doi.org/10.1186/1471-2296-11-41.

16. Miller WR, Rose GS. Toward a theory of motivational interviewing. Am Psychol. 2009;64(6):527–37.

17. Lobchuk M, Halas G, West C, Harder N, Tursunova Z, Ramraj C. Development of a novel empathy-related videofeedback intervention to improve empathic accuracy of nursing students: a pilot study. Nurse Educ Today. 2016;46:86–93.

18. Ickes W. Empathic accuracy. J Pers. 1993;61:587–610.

19. Davis MH. Empathy: A social psychological approach. Madison: Brown and Benchmark; 1994.

20. Batson CD, Early S, Salvarani G. Perspective-taking: imagining how another feels versus imagining how you would feel. Personal Soc Psychol Bull. 1997;23:751–8.

21. Ickes W. Measuring empathic accuracy. In: Hall JA, Bernieri FJ, editors. Interpersonal Sensitivity. New Jersey: Lawrence Erlbaum Associates, Inc; 2001.

22. Fitzgerald NM, Heywood S, Bikker AP, Mercer SW. Enhancing empathy in healthcare: a mixed-method evaluation of a pilot project implementing the CARE approach in primary and communication care settings in Scotland. J Compassionate Health Care. 2014;1:6. https://doi.org/10.1186/s40639-014-0006-8.

23. Mercer SW, Maxwell M, Heaney D, Watt GC. The consultation and relational empathy (CARE) measure: development and preliminary validation and reliability of an empathy-based consultation process measure. Fam Pract. 2004;21(6):699–705.

24. Halas G, Katz A, Jin D. Computer-based risk assessment: evaluating use in primary care. Electron Healthc. 2010;9(2):e10.

25. Heart and Stoke Foundation in Manitoba. The future of medicine: treating chronic disease before it starts. 2012. http://www.heartandstroke.ca/search-results-page?q=The+future+of+medicine%3A+treating+chronic++disease+before+it+starts. Accessed 7 Sept 2017.

26. Zimmerman GL, Olsen CG, Bosworth MFA. Stages of change' approach to helping patients change behavior. Am Fam Physician. 2000;61(5):1409–16.

27. Landis JR, Koch GG. The measurement of observer agreement for categorical data. Biometrics. 1977;33(1):159–74.

28. Patton M. Qualitative research & evaluation methods (3rd ed.). Thousand Oaks: Sage; 2002.

29. Lincoln YS, Guba EG. Naturalistic Inquiry. Beverly Hills: Sage Publications; 1985.

30. Ligthart SA, van den Eerenbeemt KDM, Pols J, van Bussel EF, Richard E, van Charante EPM. Perspectives of older people engaging in nurse-led cardiovascular prevention programmes: a qualitative study in primary care in the Netherlands. Br J Gen Pract. 2015;1:e-41–8.

31. Persky S, Eccleston CP. Medical student bias and care recommendations for an obese versus non-obese virtual patient. Int J Obes. 2011;35(5):728–35.

32. Poon MY, Tarrant M. Obesity: attitudes of undergraduate student nurses and registered nurses. J Clin Nurs. 2009;18(16):2355–65.

33. Cunico L, Sartori R, Marognolli O, Meneghini AM. Developing empathy in nursing students: a cohort longitudinal study. J Clin Nurs. 2012;21:2016–25.

34. Noordman J, Verhaak P, Dulmen S. Web-enabled video-feedback: a method to reflect on the communication skills of experienced physicians. Patient Educ Couns. 2011;82:335–40.

35. Ward J, Schaal M, Sullivan J, Bowen ME, Erdmann JB. Reliability and validity of the Jefferson scale of empathy in the undergraduate nursing students. J Nurs Meas. 2009;17(1):73–88.

36. Noordman J, van der Weijden T, van Dulmen S. Effects of video-feedback on the communication, clinical competence and motivational interviewing skills practice nurses: a pre-test posttest control group study. J Adv Nurs. 2014;70(10):2272–83.

37. Lane C, Hood K, Rollnick S. Teaching motivational interviewing: using role play is as effective as using simulated patients. Med Educ. 2008;42(6):637–44.

38. Cox ME, Yancy WS, Coffman CJ, et al. Effects of counseling techniques on patients' weight-related attitudes and behaviors in a primary care clinic. Patient Educ Couns. 2011;85:363–8.

39. Noordman J, van der Weijden T, van Dulmen S. Communication-related behavior change techniques used in face-to-face lifestyle interventions in primary care: a systematic review of the literature. Patient Educ Couns. 2012;8:227–44.

40. Oikarinen A, Engblom J, Kyngas H, Kaariainen M. Lifestyle counseling intervention effects on counseling quality in patients with stroke and transient ischemic attack. J Neurosci Nurs. 2017;49(3):137–41.

41. Epton T, Harris PR, Kane R, van Koningsbruggen GM, Sheeran P. The impact of self-affirmation on health-behavior change: a meta-analysis. Health Psychol. 2015;34(3):187–96.

42. DePaulo BM, Charlton K, Cooper H, Lindsay JJ. The accuracy-confidence correlation in the detection of deception. Personal Soc Psychol Rev. 1997;1:346.

43. Garner B, Sanci L, Cahill H, Ukoumune OC, Gold L, Rogers L, McCallum Z, Wake M. Using simulated patients to develop doctors' skills in facilitating behaviour change: addressing childhood obesity. Med Edu. 2010;44(7):706–15.

44. Ickes W, Stinson L, Bissonnette V, Garcia S. Naturalistic social cognition: empathic accuracy in mixed-sex dyads. J Pers Soc Psychol. 1990;59:730–42.

45. Kalish R, Dawiskiba M, Sung Y-C, Blanco M. Raising medical student awareness of compassionate care through reflection of annotated videotapes of clinical encounters. Educ Health. 2011;24(3):1–13.

46. Miller WR, Mount KA. A small study of training in motivational interviewing: does one workshop change clinician and client behaviour? Behav Cogn Psychoth. 2001;29:457–71.

47. Baer JS, Wells EA, Rosengren DB, Hartzler B, Beadnell B, Dunn C. Agency context and tailored training in technology transfer: a pilot evaluation of motivational interviewing training for community counselors. J Subst Abus Treat. 2009;37(2):191–202.

48. Rollnick S, Kinnersley P, Butler C. Context-bound communication skills training: development of a new method. Med Ed. 2002;36:377–83.

49. Mounsey A, Bovbjerg V, White I, Gazewood J. Do students develop better motivational interviewing skills through role-play with standardized patents or with student colleagues? Med Educ. 2006;40(8):775–80.

50. Fukkink RG, Trienekens N, Kramer LJC. Video feedback in education and training: putting learning in the picture. Educ Psychol Rev. 2011;23:45–63.

51. Yoo MS, Son YJ, Kim YS, Park JH. Video-based self-assessment: implementation and evaluation in an undergraduate nursing course. Nurse Educ Today. 2009;29:585–9.

52. Marita P, Leena L, Tarja K. Nurses' self-reflectio via videotaping to improve communication skills in health counseling. Patient Educ Couns. 1999;36(1):3–11.

53. Mast ME, Sawin EM, Pantaleo KA. Life of a caregiver simulation: teaching students about frail older adults and their family caregivers. J Nurs Educ. 2012;51(7):396–402.

A hermeneutic study of integrating psychotherapist competence in postnatal child health care: nurses' perspectives

Katarina Kornaros[1]* (iD), Sofia Zwedberg[2], Eva Nissen[1] and Björn Salomonsson[1]

Abstract

Background: There is a considerable prevalence of and an increasing attention to emotional problems in families with infants. Yet, knowledge is scant of how to create efficient and accessible mental health services for this population. The study qualitatively explored public health nurses' conceptions of a clinical project, in which psychotherapists provided short-term consultations and supervisions for nurses at Child Health Centres in Stockholm.

Methods: In-depth interviews with fifteen nurses. The guideline of the interviews contained open-ended questions that were analysed applying a hermeneutical approach.

Results: Four main themes crystallized; The nurses' conceptions of their psychosocial work, Trespassing on another professional role, Interprofessional collaboration at the Child Health Centre, and The nurses' conceptions of the psychotherapist's function. In a second step, an analysis that clustered the nurses' attitudes towards handling mental health problems yielded one last theme with three "Ideal types"; nurses who expressed "I don't want to", "I want to but I cannot", and "I want to and I can" (take care of families' emotional problems at the CHC).

Conclusion: The nurses appreciated the easy referral and accessibility to the psychotherapists, and the possibilities of learning more about perinatal mental illness and parent-infant interactions. For a successful cooperation with the nurses, the therapist should be a team member, be transparent about his/her work, and give feedback about cases in treatment. The study also shows how the organization needs to clarify its guidelines and competence to improve psychological child health care. The paper suggests improvements for an integrated perinatal mental health care.

Keywords: Aristotle, Child health services, Hermeneutics, Ideal type, Interprofessional relations, Nurses, Perinatal care, Psychotherapy

Background

In Sweden, "Child Health Centres" (CHC) offer tax-funded primary health care to all children between 0 and 5 years. In contrast to, for example, the UK, Sweden uses separate units ("Maternity Clinics", MVC) for prenatal health care. The MVC carries out pregnancy checks during pregnancy and prepares the parents for the birth. There is thus an overlap of the term "midwife"; in Sweden, she is only responsible up to the delivery including a one-time check-up a few weeks afterwards. The postnatal staff is called a CHC-nurse. The family chooses a local CHC and meets with the nurse, who tracks the children's weight and length and examines their developmental progress.

In 1997, the National Board of Health and Welfare [1] provided guidelines for nurses to include CHC psychosocial support to families, based on the evidence that approximately 10–15% of new mothers show signs of postpartum depression (PPD) [2–4] and about 5–10% among fathers [5, 6]. Detecting parental distress can be difficult unless a family member signals it clearly to the CHC nurse, who may then refer to psychiatric care. This procedure, however, risks stigmatizing parents with babies who seldom regard themselves as ill in a psychiatric sense [7]. Health care routines in Stockholm demand that CHC nurses receive a brief training course in the Edinburgh Postnatal Depression Scale (EPDS) [8]. Screening is offered

* Correspondence: Katarina.kornaros@ki.se
[1]Department of Women's and Children's Health, Karolinska Institutet, Stockholm, Sweden
Full list of author information is available at the end of the article

when the infant is 6–8 weeks, and the nurse talks with the mother about her questionnaire responses. This can lead to a few follow-up meetings and, if needed, a referral to an external general practitioner, psychologist, or a psychiatrist.

Psychological treatment at the CHC

Although many studies indicate substantial results of parent-infant psychotherapy (PIP) [9–11] many cases of baby worries, a term comprising parental and infant emotional distress [12], risk being excluded from primary health care. The reason is the difficulty in detecting such problems and the lack of appropriate treatment at the CHC. The roadblock is threefold; a family in need will not voice their problems clearly, the nurse will not capture the signals sensitively enough, and she will not know how and where to refer the family for professional psychological help [13, 14].

To remedy this shortcoming, a method called "Short-term Psychodynamic Infant-Parent Interventions at Child Health Centres" (SPIPIC) was developed to integrate somatic and psychological health care [12]. It has two arms; a psychotherapist supervises CHC nurses and offers families short-term treatment on the premises. Supervisions aim to inspire nurses to detect and address baby worries. The therapies of 1–5 sessions aim to help parents tackle such issues and improve their contact with the baby. One author of this study introduced the method to a group of psychoanalysts trained in adult and parent-infant therapy. The Swedish Inheritance Fund provided funding and the clinical project took place 2013–2016.

This study is part of a research project evaluating the clinical project. The overarching aim is to investigate if SPIPIC might contribute to improving postnatal mental health care. The present paper focuses on the nurse's experiences. When she observes baby worries, she is confronted with challenges; how to bring them up with parents and suggest adequate treatment. If a therapist becomes linked to the unit, the nurse needs to collaborate with him/her. Such integration of professional efforts might improve treatment quality, but factors that impede and facilitate this process need to be explored.

Methods
Aims
The study aimed to analyse CHC nurses' previous experiences of taking care of families with baby worries. And, now that a professional psychotherapist was introduced, how did they experience being supervised by her, referring cases, and collaborating with her?

Setting and sample selection
Six CHCs in Stockholm were selected to maximize the geographical and socio-economic variability. The centres hosted 3–8 nurses specialized in paediatric care, often also in public health. Each full-time nurse was responsible for about 350 children. The sampling procedure was as follows. Since we aimed to evaluate a clinical project, the interviewer (first author), approached all the involved CHCs. She asked the head nurse to supply names of colleagues who had a varying length of professional experience and professional positions. This resulted in fifteen nurses being interviewed, of which six were head nurses. All interviews were face-to-face. An unknown number declined to participate due to time constraints. The unknown number is due to the interviewer's non awareness about how many nurses had been asked to participate. Yet, she got information about nurses rejecting the proposition. All participants were female, had Swedish background and their average age was 53 (35–65) years. Interviews took place during the end of the research project, January–May 2016. They were conducted by the first author who had profound experience in qualitative interviewing.

Procedure
Interviews took place in each nurse's consulting room. First, the interviewer went through the study aims and clarified routines of confidentiality. Characteristics about the interviewer was brought up before the interview started, such as reason for doing the research and personal goals. Participation was voluntary and if a nurse decided to leave the study, data would be deleted. All nurses consented by signing an agreement. Interviews lasted 1 hour and were audio-recorded and transcribed verbatim. The interview format was built on 14 questions concerning the nurses experience of perinatal mental health [PMH] and the clinical project. They were created by the first author and posed in an order that suited the topics broached by the nurse. When relevant, the interviewer could probe further into one area. Field notes were made at some occasions. Below are the interview questions:

1. Which were your expectations of the clinical project?
2. What kind of education do you have?
3. Have you felt any lack of any competence in your work?
4. How do you feel the collaboration with the psychotherapist worked?
5. Describe what happened in the supervision by the psychotherapist.
6. How did you experience the supervision?
7. How do you observe parents with emotional problems?
8. Tell me how you reason when you meet parents with babies who do not address that they need psychological help, yet you identify their problem.

9. Tell me if you experience that your ability to detect parents and children with emotional problems has changed during the project?
10. How do you experience bringing up questions about mental health with the parent(s)?
11. "What kind of" parents did you refer to the psychotherapist?
12. Did you mention to all parents you met that the therapist was working at the CHC?
13. How did you handle these cases before the psychotherapist was available here?
14. Does the project conform with your expectations?

Data analysis

The analyses were based on philosophical hermeneutics [15], which presupposes that any interpretation of texts, words, or behaviours is created out of the respondent's verbal and non-verbal testimonies as well as the researcher's preconceptions. In the Geisteswissenschaften [16] or human sciences, of which this study is an example, the interpreter acknowledges his subjectivity and considers it essential for his/her interpretation. Interpretations will thus depend on the individualities of respondent and interviewer and will, accordingly, not reflect universal laws. Knowledge emerges in a dialogue based on equality between interviewer and informant in that both are human subjects [17]. True, analysing a text, in contrast to an interview, entails no dialogue but the interpreter maintains an internal discourse with the text and uses self-reflection to reach a deeper understanding. Each author of the paper, one social worker, two midwives, and one child psychoanalyst, applied this procedure to the interview texts and the group met regularly to discuss the material and the interpretations. We did not use any qualitative software since, in our opinion, it is more appropriate for example in content analysis. Our hermeneutic analyses were based on an interaction between discussions in the group and recourse to the interview transcripts.

The group analysed recurrent statements in the nurses' comments and sought to detect their underlying meanings and collected them into themes that were labelled. This inductive analysis [18] was later complemented by an abductive approach [19, 20] of identifying Ideal types. Abduction involves forming conclusions from the information that is known. This procedure aimed at "making sense of data" ([20], p. 5) and at enabling further theorizing on the nurses' attitudes in handling emotional family problems. Ideal types was introduced in sociology [21] and later in psychotherapy research [22, 23]. The researcher extracts concise descriptions out of each case and clusters observable phenomena and concepts in an interpretative or exploratory schema [22]. The clustering combines objective observations and the interviewer's subjective emotional reactions to the interviewee [24].

Results

All names contained in the result section are pseudonyms and have been changed to ensure the anonymity of study participants. Nurses from one CHC have identical initials, for example, Thea and Tora from CHC-T. The hermeneutic analysis crystallized four main themes. In a second step, an analysis that clustered the nurses' attitudes towards handling mental health problems yielded one last theme.

The nurses' conceptions of their psychosocial work

Many nurses mentioned that health care organization had changed the last decades, with ensuing alterations in their duties. This created a tension between their previous medical training and today's tasks, which increasingly concern psychological problems.

Dina: "I miss working with medical health care here (...). When the family doctor reform was instituted, all casualties disappeared. Earlier, we could get burns, wound dressing, suture removal and all that. It disappeared! Now they visit the family doctor instead."

(The family doctor reform implied that all citizens should have the opportunity to choose a personal general practitioner). Nurses also described that this change meant that they must shift focus from the child to the parents. They reported that today's parents need to be confirmed, their agenda is crammed, and they must achieve and compare themselves with others. Nurses felt they had become more of a "grandmother" or a "speaking partner".

Paulina: "The number of families who feel mentally ill is incredibly larger than ten years ago.... A huge difference! One would think that today, every family is in a bad emotional state... Once you get a family without any worries, you almost think it's a bit unusual."

Some nurses pointed out that conversations during coffee breaks often revolved around distressed families and they deplored not finding time for exchange and reflection during working hours. Cleo missed time for reflection during supervisions:

"What will happen to me as well when I meet this mother who is so worried about her child (...) How do I feel then, how worried am I? How scared am I? What do I bring with me home? These are things I would like to leave behind at supervisions!"

Many nurses regarded the EPDS screening 6–8 weeks after childbirth as indispensable for capturing emotional issues. It helped them raise matters about mental illness in a less intrusive way. Most of them regarded the questionnaire score as a major source of understanding the mother's emotional well-being. However, proceeding to suggesting to the mother some counselling sessions based on the EPDS responses, felt cumbersome.

> Thea: "It gets to an entirely different level when you're screening [EPDS]. Afterwards [when the results are discussed with the mother], you must have something to offer! We don't have any therapeutic education or anything like that, but we have built on experience, quite simply, and if you don't have that... then it must be hard!"

Some nurses abstained from EPDS-screening for mothers with insufficient knowledge of Swedish, or those who were problematic cases or difficult to identify, because they felt overloaded. They knew that these families needed psychotherapeutic help but did not refer them. They felt they had enough work to manage the usual tasks in time. The nurses also felt they needed more knowledge about parent-infant psychology and wanted introductory psychotherapy training. Some thought paediatric nursing education needed to be modernized.

> Tanja: "Is [parental support] our job today? What does our education look like? There's very little of [psychological issues] in our training. They may need to change [education] because it feels there will be more and more of this field. And then you would of course need to have someone like Therese [the therapist] (...) to guide [us]; is this [case] healthy or not healthy?"

Other nurses did raise psychological issues directly rather than waiting for the EPDS-screening or an explicit statement by the parent. Ebba "talked to herself" about how to interact with and address every family. Cleo used mother-infant interaction massage to discern attachment problems in the dyad.

> Cleo: "In a group with parents (...) I can see someone with vast interaction difficulties, and I can ask [the mother]: 'Is it difficult being close to the child this way?' Maybe one mother always turns her child away from herself, and the child is turning outwards, away from her."

In our interpretation, nurses who missed the medical tasks they had been trained in focused on the child's physiological development and referred psychosocial problems instantly to the therapist or other professionals. They felt dismissed having been withdrawn from duties they felt capable of handling, such as ordinary medical problems. Instead, they felt forced to work with psychosocial issues, where they felt less competent. Others, who had changed focus or who had not previously worked according to the traditional medical role, deplored that they did not have the knowledge to work deeper with psychological problems.

Trespassing on another professional role

Many thought that addressing the mother about her mental health was a sensitive topic. Hence, they separated the task of capturing her emotional problems from the therapist's task of treating them. If this was not a possible option, many considered crossing this line to be an act of trespassing on another professional role.

Sara felt secure as a CHC-nurse but when encountering a sad mother in a EPDS-screening, she felt insecure and that she was "stepping into the therapist's shoes". Despite her training, she had not carried out EPDS-sessions for 15 years because she had felt like a "semi-psychologist" and "a little bluffer". The reason for such feelings was not any lack of professional experience. Rather, some nurses felt they did not have anything new to say to the parent in the EPDS-sessions. When touching anxiety-provoking topics, they feared they might open up reactions they could not handle.

> Erika (pretending to talk to a mother): "'Okay, you're afraid to leave your home, because you're afraid someone will follow you, push your stroller out in the street and harm your baby'. I can't explain WHY she has such thoughts! I can't suggest what she can do. Then something else needs to be added."

We interpret that Erika was stuck in a demand to offer the mother advice and suggestions. She was more familiar with having an active, advisory role and less trained in listening to and containing the parents affects, which was felt as trespassing on therapist territory. Having a psychotherapist at the CHC bridged this dilemma. She was now seen as a haven of wisdom and a relief for the nurse. Cases could be remitted to her and the therapist often received the cases without any reserve, which made them refer on a broader and less selective scale. Cases that were previously difficult to identify, or those which gave the nurse a "lump in the stomach", could now be referred on a looser basis.

> Cleo: "Some of my parents may not seem to be in a very bad mood or do not score very high on the EPDS. Yet, in our conversations I may find out that they are worried after all and are not feeling very well. And then I have told them that they have an opportunity to meet with a psychotherapist here".

Interprofessional collaboration at the child health Centres

Two CHC groups, positive and critical, crystallized. Ebba called the therapist "a godsend", caring, structured, and involving the team in treatment decisions. Supervisions were regular, and the therapist provided transparent feedback about referred families. In our interpretation, Ebba addressed transparency in two ways; the therapist was open to the nurses' points of view and, concretely, left her door open whenever possible. This also resulted in an open attitude between Ebba and the parents. She felt at ease asking the parents about therapies. At CHC-P, Pella described the therapist's transparency:

> "It is more enjoyable and easier to work with someone who completely trusts our confidentiality! She probably does, otherwise she wouldn't tell us everything she's actually doing! (...) We are all bound by professional secrecy. I think it's OK that she tells us everything when we ask for it. Such an approach inspires confidence, rather than someone saying, 'No, I can't tell you about it'."

Sara had different experiences. The therapist Sonya was kind but "closed". Sara received no information about referred families, since Sonya did not divulge anything. Supervisions took place monthly, but Sara felt they were "so-called supervisions", since the therapist did not talk about the referred families. Sara called them "conversations about travelling and weather". She requested clear rules of transparency and secrecy, trust in everyone's competence, and focus on the families.

> Sara: "I don't know if Sonya wants to maintain confidentiality, maybe out of considerations of secrecy? I haven't actually asked her, because when I asked about referred parents... [short pause] I didn't get to know very much. I have respected that and thought she probably doesn't want to say anything. Perhaps it's right but it offers me less."

One interpretation is that Sonya came from another professional context as a private practitioner and was used to sharing information more restrictedly, which clashed with the CHC culture. Nevertheless, the nurses appreciated her clinical work. The nurses were accommodating because they feared losing Sonya. Instead of bringing up the problems with her, they worked in parallel with her and found their own ways of complementing her administrative routines and secrecy.

On CHCs with less satisfactory supervisions and contacts with the therapist, parental discontent with therapy was interpreted as proof of the therapist's failure. Still, no nurse raised such topics with the therapist. At CHCs where nurses were satisfied, discontent was brought up even though it was awkward. Pella informed the therapist about a dissatisfied parent:

> "I must admit it was embarrassing, because in my eyes she's good. You are working together, after all, she's here once a week, we have supervision with her so she feels like a colleague. Such things are always tough to raise with a colleague".

The nurses' conceptions of the psychotherapist's function

Overall, nurses had vague ideas about how therapies were performed. At CHCs where supervisions were felt to be unsatisfactory, this added to the dissatisfaction and made nurses refer less to the therapist. In centres where supervisions worked well and the therapist was perceived as a team member, the "mystery" surrounding therapies was unimportant for their trust in her. In addition, these therapists gave some insight into how treatments were performed. In general, nurses were positive about the treatment model per se, even the ones who felt critical of the local psychotherapist.

> Pella (positive of the local therapist): "It would be wonderful if this ended up being a project and became part of general child health care (...) especially in socio-economically burdened areas".

Referrals to other units were expressed as time-consuming, since it implied an obligation to convince a professional that their patient was a case for them. In the case of GP consultations, some nurses felt the doctors did not have the necessary qualification. Thus, a local therapist made work more flexible and help more accessible. Families came for regular nurse calls followed by a therapy session. If the nurse was considering therapy for the family member(s), she could ask questions to the therapist, get immediate answers, and refer the family.

> Tanja: "Sometimes, suggesting another unit to the family meets with a huge resistance. They seem to think it's too much psychiatry and a harder step to go somewhere else. Here [to the CHC] they come anyway!"

Most parents were referred to the therapist because they brooded on their parental role and felt lonely and uncertain when interacting with the baby. Though many had a psychiatric history, such specialist units did not consider them as "their cases". The nurses worried that their emotional states could affect the infant negatively and emphasized the importance of early intervention. Prior to the project, it had been difficult to implement this family approach at the CHC. In CHCs with many immigrants, nurses had difficulties in understanding the family member's state due to language barriers, attitudes towards mental illness, and lack of familiarity with psychotherapy.

> Pella: "It is a bit of our 'mourning [problem] child', or I think, it should be all of Sweden's mourning child in some way. What do we do with [immigrant families] who do not crack all the [cultural] codes?"

Attitudes to taking care of psychological problems: Ideal Types.

The themes reported above resulted from analyses of the interviews; the nurses' comments were grouped inductively into themes. Afterwards, we also analysed in another direction; nurses were clustered into Ideal Types according to their attitudes towards handling psychological problems. Three types emerged.

Ideal type 1: "I don't want to"

> Tora: "I am a CHC nurse. That's what I am! I have great tools for what I should be able to perform and for what my competence is supposed to include (...). There are limits to which dialogues we CHC-nurses can have with the parents. We are not therapists and we are not educated for it and then one should feel the limit of what a CHC visit implies".

We interpret this nurse to be unwilling to expand her professional role to include working with mental health problems. She has decided not to work with what she feels amounts to a trespassing on another profession's duties.

Ideal type 2 "I want to but I cannot"

> Sandra: "This mom is so worried about every little thing. She had difficulties letting go of the child. In itself, that need not lead to a long-term psychological contact. It usually lights up at three-four months. I usually try to see if I can solve it myself as a nurse. But I felt nothing happened after our counselling meetings and phone calls... so I asked Sonya for an appointment. I couldn't handle the mother's worries."

The nurse has understood that this mother is worried and has started consultations but feels she lacks skills to deepen the dialogue. She tries to understand the mother, but when she perceives that the mother's worries do not

diminish, her own worries about the mother increase. She questions her own capability of handling maternal worries.

Ideal type 3 "I want to and I can"

> Ebba: "I have a supplementary assignment at CHC with groups of depressed mothers (...). I try with the help of infant massage and such to promote interaction and find the joy too! (...) Some [mothers] who are depressed can be very self-absorbed and need help opening up to see their little 'Charlie'.

We interpret that the nurse has an interest and feels she can supervise such groups. She has noted that the mothers are self-absorbed and has found a solution to guide them to better understand their babies. She facilitates maternal self-insight by including the baby in the interaction.

Discussion

This paper investigated nurses whose working place, Child Health Centres, had been provided with a psychotherapist through a clinical project. It integrated routine health care with qualified brief psychotherapy and aimed to enhance the competence and the incentive among nurses to handle perinatal psychological problems. It thus viewed the *nurse as a key person* in perinatal psychological health care. The discussion will cover [1] our study's contribution to existing research on midwives' and nurses' attitudes to, and difficulties in dealing with, perinatal emotional issues, [2] the interview findings within an Aristotelian conceptual framework, and [3] conclusions from the interviews on how to organize and educate perinatal health care providers in ways that integrate medical and psychological perspectives.

Comparison with other nursing studies

Some studies have focused on midwives' and nurses' attitudes to perinatal psychological problems. London midwives [25] indicated their willingness to take responsibility but they lacked confidence and knowledge. Many did not know about the "high incidence of perinatal mental health problems [and] the signs and symptoms of some of the most serious perinatal mental illnesses" (p. 334). Two studies of Australian midwives [13, 26] yielded similar findings. To improve the situation, Ross-Davie et al. [25] recommended better training and "adequate staffing levels and the provision of specialist perinatal mental health service for onward referral" (p. 334). McCauley et al. [13] suggested "improved liaison with other disciplines, [such as] a perinatal mental health nurse specialist or practitioner" (p. 792). Such a procedure was instituted in a Dublin project [27]. This differs from our project's placement of a psychotherapist at the CHC, who used her expertise in treating parents and supervising nurses. We believe this is advantageous since depressed parents, as well as their nurses, are burdened by the fear of stigmatization when referred to other units. A therapist on the premises conveys, together with the CHC nurse, that *mental health issues are a natural and integral part of parenthood*. Also, a therapist's expertise covers not only symptoms of emotional suffering but also how to create a fruitful dialogue with the patient. The need to deepen midwives' skills in handling parental distress was shown by Rollans and co-workers [14]. They investigated qualitatively what took place at antenatal booking visits, in which midwives were required to make a routine psychosocial assessment. Their unfamiliarity was indicated by the many who read out the questions from their computer screen at the end of the visit, a procedure that might impact negatively on the future mother's "comfort in disclosing her concerns and on her relationship with midwives and the maternity service" (p. 6). Midwives should thus be given "opportunities to discuss their own experiences of listening and responding to women's trauma experiences" (p.7).

In our project, such opportunities were supposed to be given through the therapist supervisions. When such collaboration did not work well it was not at firsthand, in contrast to the London study [25], due to lack of knowledge of symptoms of perinatal distress and disorder. In fact, nurses in our project knew about such issues but were embarrassed when broaching them with the parents. This was reflected in several themes in the qualitative analysis, for example, that such dialogues with a parent felt like "trespassing" on the therapist's profession. Her presence on site was much appreciated, but some nurses felt uncertain of how to utilize this opportunity. Judging from the interviews, a similar unfamiliarity probably existed among those therapists who seemed to have difficulties with maintaining professional secrecy while simultaneously being open with the nurses. This question will be further investigated in an upcoming interview study with the therapists.

Turning to our Ideal Types, we suggest that the one named "I want to but cannot" corresponds with many nurses in the studies from London and Australia. We found one reason behind such attitudes; the recent paradigm shift in health care, which deeply affected the nurses' views of professional roles and pride; from medical tasks focusing on the child to a psychosocial family perspective. This made them feel uncertain about their professional duties. This finding might correspond with an argument in a British study [28] that nursing education has not realized that integrating knowledge in psychology, biology, and sociology is essential to promote holistic care. Possibly, when some nurses complained about insufficient time to counsel parents and reflect with colleagues, this might not only reflect

hard facts but also uncertainties about their new professional role. When they were helped in this by the therapist they valued it greatly, whereas other nurses felt supervisions were unsatisfactory and unnecessary. Such differences did not relate to the therapists' *clinical* skills but to her *openness* vis-à-vis the nurse team and her unclear ways of leading the supervision sessions. Too much attention was being paid to maintaining patient secrecy, and some therapists seemed unfamiliar with chairing the sessions. In contrast, their skills with patients were seldom questioned by the nurses. Everyone appreciated the clinical resource – although they knew little about the content of the therapies. Problems rather arose in the area of therapist-nurse *collaboration*.

An Aristotelian framework

To further understand the nurses' problems in handling baby worries, and to substantiate the validity of the Ideal types, we will discuss our results in line with Aristotelian epistemological concepts; *phronesis, techne,* and *episteme* [29]. *Phronesis* implies judgement based on practical wisdom and reflection used to approach the current situation. It has also been described as "gut feeling" or "tacit knowledge" [30, 31]. Skerrett [32] applies it to psychotherapeutic work and points out that to Aristotle, "our social practices constantly demand choices, such as how to be fair, how to take a risk, how to determine a course of action (...) Making the best choice demands wisdom" (p. 49). Phronesis also implies self-control, justice and courage. In Aristotle's ([33], p. 95) own words, phronesis "is a true and reasoned state of capacity to act with regard to the things that are good or bad for man". To illustrate, when a nurse sets out to consider a patient's emotional state before inoculating, she applies phronesis.

Techne refers both to a technology adapted for a particular task and to a craft, for example, all the practical details involved in a vaccination; the procedure is the same regardless of the patient's physical and emotional condition. *Episteme*, finally, refers to the logic behind an action. A nurse who decides, prior to a vaccination, to investigate if a child is infected applies episteme based on the general knowledge that it may be perilous to inoculate a sick child. The research that yielded such conclusions also took place within this paradigm.

To obtain a clinical knowledge that is as all-encompassing and profound as possible, it is essential to combine the three Aristotelian roads. Constrictions arise when one excludes or obfuscates any of them. In the Western health care paradigm, techne and episteme are viewed as essential for increasing knowledge and developing treatment methods. One example of the bias on episteme and techne was found in a Swedish study [34] comparing how nurses described their behaviour in parental groups with how they performed in video-recorded sessions. Despite their belief in the contrary, they tended to act as experts and leave little time to parents for discussions and reflection. The latter attitude seems much needed especially with parents with emotional problems. Similarly to the conclusions by Berlin et al., we believe that the therapists' supervisions are essential to help the nurses develop in such a direction.

In contrast to techne and episteme, phronesis has not gained equal respect. It implies that we deliberate on the unique case, whereas episteme involves demonstration of the general. Therefore, only the latter paradigm has acquired the reputation of providing better treatment evidence. When taking care of patients, phronesis contributes by meeting the criteria of the individual. To substantiate, we bring in a phenomenologic study [35] where first-time mothers were interviewed about their experiences of support from the nurse. They appreciated moments when she showed patience with the mother, remained with her in difficult moments, and gave proactive support. Such behaviour seemed to reflect the nurse's identification with the mothers, an attitude of "I know how it once was to be an inexperienced mother", in other words one of phronesis. We argue that the panic and helplessness among the mothers in this study were similar to what an anxious or depressed mother may feel when being alone with her baby. We also claim that their nurses were able to use phronesis with them.

As a counterargument, one might claim that an attitude of phronesis will be attained as the nurse's experience grows. Benner [36] describes the nurse's gradual development to become an expert in her profession. A newly graduated nurse sticks to settled rules and routines, but with increased experience she can become more independent and trust her intuition. In Aristotelian terms, she has moved from a one-sided reliance on techne and episteme to including more of phronesis. Phronesis certainly needs time to develop, but the paradox in our study is that all nurses had a long professional experience. We suggest several factors that seemed to stunt their reflection, empathy and curiosity of the young families' dilemmas; organizational factors, lack of training, and a change in today's health care paradigm compared with the one prevailing during their training. As Kinsella and Pitman [37] point out, today's medical education and politics prioritize "instrumental values", a term close to techne. When the aims of phronesis, techne, and episteme conflict and this remains unacknowledged, problems will arise. Phronesis also implies to sometimes work in an atmosphere of uncertainty and even bewilderment, whereas in techne and episteme the answers seem more obvious. This conflict emerged in the attitudes among our nurses towards the EPDS-questionnaire. Like in other studies [30, 38], it was perceived as a user-friendly instrument. Nevertheless, many nurses feared handling the ensuing EPDS-sessions. Their

apprehension of trespassing made them avoid talking about mental illness with the parents.

We wish to also interpret the ideal types in terms of the Aristotelian concepts. Type 1 nurses, "I don't want to", preferred to work with medical issues, instead of maintaining a holistic perspective of the family. They acknowledged psychological issues but delegated them directly to the "expert" psychotherapist. They did intuit emotional problems in the family but abstained from talking about them, seemingly because they should be addressed by professionals possessing relevant techne and episteme. Some acknowledged that personal life experiences had provided them with wisdom but claimed this was not possible to apply in conversations with the families. Thus, in not making full use of their phronesis, their "personhood", "a crucial element in accomplishing the goals of medicine" ([39], p. 321) receded in the background.

Ideal type 2 nurses, "I want to but cannot", believed treatment of mental illness requires an "unknown" mode of techne and episteme. They applied it to some extent but dared not to delve deeper. They devalued the very phronesis they felt they possessed. Ideal type 3, "I want to and I can", seemed to find a balance in tasks demanding mostly techne and episteme (nutrition advice, weighing and measuring) and phronesis (handling EPDS-sessions and maintaining dialogues with the families).

Phronesis also implies *ethical considerations*. The nurses' dilemma can be described in terms of "moral distress" [40, 41]. This concept covers situations when a professional knows the right thing to do, but the institution makes it difficult to do what s/he knows is best. Tiedje [41] highlights the risks when moral distress is not acted upon; it can overwhelm the nurse's coping resources. Tiedje recommends a coach who listens, guides and sorts out the professional and emotional dilemmas. The therapists in our project seemed to assume this function in structuring supervisions and increasing the nurses' psychological understanding. Moral distress can also be countered by courage [40], and the supervisors seemed to embolden nurses to bring up emotional problems with the parents.

Perinatal health care organization and education
In this area, we emphasize the paradigmatic shift in nursing duties in recent years. Apart from differences between individual municipalities and county councils [42], we discovered "local CHC cultures" regarding attitudes towards psychological care. Paradoxically, this homogeneity at each CHC risks creating heterogeneity for families needing psychological help; they might not obtain adequate care if their needs fall outside the local culture.

Another finding is that the health care organization, though it demands nurses to focus on psychosocial issues, does not systematically train them in this. Perhaps, the organization does not clarify whether nurses should work according to the attitudes mirrored by the Ideal types 1, 2, or 3. When nurses declared they felt congested with duties and professionally disregarded, we interpret this to reflect their dissatisfaction with the gap between training and the organization's requirements.

The psychotherapist's patency and accessibility vis-à-vis the nurses seemed crucial for the group dynamics during supervisions. Nurses wanted her to lead yet also be a team member. Therapists were different, which led to divergent attitudes towards psychosocial issues among the CHCs. In general, the nurses' views of the therapist depended on the head nurse's attitudes towards her and the supervisions, but she rarely understood her importance in this.

Despite some nurses' critique, they considered the therapist a needed resource. We suggest two interpretations; the nurses were eager to receive another therapist in the future and they also feared being openly critical of her. The nurses' reluctance to criticize her was perhaps akin to their unwillingness to confront the health care organization with their discontent with the lack of time for reflection in peer group discussions and supervisions.

If a nurse seeks support for a mother from the Swedish psychiatric health care's "first line psychiatry" [42], which is a low-level form of psychiatric care often instituted at GP clinics, this implies a detour in the referral process. The nurse interviews allow for an interpretation that integrating a psychotherapist at CHC implied faster referral and greater accessibility of specialised parent-infant treatment and, in addition, interchange of information between therapists and nurses.

As for immigrant families, they constituted a specific challenge in that the nurses felt a lack of cultural competence. This made them sometimes avoid bringing up such perceived problems with the family involved. This finding corresponds to previous research [30, 43]; the Swedish Child Health Care organization lacks competence and guidelines to deal with mental illness among immigrant families. Also, our therapists seemed unfamiliar with encountering patients from other cultures than their own. In today's increasing immigration, we can expect mental illness to become more frequent among newcomers. Therefore, it is of importance to detect these problems and handle them at an early stage in a professional way.

Limitations

The informants were sometimes recruited by the head nurse, which brings about the issue of voluntary participation. Possibly, some participants felt persuaded by her to be interviewed, but the interviewer emphasized that participation was voluntary and that one could withdraw at any time without the head nurse being informed. Perhaps, recruitment involved a bias in that the head nurse would only ask nurses whom she appreciated. If any such bias existed, it was hard to control for.

The hermeneutic analytic method, with its emphasis that the interpreter's subjectivity forms part of the basis of the interpretation, raises the question of trustworthiness [44], including external validity. To maximize the level of trustworthiness, we created a group of four interpreters who worked, first individually and then together to reach reasonably coherent interpretations.

Conclusions

Instituting early interventions for families with mental health problems is crucial for optimizing the child's development. Psychotherapeutic interventions have proven to be effective in such situations. The challenge is how to detect these persons, talk with them about it, and offer high-quality care. We have evaluated one model where the psychotherapist was integrated with regular health care at the CHC. In general, nurses were positive and wanted it to be permanent due to the effective remittance procedure and easy accessibility, and the possibilities of learning more about perinatal mental illness and parent-infant interactions. This is urgent especially for nurses who either have little interest in PMH or are vigilant about such issues but feel poorly equipped to deal with them. For a successful cooperation with the nurses, the therapist should be a team member, be transparent about his/her work, and give feedback about cases in treatment. The study also shows how the organization needs to clarify its guidelines and competence to improve psychological child health care. It also needs to improve education in cultural competence regarding immigrant families. This applies both to nurses and therapists.

Abbreviations
CHC: Child Health Centres; EPDS: Edinburgh Postnatal Depression Scale; PIP: Parent-infant psychotherapy; PMH: Perinatal Mental Health; PPD: Postpartum depression; SPIPIC: Short-term Psychodynamic Infant-Parent Interventions at Child Health Centres

Acknowledgements
We wish to thank the CHC-nurses who generously gave their time to participate in this study. The study was supported by Karolinska Institutet and the following foundations: Bertil Wennborgs Stiftelse, Clas Groschinskys minnesfond, Helge Ax:son Johnsons stiftelse, Stiftelsen Solstickan, and Kempe-Carlgrenska fonden. We thank them all.

Funding
Bertil Wennborgs stiftelse; Clas Groschinskys minnesfond; Helge Ax:son Johnsons stiftelse; Karolinska Institutet; Stiftelsen Solstickan, Kempe-Carlgrenska fonden.

Authors' contributions
The first author (KK) interviewed the participants and listened through the transcribed material. All authors (KK, SZ, EN, BS) analysed the data, read and approved the final version of the manuscript. Major contributors in writing the manuscript were authors KK and BS.

Competing interests

The authors declare that they have no competing interests.

Author details

[1]Department of Women's and Children's Health, Karolinska Institutet, Stockholm, Sweden. [2]Sophiahemmet Högskola, Stockholm, Sweden.

References

1. Socialstyrelsen. Stöd i föräldraskapet (Support in parenthood) SOSFS 1997: 161. Stockholm: Socialstyrelsen (Swedish National Board of Health); 1997.
2. Gaynes BN, Gavin N, Meltzer-Brody S, Lohr KN, Swinson T, Gartlehner G, et al. Perinatal depression: Prevalence, screening accuracy, and screening outcomes Evidence Report/Technology Assessment AHRQ Publication 2005; 119(05-E006–2).
3. O'Hara MW, Swain AM. Rates and risk of postpartum depression-a meta-analysis. Int Rev Psychiatry. 1996;8(1):37–54.
4. Wickberg B, Hwang CP. Screening for postnatal depression in a population-based Swedish sample. Acta Psychiatr Scand. 1997;95(1):62–6.
5. Johansson M, Svensson I, Stenström U, Massoudi P. Depressive symptoms and parental stress in mothers and fathers 25 month after birth. J Child Health Care. 2016;21(1):65–73. https://doi.org/10.1177/1367493516679015.
6. Paulson JF, Bazemore SD. Prenatal and postpartum depression in fathers and its association with maternal depression: a meta-analysis. JAMA. 2010; 303(19):1961–9.
7. Stern DN. The motherhood constellation: a unified view of parent-infant psychotherapy. London: Karnac Books; 1995. 229 p
8. Cox J, Holden J, Sagovsky R. Detection of postnatal depression: development of the 10-item Edinburgh postnatal depression scale. BJPsych. 1987;150:782–6.
9. Cohen NJ, Lojkasek M, Muir E, Muir R, Parker CJ. Six-month follow-up of two mother-infant psychotherapies: convergence of therapeutic outcomes. Infant Ment Health J. 2002;23(4):361–80.
10. Murray L, Cooper PJ, Wilson A, Romaniuk H. Controlled trial of the short- and long-term effect of psychological treatment of post-partum depression. 2. Impact on the mother–child relationship and child outcome. BJPsych. 2003;182(5):420–7.
11. Salomonsson B, Sandell R. A randomized controlled trial of mother-infant psychoanalytic treatment. 1. Outcomes on self-report questionnaires and external ratings. Infant Ment Health J. 2011;32(2):207–31.
12. Salomonsson B. Psychodynamic interventions in pregnancy and infancy: clinical and theoretical perspectives. London: Routledge; 2018.
13. McCauley K, Elsom S, Muir-Cochrane E, Lyneham J. Midwives and assessment of perinatal mental health. J Psychiatr Ment Health Nurs. 2011; 18(9):786–95.
14. Rollans M, Schmied V, Kemp L, Meade T. 'We just ask some questions...' the process of antenatal psychosocial assessment by midwives. Midwifery. 2013; 29(8):935–42.
15. Gadamer HG. Truth and method. 2nd ed. London: Continuum; 1975/1989.
16. Dilthey W. Introduction to the human sciences. Makkreel R, Rodi F, editors. Princeton, NJ: Princeton University Press; 1989.
17. Gill S. "Holding oneself open in a conversation" – Gadamer's philosophical hermeneutics and the ethics of dialogue. J Dialogue Stud. 2015;3(1):9–28.
18. Thomas DR. A general inductive approach for analyzing qualitative evaluation data. Am J Eval. 2006;27(2):237–46.
19. Kloesel C, Houser N, editors. The essential Peirce, vol. 2: 1893–1913. Bloomington: Indiana University Press; 1998.
20. Tavory I, Timmermans S. Abductive analysis: theorizing qualitative analysis. Chicago: University of Chicago Press; 2014.
21. Weber M. Die "Objektivität" sozialwissenschaftlicher sozialpolitischer Erkentnisse ("objectivity" in social science and social politics). Gesammelte Aufsätze zur Wissenschaftslehre. Tübingen: Mohr; 1904.
22. Kächele H, Schachter J, Thomä H. From psychoanalytic narrative to empirical single case research. New York: Routledge; 2009.
23. Wachholz S, Stuhr U. The concept of ideal types in psychoanalytic follow-up research. Psychother Res. 1999;9(3):327–41.
24. Lindner R, Fiedler G, Altenhofer A, Götze P, Happach C. Psychodynamic ideal types of elderly suicidal persons based on counter transference. J Soc Work Pract. 2006;20(3):347–65.
25. Ross-Davie M, Elliott S, Sarkar A, Green L. A public health role in perinatal mental health: are midwives ready? Br J Midwifery. 2006;14(6):330–4.
26. McCann T, Clark E. Australian bachelor of midwifery students' mental health literacy: an exploratory study. Nurs Health Sci. 2010;12:14–20.
27. Madden D, Sliney A, O'friel A, McMackin B, O'callaghan B, Casey K, et al. Using action research to develop midwives' skills to support women with perinatal mental health needs. J Clin Nurs. 2018;27(3–4):561–71.
28. Mowforth G, Harrison J, Morris M. An investigation into adult nursing students' experience of the relevance and application of behavioural sciences (biology, psychology and sociology) across two different curricula. Nurse Educ Today. 2005;25(1):41–8.
29. Garefalakis J. Paideia: Om bildningens historiska rötter (paideia: on the historical roots of "Bildning"). Riga: HLS Förlag; 2004.
30. Borglin G, Hentzel J, Bohman DM. Public health care nurses 'views of mothers' mental health in paediatric healthcare services: a qualitative study. Prim Health Care Res Dev. 2015;16(5):470–80.
31. Belle MJ, Willis K. Professional practice in contested territory: child health nurses and maternal sadness. Contemp Nurse. 2013;43(2):152–61.
32. Skerrett K. We-ness and the cultivation of wisdom in couple therapy. Fam Process. 2016;55(1):48–61.
33. Aristotle. *Nicomachean ethics*. Kitchener, Ont.: Batoche Books; 1999.
34. Berlin A, Rosander M, Frykedal KF, Barimani M. Walk the talk: leader behavior in parental education groups. Nurs Health Sci. 2018;20:1–8.
35. Hong TM, Callister LC, Schwartz R. First-time mothers' views of breastfeeding support from nurses. MCN Am J Matern Child Nurs. 2003;28(1):10–5.
36. Benner, P (1984) From novice to expert: Excellence and power in clinical nursing practice. AJN: Dec 1984, Vol 84, Issue 12, pp 1480.
37. Kinsella EA, Pitman A. Engaging phronesis in professional practice and education. Phronesis as professional knowledge. Rotterdam: Sense Publishers; 2012. p. 1–12.
38. Rush P. The experience of maternal and child health nurses responding to women with postpartum depression. Matern Child Health J. 2012;16(2):322–7.
39. Boudreau J, Fuks A. The humanities in medical education: ways of knowing, doing and being. J Med Humanit. 2015;36(4):32136.
40. Gallagher A. Moral distress and moral courage in everyday nursing practice. Online J Issues Nurs. 2011;16(2):1B.
41. Tiedje LB. Moral distress in perinatal nursing. J Perinat Neonatal Nurs. 2000;14(2):36–43.
42. Kartläggningsrapport. Uppdrag Psykisk Hälsa. Kartläggningsrapport: Första linje för barn och ungas psykiska hälsa. En kvantitativ beskrivning utifrån data insamlad mars-september 2014. (Report: First line mental health of children and adolescents. A quantitative description based on data collected March-September 2014). Retrieved 180520. Available from: https://www.uppdragpsykiskhalsa.se/fl/.
43. Berlin A. Cultural competence in primary child health care services - interaction between primary child health care nurses, parents of foreign origin and their children. Stockholm: Karolinska Institutet; 2010.
44. Lincoln YS, Guba EG. Establishing trustworthiness. Naturalistic inquiry. London: Sage; 1985.

18

Non-application of the nursing process at a hospital in Accra, Ghana

Joana Agyeman-Yeboah[1]*⊙ and Kwadwo Ameyaw Korsah[2]

Abstract

Background: Registered nurses in Ghana are trained to plan the care that they provide to their patients in a systematic and organized manner. This scientific approach to care is known as the nursing process. There is evidence that the nursing process is not being practised by professional nurses in Ghana, as expected. This research seeks to explore what informs nursing interventions in the clinical area.

Methods: A qualitative study was conducted with ten registered nurses; and this was descriptive in nature. One-on-one interviews were conducted with the research participants, as a means of collecting the data. A semi-structured interview guide was used as the data-collecting tool. The collected data were analysed by using latent-content analysis. Three main themes emerged from the data analysis.

Results: It was found that registered nurses did not plan their nursing care. The care that the nurses provided was based on routine nursing care and doctors' orders, both verbal and non-verbal; or written communication were the means whereby the care was provided; and that was communicated among the nurses.

Conclusion: Registered nurses are taught the nursing process; and they are expected to implement the acquired knowledge in the clinical area. The failure of nurses to practise the expected standard of care results in their relying on the decision of other health-care professionals, such as doctors. This makes registered nurses appear to be assistants to doctors. We, therefore, conclude that nurse leaders must supervise nurses to put into practice what they were taught during their training; so that they can have professional autonomy in their practice as nurses. It is also suggested that nurses must show evidence of using the nursing process in their daily work by the use of the nursing care-plan form.

Keywords: Nursing process, Nursing care-plan, Non-usage, Nurses

Background

Registered nurses are expected to be able to identify the client's health problems, with the intention of preventing, protecting and promoting the wellbeing of the patient. Whatever help the patient may require, in order for his or her needs to be met, be it physical, social, economic, or psychological; while he or she is undergoing some form of medical or surgical treatment, it is the nurse's responsibility to see to it that these needs are met – either directly by his or her own activity, or indirectly by calling in the help of other healthcare professionals [1]. The nursing process provides a framework that can be used in all nursing situations [2].

It has been defined as an orderly, systematic manner of determining the client's health status, specifying those problems, which have been defined as alterations in human needs; and making plans to solve them – and implementing the plan, as well as evaluating the extent to which the plan was effective in promoting optimum wellness and resolving the problems identified [3].

According to Carpenito-Moyet [4], "The nursing process and [the] nursing diagnoses are often a visible subject in each course syllabus; but in reality, classroom teachings and discussions are focused predominantly on medical diagnoses. Nursing students are therefore guided by their tutors to learn how to make

---
* Correspondence: joanaagyemanyeboah@outlook.com
[1]International Maritime hospital, Tema, Ghana
Full list of author information is available at the end of the article

medical diagnoses; and they are left on their own to learn nursing diagnosis. Thus, in the end, medical diagnoses guide their practices, leaving nursing diagnoses as only an unpleasant memory. Often, the nursing tutors teaching the nursing process do not understand nursing diagnoses; and therefore, do not embrace, value, or teach them. A lot of students spend hours creating care plans by copying from textbooks, without learning the critical thinking skills needed for the analysis of the data they have obtained; hence, the nursing diagnoses have no relevance to them; and they remain irrelevant to them after graduation" (P. 126). It is evident that nurses find it difficult to implement the nursing process; because some professional nurses do not quite understand it [5].

A study conducted in Ghana on factors that influence clinical utilization of the nursing process found that, registered nurses were not formulating, or stating the nursing diagnosis. They carried out various nursing interventions that were not based on the nursing diagnosis. They were also not evaluating the rendered care; thus the nursing process in totality was not being implemented [6]. If professional nurses in Ghana are not implementing the nursing process, what then informs their practice? The purpose of this study was to explore and describe the extent to which registered nurses working at the 37th Military Hospital implement the nursing process in the clinical area.

Methods

The study aimed to explore what informs nursing interventions in the clinical area. A qualitative research design was employed, which was descriptive in nature. This design gave the participants the opportunity to express their opinion on the situation being studied. The study was conducted at the 37 Military Hospital. This is a 400-bed hospital located in Accra, the capital of Ghana. The participants consisted of five nursing officers, two senior staff nurses and three staff nurses. Their ages ranged from 27 years to 41 years; and the range of the years that they have been working was from 4 years to 9 years. The male-to-female ratio of the participants was 1:9.

The participants were selected by using the purposive-sampling technique. Arrangements were made with those who expressed interest in the research. The researcher met them; and they were briefed about the research. They were informed about the purpose of the study; and how the data would be collected from them. They were assured of their confidentiality. How the data would be managed was also explained to them. They were informed that their participation in the research would not affect their employment in the hospital. Their right and freedom to withdraw from the study, at any time, was explained to

them. The research participants were also given the opportunity to ask any questions to clarify any issues related to the study.

Those willing to participate in the study were given the consent form to read; and further explanation was given on what was stated in the form. Those who accepted to participate in the study were allowed to sign the consent form. They were given a copy of the signed consent form to keep. An arrangement was made with the participant for a convenient time and place for the interview.

A semi-structured interview guide was used as the data-collecting tool (attached as an Additional file 1) This interview guide was first piloted in a public hospital in Accra, in order to test the validity of the tool. After the pilot study, the interview guide was slightly amended.

The participants were interviewed until the tenth participant, after which no new information was forthcoming. The data analysis was done concurrently with the data collection. The researchers observed from the data analysis that no new themes or concepts were emerging from the interview; and therefore, the researchers stopped the interviews. The interviews were recorded on a voice recorder with the permission of the participants; and points on key issues were also written down as part of the field notes during the interview. Each interview lasted for approximately forty-five minutes to one hour. The data in this study were analysed by using latent-content analysis [7].

Immediately after the interview session, the recorded interviews were replayed and transcribed verbatim. The data were then coded; and during the coding, the data were read by the researcher several times. Sections of the text were highlighted; and comments were made regarding anything that was striking. These comments included overall impressions; and points of interest were written in a margin created at the right side of the sheets. After coding, the data were organised with related codes; and they were put into categories [7]. The coding and analysis of the data was done by an independent coder.

Consensus was reached between the researchers and the independent coder, before the themes were finalized. A label was given to each category. Once the data were categorized, a summary for each of the categories was written. How the categories relate to each other was carefully analysed; and then the themes were developed.

Results

Three main themes emerged from the data analysis. These were: nursing care is not planned by nurses; alternatives to the nursing care plan and means of communicating nursing care. Two of the main themes had their respective sub-themes. These are described below:

Nursing care is not planned by nurses

Unplanned nursing care was a major theme that emerged from the analysis. By this it is meant that nursing care is provided to the patient, without any formal care plan as a guide. Nurses stated they knew they must plan care; but they did not do it. Instead, they provided nursing care, based on what they perceived the patient needed at that time. Some nurses stated that this lack of formal plan of care was due to the high patient–nurse ratio and the inadequate time available. This was expressed by one participant as follows:

> "We actually do not have a plan per se, when we admit a patient, we do not plan the care of the patient right on admission. I think what we do is that from time-to-time, we meet the needs of the patient, as time goes on, or when the need arises; but ideally, we are supposed to plan the patient care, according to the diagnosis and treatment of the patient."

Another participant also felt that they were not able to plan the care of the patient; because they needed to care for a lot of patients at a particular time; hence, they do not get the necessary time to plan the care; although they are aware that planning of the care is the correct thing to do. One of them stated it in this way:

> "Ideally, we are supposed to use the nursing-care plan; but because of the low nurse-to-patient ratio, we do not get the time to do that. We usually care for the patient and what their needs are immediately; but we do not use the nursing process."

It was evident from the data analysis that, when a patient comes for admission to the ward, the nurses do not plan the care of that patient with the patient. Instead, just as they decide the overall care for the patient, they again use their discretion. One participant indicated it this way:

> "As for the planning, it is not done; it is just that when the patient comes on admission, we use the admission books like the nurses' notes, the temperature, pulse and respiration chart; and then we follow the doctor's orders from the folder; and we also use our discretion to nurse the patient."

Although no planning is made in relation to the care that the patient receives; some of the participants did not really see this as a problem. They indicated that it was a nation-wide situation; and that it was not peculiar to the institution in which they work. One of the participants expressed his view by stating that:

> "I will say even in this hospital, I don't know whether we even plan the care. Planning is not done; we really care for the patient, but not with the care plan. I think the problem is not just with the 37 Military Hospital; but I think it is a nation-wide problem. The nursing process in actual fact is not being used well in Ghana. I think it is a foreign concept; and also the high patient to nurse ratio is a contributing factor."

The above statement from the participants reveals that they are aware of the existence of the nursing-care plan. They are also aware that they are supposed to plan the care of the patient; but they are not doing it.

Alternatives to the nursing-care plan

This theme describes what nurses actually depend on to care for the patient instead of developing and using the care plan. Two sub-themes emerged: (a) care based on nursing routines; and (b) care based on the doctor's orders.

Care based on nursing routine

Some of the participants indicated that the care that they provide to the patient is based on the daily routine care that they normally provide for all the patients, regardless of their medical diagnosis. This was how a participant stated it:

> "We do the normal routine nursing care, like checking the temperature, blood pressure and serving of medication; and if the patient needs any more care, the patient would call; and we would then attend further to the patient."

From the experiences that the nurses had, they knew what was normally done for the patients during the morning, afternoon or the night shift; hence when the nurses come to work, they go strictly according to the daily routines. For patients who are able to verbalize their problems and request particular care; the nurses would attend to these requests and try to meet their needs. One of the participants had this to say:

> "In the morning we take over from the night staff by moving from bed to bed; and if along the line there is any special plan about a specific client that we need to be notified, the night staff do that. If we need to bring that to the attention of the doctor, we do that; and we also do the bed-making; we tidy up the ward; and we then carry on with the other daily routines, such as the dusting of the ward, as well as the nurses' station."

Another participant with a similar view stated:

"Depending on the shift in which you are coming; if it is in the morning shift, you know you have to prepare the patient for the ward rounds, feed those who cannot feed themselves, serve medications; and sometimes even sit by the patients and converse with them. If you come for afternoon shift too, the routines are the serving of medications, talking with the patients, turning those who are bed-ridden, or feeding them when necessary."

The nurses were aware of what they were expected to do for the patient, as a routine activity, depending on the shift in which they are working. These routine activities were not formally planned, nor based on the specific needs of the patient; but they were carried out as a daily formality, irrespective of the patient's condition. Patients who were able to verbalize their problems receive the necessary care to assist them in solving their problem.

Nursing care based on doctors' orders

The participants indicated that they depend on the orders or the instructions given by the doctor, as stated in the patient's folder, in order to care for the patients. They follow these instructions to provide the care of the patient, instead of, as one participant noted, critically thinking about the presenting complaints of the patient and then planning care that will be holistic and individualized, depending on the health needs of the patient. This tends to make the nurses dependent on the doctors. A participant passionately expressed this as follows:

"I have also observed that our seniors see themselves as subordinate to the doctors; so they tend to follow whatever the doctors say, instead of them actually thinking critically, to be able to analyse things and to do what is right for the patients. This, therefore, does not actually cause the nurses to think, and then to use all that they were taught in school."

The participants pay particular attention to what the doctors write in the patient's folder; and they then follow those instructions strictly. This was how a participant expressed it:

"When a patient comes to be admitted, after the admission, I think; whatever the medical instructions, which have been given or the medical orders, are implemented."

Although the nurses followed strictly what the doctors have written in the patient's folder, one of the participants saw the practice of taking orders from the doctors and not planning the care by coming out with

nursing orders to guide the nursing care, as not being good for the nursing profession. He believed that nurses are expected to have their own nursing orders, as well as implementing the medical orders. He stated:

"That is why I am saying that the nursing we are practising now is more dependent on medical orders than nursing orders, which is not always too good for the profession."

Adherence to the daily routines usually performed by the nurses and the implementation of medical orders stated by the doctors in the folder were the two main alternate means, which the participants stated that the nurses uses instead of the nursing care plan. There were some perspectives put forward that nursing care could have been more client specific; and furthermore, it could focus more specifically on addressing the identified health problems; so as to meet the needs of the patient holistically.

Means of communicating nursing care

This theme describes the various means by which nurses communicate the care provided to the patient with one another, as well as how they document what is yet to be done for the patients. Two sub-themes emerged from this theme; and they were: (a) verbal communication and (b) non-verbal, or written communication.

Verbal communication

The participants indicated that they do not plan the care of the patient, but nursing interventions that have already been carried and are yet to be implemented, they communicate verbally with each other. This occurs during the handing over of care from one shift to the next. At change of shift, they verbally tell the incoming nurses what has been done for the patients. One of the participants explained this as:

"During the handing over, communication of the rendered care is done orally, but the in-coming nurses also read through the notes written in the changes book, before we start the handing over. The out-going nurses will tell the in-coming nurses whatever care that has been rendered to the patients in their absence."

Another participant also indicated that:

"We do that orally; as we change over from one shift to the other. All reviews made by the doctors are documented in the changes book. We hand it over orally to the in-coming nurses; but it is also recorded in the changes book, as well."

The verbal communication was not only used to throw more light on what has already been done for the patient and documented. It was also used to tell the incoming nurse of things that are supposed to be done for the patient. This was evident in the comments of one of the participants, who developed a strategy to note the verbal information down, in order for him not to forget:

"I have a notebook; in which I document all the information that is handed over to me. If I am not able to attend to the needs of all the patients; then I hand over what could not be performed to the in-coming nurse. But it is not documented in the care plan, which would have been easier for the incoming nurse to know what has already been done and what is yet to be done, which would have enhanced the continuity of care."

Verbal communication was used by the nurses to communicate documented and undocumented nursing care; but this was not done with the use of the nursing care plan.

Non-verbal or written communication

It was expressed by the participants that all the nursing care provided by the nurses is supposed to be documented in the nurses' notes, the changes book, and the 24-h report book. These are expected to be read by the incoming nurses, to enable them have an idea of what has already been done for the patient in the previous shifts; and also to be informed about what they are supposed to do for the patients, and at what time. One of the participants had this to say:

"The care provided is written in the changes book for the in-coming nurse to read. During the handing over, the nurse is told what has already been done, and what is yet to be done."

Another participant also expressed it as follows:

"We write every procedure we do for the patient in the nurses notes and in the changes book; so when new nurses come or somebody comes in the afternoon to take over from me, the person reads the changes book and the nurses' notes at the nurses' station, goes through everything to see what has been done for the patients in his or her absence, before going round to say hello to the patients."

One other participant stated that:

"We usually write notes on patients in the changes book and in the nurses' notes. This informs the incoming nurse of what has been done for the patient and the things that are pending or yet to be done for the patient."

The care provided by the nurses is documented in the nurses' notes, the changes book and the 24-h report book. The care that is yet to be provided is at times not documented; but verbally handed over. If the nurses were using the nursing care plan, the rendered care would have easily been documented on the care plan; and what was yet to be carried out would have been stated under the nursing orders, which would have made the handing over procedure easy; and this would also have ensured continuity of care.

Discussion

The purpose of the study was to explore what informs nursing interventions in the clinical area; since the nurses were not using the nursing process. The participants comprised 9 females and 1 male. This outcome was not surprising, because of the highly dense population of females in the nursing profession in Ghana than males. However, this observation was in sharp contrast to that made by Auerbach, Buerhaus, Staiger and Skinner [8]. The findings from this current study revealed that, the nurses in the study stated they knew they must use the plan care; but they did not do so. In addition, they did not plan the care of the patients; instead, they provided nursing care based on what they perceived the patient needed at that time; and they decided the overall care for the patient by using their own discretion. The perception of the nursing process as a foreign concept might have also affected their non-utilization thereof.

Unlike the findings from an earlier study by Hayrinen, Lammintakaren and Saranto [9], the planned or performed nursing interventions were documented by using the nursing-process model. A systematic review on nursing diagnosis, interventions and outcome, application and input on nursing practice reported that nursing diagnoses are commonly found in nursing practice [10]. What Hayrinen, Lammintakaren and Saranto [9] and Muller-Staub, Lavin and Needham [10] are saying seems to be pointing at a common issue regarding the documented use of the nursing process in patient care, which is generally accepted as a scientific way of planning and implementing patient and client care by professional nurses [11].

This is in sharp contrast from the findings of the current study, which has noted that the nurses provided nursing care to patients, based on their own discretion or preference that appears to be intuitive or instinctive in nature grounded on knowledge and experiences in practice by the nurses. This may be seen as an insentient or unconscious awareness of reasoning and cognition [12]. As researchers who have also practised as professional nurses for over 17 years, we have experienced this phenomenon of intuitive reasoning among nurses during patient care in selected hospitals in Ghana, in which we have worked.

The study also revealed that nurses normally provided daily routine care for all the patients, irrespective of their medical diagnosis. These routine activities were not formally plan-based on the specific needs of the patients; and those patients who were able to verbalize their problem received care to assist in solving their problem. The participants' care that they provided to their patients was based on the medical orders, or the instructions stated in the patient's folder by their doctors. This assertion is similar to the findings of Carpenito-Moyet [4], who reported that nurses are perceived as assistants to the doctors; but not as professionals in their own right.

The nurses in this context exclusively focused on the problems of the patients that are associated with medical diagnosis or treatment; hence, failing to embrace professional nursing. From the researchers' clinical experiences, nurses follow the medical orders of doctors to the last; and at times, they are unable to provide any better care to patients who in a specific day were not reviewed by their medical doctors. Hence, the nurses do not take the initiative in patients' care; as professionals are expected to do.

The findings from this study also revealed that the participants documented the nursing care provided to the patients in the nurses' notes, the changes book and the 24-h report book, but not in the nursing care plans. Since there is no plan on the care, there is no documentation on the next care to be received by the patients. Verbally, these unplanned cares are handed over to the next shift. What then happens if the outgoing nurse forgets to inform the incoming nurse of this undocumented care? Implementation of the nursing process and the dutiful use of the nursing care plan is therefore very crucial in professional nursing practice; and it should not be trivialized by nurses.

Limitations of the study

The study was conducted in only one Hospital; and consequently the findings could be specific to only that hospital. The findings from this current study could also not be generalized, due to the qualitative nature of the research design.

Recommendations

Based on the findings, we recommend the following

- Nursing administration should put measures in place to ensure that the nurses are well supervised, in order to practise what they have been taught from school. For instance, the principles underlying "nursing audit" may be applied in hospitals, in which

nursing administrators may be tasked to visit hospital wards on a regular basis, in an effort to appraise the patient care rendered by nurses with particular reference to the application of the nursing process among other nursing interventions. Nursing audit is a thorough evaluation and assessment of designated or particular clinical accounts by qualified professional nurses; or it is an assigned duty for the personnel to appraise the value and worth of the nursing care rendered to the patients/clients [13].

- During the handing over of the care rendered to the patients by the nurses, the care plan should be a means of communication and it should be part of the patient's folder. Since the care plan would have the client's health problem, the nursing diagnosis, the outcome criteria, the nursing orders and the nursing interventions documented, the incoming nurse at a glance of the care plan will have an idea of the interventions that have already been carried; out and what is yet to be carried out. Additionally, the extent to which the objectives set to address the clients' problem have been achieved would also be documented in the care plan. This would also help to avoid any repetition of the care that did not assist in meeting the outcome criteria of the patient.

- Nurses must show evidence of using the nursing process, in order to qualify them for promotion to the next level in their career. If this is enforced, nurses would be compelled to practise what they were taught in nursing school; and this would also contribute to the promotion of standards in the nursing profession.

- Nursing lectures should receive in-depth training on strategies to transfer the knowledge on the concept of the nursing process to student nurses in such a way that implementation of the concept after school does not just become a challenge.

- There should be further studies done in other parts of the country on the non-utilization of the nursing process to ascertain the greater picture of the problem in the country as a whole.

Conclusions

Professional nurses in Ghana's non-usage of the nursing process is worrying; since they are not implementing theoretical knowledge in the clinical setting. The failure of nurses to practise the expected standard of care results in them relying on the decision of other health-care professionals, such as the doctor, thereby making nurses appear as mere assistants to doctors. We therefore conclude that nurse leaders must supervise nurses to put into practice what they were taught during their professional training; so that they can have professional autonomy in their practice as nurses.

Abbreviations
IRB: Institutional Review Board

Acknowledgements

We are grateful to all the professional nurses who participated in this study. Additionally, we appreciate the support from the management of the study hospital.

Funding

No funding was obtained for the study.

Authors' contributions
JAY conceptualised the study, collected the data and conducted the data analysis. KAK assisted with the conceptualisation and the data analysis; and supervised the writing up of the study. JAY drafted the manuscript, KAK assisted in finalising the manuscript for publication. All authors have read and approved the manuscript.

Competing interests
The authors declare that they have no competing interest.

Author details

[1]International Maritime hospital, Tema, Ghana. [2]School of Nursing, University of Ghana, P. Box LG43, Legon, Ghana.

References

1. Tomey AM, Alligood MR. Nursing theorists and their work. 9th ed. USA: Elsevier; 2017.
2. Parahoo K. Nursing research: principles and issues. 3rd ed. UK: Palgrave Macmillan; 2014.
3. Adejumo PO, Olaogun AA. Nursing process: a tool to holistic approach to nursing care. West African J Nursing. 2009;20(1):34–5.
4. Carpenito-Moyet LJ. Invited paper: teaching nursing diagnosis to increase utilization after graduation. Int J Nurs Terminol Classif. 2010;21(3):124–33.
5. Ogboukiri GU. Challenges facing nursing practice in Kadura, Nigeria. 2008. Retrieved July, 15, 2011 from.crhronline.org.
6. Agyeman-Yeboah J, Korsah AK, Okrah J. Factors that influence the clinical utilization of the nursing process at a hospital in Accra Ghana. BMC Nurs. 2017;16(30):1–7.
7. Mayan MJ. Essentials of qualitative inquiry. California: Left Coast Press Inc; 2009.
8. Auerbach D, Buerhaus P, Staiger D, Skinner L. Data brief update: current trend of men in nursing. In: Centre for interdisciplinary health-workforce studies; 2017.
9. Hayrinen K, Lammintakanen J, Saranto K. Evaluation of electronic nursing documentation--nursing process model and standardized terminologies, as keys to visible and transparent nursing. Int J Med Inform. 2010;79(8):554–64.
10. Muller-Staub M, Lavin MA, Needham I, Achterberg TV. Nursing diagnoses interventions and outcomes – application and impact on nursing practice: systematic review. J Adv Nurs. 2009;56(5):514–31.
11. Afolayan JA, Donald B, Baldwin DM, Onasoga O, Babafemi A. Evaluation of the utilization of nursing process and patient outcome in psychiatric nursing: case study of psychiatric hospital Rumuigbo, Port Harcourt. Adv Appl Sci Res. 2013;4(5):34–43.
12. Senanayake T. Intuition in nursing practice – knowledge, experience, and clinical decision-making. Thesis submitted to Arcada University of Applied Sciences in partial fulfilment of the award of a Nursing Degree 2017.
13. Mykkanen M, Saranto K, Miettinen M. Nursing audit as a method for developing nursing care and ensuring patient safety. 11th International Congress on Nursing Informatics. 2012: June 23–27 Montreal Canada.

19

Quality of nursing work life and turnover intention among nurses of tertiary care hospitals in Riyadh

Bayan Kaddourah[1], Amani K. Abu-Shaheen[2] and Mohamad Al-Tannir[2*]

Abstract

Background: Nurse turnover has a negative impact on the ability to meet patient needs and provide a high quality of care, which may create more stress on other staff due to increased workloads. This can lead to critical changes in the behavior of nurses towards their jobs resulting in low work satisfaction, low productivity, and leaving the organization. Thus, this study aimed to assess the quality of nursing work life (QNWL), to explore the nurses' turnover intention and to examine the correlation between QNWL and nurses' turnover intention.

Methods: A cross-sectional survey was conducted on nurses with at least 1 year of nursing experience at two hospitals selected randomly from Riyadh, Saudi Arabia: King Fahad Medical City and King Faisal Specialized Hospitals. Data were collected using a self-administered questionnaire comprising four sections (Brooks' survey of QNWL, Anticipated Turnover Scale (ATS), open-ended questions and demographic characteristics).

Results: A sample of 364 nurses was recruited. Results proposed that the participants were dissatisfied with their work life (54.7%), with almost 94% indicating a turnover intention from their current hospital. Moreover, 154 (93.3%) out of 165 nurses who reported satisfaction with QNWL indicated the intention to turnover. The correlation between QNWL and ATS for binary variables was too week ($r = -0.024$) and statistically not significant ($p = 0.206$).

Conclusion: The QNWL and nurse turnover are challenging issues for healthcare organizations because of its consequences and impact on patient care. Our study provided critical findings low indication satisfaction of nurses with their QNWL and a high turnover intention. The results of this study could be used as a nexus for the development of regulations and practical strategies to enhance QNWL and to decrease the turnover.

Keywords: QNWL, Nursing, Nurses' turnover, Saudi Arabia

Background

Health organizations in many countries have faced some difficulties like shortage of health experts, and increase the turnover rate, especially amongst nurses. Nurse turnover has a negative impact on the ability to encounter the patient needs and deliver high standards of care [1]. Additionally, the turnover of nurses leads to insufficient staffing, which increases the workloads and stress on other staff [2–4]. Consequently, this may lead to serious variations in nurse's behavior towards their jobs causing low work satisfaction and productivity, and then shifting to another organization. As well, insufficient nurse staffing leads to poor patient outcomes, like increased patient mortality and infection rates error rates might be increased [5, 6]. The previous research in the health field has concentrated on answering these issues and their related causes [4, 5]. Some studies have shown the impact of quality of work life on the commitment of nurses and other health professionals [4, 7, 8]. The quality of nursing work life (QNWL) defined as the degree to which registered nurses can satisfy important personal needs through their experiences in their work organization while achieving the organization's goals [9]. Evaluating QNWL permits organizations to realize how challenges in work environments affect nurse's job satisfaction and commitments [10]. The high quality of work life is

---

* Correspondence: maltannir@kfmc.med.sa
[2]Research Center, King Fahad Medical City, Riyadh, Saudi Arabia
Full list of author information is available at the end of the article

crucial for organizations to appeal to new employees and maintain their workforces. However, reliable information on the quality of work life and turnover intention of nurses is limited in Saudi Arabia. In an in-depth review of literature proposes that there is a remarkable increase in the rate of nurse organizational turnover supplemented via an insignificant increase in nursing resource [7, 9]. In Saudi Arabia, nurses come from different countries, some of which may be unharmonious with the culture of Saudi Arabia. The previous study reported that non-Arabic speaking nurses are at a shortcoming as care providers for people in public because of the language barrier and cultural variances [11]. Such challenges for nurses alongside other causes linked to the organization generate a high level of stress which adversely affects the quality of their working life. Another study conducted by Alhusaini and Alamri et al. indicated that the majority of foreign nurses move to industrialized countries after attaining enough experience [12, 13]. In consequent of, competition to attract competent nurses, Saudi Arabia might miss experienced nurses who may choose to work with other establishments that deliver right working environments. It is integral for a policymaker to assess their quality of work life and to understand their organizational and career intentions, which may improve the nurses' work satisfaction and productivity, which subsequently improve the health services being delivered to their patients. Thus, the objectives of this study were to assess the QNWL, to explore the nurses' turnover intention and to examine the correlation between QNWL and nurses' turnover intention.

Methods

Study design and settings

A cross-sectional survey was conducted at two out of four tertiary hospitals in Riyadh city, Saudi Arabia. The hospitals were selected randomly: King Fahad Medical City (KFMC) and King Faisal Specialized Hospitals (KFSH) from March 2015 to March 2016.

Study participants and sampling

Nurses with at least 1 year of nursing experience in various clinical settings at KFMC and KFSH were eligible to participate in this study. Nurses working at different shifts were selected randomly from the two hospitals by a quota-based sample, after obtaining written informed consent form from each participant. Data were collected by administering self-reported questionnaires in the English language as it is the main using language for the staff in the hospital and they studied nursing in the English language.

Participants were provided with the study package which included the cover letter, questionnaire, and an envelope. Moreover, participants were received a reminder by the study coordinator to fill and put the completed survey in a large labeled envelope and then return them to the hospital mail service ensuring anonymity and confidentiality.

Data measurement

Two instruments were used to answer the objectives of this study: Brooks' survey of QNWL and anticipated turnover scale (ATS). The developers of the research instruments granted permission to use their questionnaires.

The QNWL is a self-administered questionnaire which encompasses 42 items in four subscales which are work life/home life, work design, work context and work the world. The work life/home life dimension is the interface between the nurses' work and home life. The work design dimension is the composition of nursing work and describes the actual work that nurses perform. The work context dimension includes the practice settings in which nurses' work. Finally, the work world dimension is defined as the effects of broad societal influences and changes in the practice of nursing [14]. The instrument asks respondent nurses how much they agree or disagree with each item on a 6-point scale, '1' indicating 'strongly disagree' and '6' indicating 'strongly agree'. Responses with means ≤4.2 were considered as an indication of dissatisfaction of respondents towards the quality of work life. The reliability of the scale is 0.90 and construct validity is 0.89 [9].

The ATS is a 12-item self-administered questionnaire. It was created by Hinshaw and Atwood to investigate the turnover intention amongst nurses. It measures the employees' attitudes and perceptions of the probability of terminating their current job [15]. The ATS instrument is a 7-point Likert scale ranging from 'agree strongly' to 'disagree strongly' [15]. The instrument's items were related to an employee's anticipated length of time to leave and certainty of leaving the job. The total score was obtained by calculating the sum of all items in the scale divided by the number of items in the scale. Greater scores reveal a more intent to leave the current job. Responses with means > 3.5 were reflected as a sign of turnover intention [16]. The internal consistency reliability estimated with Cronbach's α was 0.84 [17].

As well as, the QNWL and ATS scales; demographic data (age, gender, marital status, family members living in KSA, having children, primary family caregiver, total years of nursing experience, total years of nursing experience in Saudi Arabia, current nursing position, total years working in the current position, monthly income, having additional financial benefits) which may affect the findings were also collected from the study participants. Demographic characteristics exhibit independent effects: therefore, they must be considered as contributors to turnover [18].

The study assumes a correlation between work-life related factors, nurses' demographic characteristics, quality of work life (QWL) level and turnover intention. QWL is influenced by work-life factors as reported by Brooks and Anderson [9] as well as demographic factors, which might lead either too high or low level of QWL, which can seriously change the behavioral intention of the nurses.

Pilot study

The pilot study was conducted to test the clarity and time taken to fill out the questionnaire. Seventeen ($N = 17$) nurses from one hospital participated. According to the participants' recommendations some modifications were made to the questionnaires. Based on the pilot study, the results showed that for QNWL and its dimensions, Cronbach's' α were 0.89 for QNWL and 0.90 for the ATS.

Sample size estimation

The sample size was calculated using the Raosoft online sample size calculator with 5% margin of error and a 95% confidence interval. Based on results from the pilot study, the prevalence of turnover intention was estimated at 32%, which allowed us to calculate the needed sample size of 365 subjects.

Statistical analysis

All data was entered and analyzed through statistical package SPSS version 22. Categorical variables were presented in frequencies and percentages. Whereas, continuous variables like all test scores ATS and QNWL were expressed as mean (S.D). Cronbach α test was applied to assess the internal consistency of QNWL and ATS. Independent sample t-test/ANOVA was used to determine the mean score of ATS and QNWL with demographic characteristics of the survey's participants. A bivariate stepwise logistic regression analysis was performed to identify the factors that might be associated with ATS score. P-value < 0.05 two-tailed was considered as statistically significant.

Results

A representative sample of 400 nurses was invited to participants in this study, out of whom 364 nurses were recruited (response rate is 91%). Respondents' demographic characteristics were presented in Table 1. A total of 329 (90.4%) of respondents were females. Two hundred thirty 236 (64.8%) nurses are married, and 149 (40.9%) respondents had family members living in KSA. The majority of participants 198 (54.5%) had between 1 to 5 years of clinical experience in Saudi Arabia and were Filipino 206 (56.6%).

According to ATS criteria of cutoff (> 3.5) intent to leave the current position, our data shows that 94% of participants were willing to leave the current job. Moreover, QNWL criteria of cutoff (≤ 4.2) satisfaction towards the QWL revealed that 54.7% of participated nurses were dissatisfied with the quality of work life. There is no significant difference between the answers given by the respondent's

nurses were working in different departments in the two different hospitals.

Table 2 shows the association of demographic characteristics with the cut off levels of the QNWL and ATS scales. The majority of male nurses 21 (60%) were satisfied with the QNWL than females 144 (43.8%). Among the age group, the majority of nurses were dissatisfied with the QNWL except in the age group 31–40 years. Moreover, about 75 (61.5%) of the never married nurses were dissatisfied with the QNWL compared to 120 (50.8) who were married. The majority of nurses with associate degree 4 (80) and those with less than 5 years of experience were reported dissatisfaction with QNWL. Nurses with a monthly income of more than 15,000 SAR 3 (100%) were all satisfied with QNWL. Overall, a significant difference was found between satisfactory nurse status and total years of nursing experience ($p = 0.025$), total years of nursing experience in Saudi Arabia ($p = <$ 0.001), and monthly income ($p = 0.005$). However, further logistic regression analysis showed that nurses who have been working in Saudi Arabia between 11 and 15 years were the only satisfied ($p = 0.006$) with QNWL among other nurses. Also, nurses with monthly income less than 5000 and 5000–10,000 Saudi Riyal were found to exhibit an effect on nurses' satisfaction ($p = < 0.001$; for both) about QNWL.

Regarding the anticipated turnover intention, the majority of males 30 (85.7%) and females 312 (94.8%) have the intention to turnover. Moreover, the vast majority of nurses at their different demographic characteristics have reported the intention to turnover. Also, the statistically significant difference was only found between nurse intention to turnover with gender ($p = 0.031$) and total years working in the current position ($p = 0.002$). Nevertheless, logistic regression analysis showed that charge nurse position ($p = < 0.001$) and total years working in the current position ($p = 0.017$) were found to exhibit an effect on nurses' intention to turnover (Table 2).

Table 3 shows that among the 199 nurses who were dissatisfied with the QNWL, about 188 (94.5) of them have the intention to turnover. Moreover, 154 (93.3) out of 165 nurses who reported satisfaction with QNWL indicated the intention to turnover. The correlation between QNWL and ATS for binary variables was a week ($r = -0.024$) and statistically not significant ($p = 0.206$).

Discussion

This study provides an initial step in understanding the work life of nurses in tertiary care sitting and shed light on an important topic which if not assessed and well managed by an organization might have a negative impact on the ability to meet the patient needs and deliver high standards of care. Our study revealed that the majority (54.7%) of respondents was dissatisfied with their

Table 1 Demographic characteristics of respondents

Characteristics	Categories	n (%)
Gender	Female	329 (90.4)
	Male	35 (9.6)
Age Group	22–30	179 (49.2)
	31–40	132 (36.3)
	41–50	45 (12.4)
	> 51	8 (2.2)
Marital Status	Married	236 (64.8)
	Single	122 (33.5)
	Widowed	3 (0.8)
	Divorced	3 (0.8)
Nationality	Filipino	206 (56.6)
	Indian	106 (29.1)
	Saudi	9 (2.5)
	Jordanian	7 (1.9)
	others	36 (9.9)
Family members living in KSA	Yes	149 (40.9)
	No	215 (59.1)
Having children	Yes	162 (44.5)
	No	202 (55.5)
Primary family caregiver	Yes	103 (28.3)
	No	261 (71.7)
Education level	Associate Degree	5 (1.4)
	Diploma	81 (22.3)
	Bachelor	275 (75.5)
	Master's Degree	3 (0.8)
Total years of nursing experience	1–5	88 (24.2)
	6–10	58 (15.9)
	11–15	149 (40.9)
	>15	69 (19)
Total years of nursing experience in Saudi Arabia	1–5	198 (54.5)
	6–10	42 (11.5)
	11–15	100 (27.5)
	>15	24 (6.6)
Current nursing position	Staff Nurse	334 (91.8)
	Charge Nurse	25 (6.9)
	Others	5 (1.4)
Total years working in the current position	≤5	201 (58.5)
	>5	151 (41.5)
Monthly income (SR)	< 5000	200 (54.9)
	5000–10,000	153 (42)
	11,000 – 15,000	8 (2.2)
	>15,000	3 (0.8)
Having additional financial benefits (e.g. housing allowance)	Yes	151 (41.5)
	No	213 (58.5)

Table 1 Demographic characteristics of respondents *(Continued)*

Characteristics	Categories	n (%)
ATS cutoff	≤ 3.5	22 (6.0)
	> 3.5	342 (94)
QWL Cutoff	≤ 4.2	199 (54.7%)
	> 4.2	165 (45.3%)

SR Saudi Riyal

work life and 94% have turnover intention. Our result is higher than reported in previous studies on nurses' turnover intention. A study carried out by Brooks et al., to assess the QNWL of staff nurses using the same scale reported nursing dissatisfaction with their work life [17]. In Saudi Arabia, a study conducted by Almalki et al., on 508 primary health care nurses, reported that the participants were dissatisfied with their work life, with nearly 40% showing a turnover intention [19]. In Sweden, a prospective study on 1417 nurses showed that every fifth nurse intended to leave their profession after 5 years [20]. In a study based on 6469 hospital nurses in seven European countries, reported that nurses have reward frustration with higher turnover intentions [21]. Our results were critical and alarming, however, these findings could be explained by the fact that the majority of the nurse in the study sites were expatriate nurses from different countries.

Previous studies reported monthly income, length of work experience, and organization tenure as important predictors of employees' satisfaction with QWL [22, 23]. Our results showed that total years of nursing experience, total years of nursing experience in Saudi Arabia, and monthly income significantly affect nurses' satisfaction about QNWL. This could be explained by that nurses with more work experience have more stability in their job and thus experience a better QNWL. However, previous studies conducted by Nayeri et al. and Boonrod revealed that they could not found a significant association between QNWL and the length of work experience [24, 25].

Consistent with previous studies our results showed that gender, total years working in the current position were also affecting nurses' intention to turnover [17, 24]. While, other studies reported no relationship between gender and employees' intention to leave their work [25, 26].

Although previous studies confirmed the significance of family to the view of the nurses to their QNWL [1, 17], the results of the present study showed no significant association between QNWL and neither family member living in KSA nor marital status. Similarly, two studies have also found that QWL has no significant relationship with marital status [23, 24].

In the present study we examined the correlation between QNWL and ATS. Although the work context

Table 2 Association of demographic characteristics with QNWL and ATS

		QNWL			ATS		
		< 4.2 n(n)	≥ 4.2 n(n)	p value	≤ 3.5 n(n)	> 3.5 n(n)	p value
Gender	Male	14 (40)	21 (60)	0.067	5 (14.3)	30 (85.7)	0.031*
	Female	185 (56.2)	144 (43.8)		17 (5.2)	312 (94.8)	
Age Group	22–30	107 (59.8)	72 (40.2)	0.071	8 (4.5)	171 (95.5)	0.196
	31–40	61 (46.2)	71 (53.8)		12 (9.1)	120 (90.9)	
	41–50	25 (55.6)	20 (44.4)		1 (2.2)	44 (97.8)	
	> 51	6 (75)	2 (25)		1 (12.5)	7 (87.5)	
Marital Status	Divorced	2 (66.7)	1 (33.3)	0.259	0 (.0)	3 (100.0)	0.218
	Married	120 (50.8)	116 (49.2)		15 (6.4)	221 (93.6)	
	Single	75 (61.5)	47 (38.5)		6 (4.9)	116 (95.1)	
	Widowed	2 (66.7)	1 (33.3)		1 (33.3)	2 (66.7)	
Dependent Children	Yes	91 (56.2)	71 (43.8)	0.606	8 (4.9)	154 (95.1)	0.428
	No	108 (53.5)	94 (46.5)		14 (6.9)	188 (93.1)	
Education Level	Associate Degree	4 (80)	1 (20)	0.682	1 (20.0)	4 (80.0)	0.252
	Bachelor Degree	149 (54.2)	126 (45.8)		19 (6.9)	256 (93.1)	
	Diploma	44 (54.3)	37 (45.7)		2 (2.5)	79 (97.5)	
	Master's Degree	2 (66.7)	1 (33.3)		0 (.0)	3 (100.0)	
Total years of nursing experience	1–5 years	60 (68.2)	28 (31.8)	0.025*	4 (4.5)	84 (95.5)	0.706
	11–15 years	28 (48.3)	30 (51.7)		4 (6.9)	54 (93.1)	
	6–10 years	73 (49)	76 (51)		8 (5.4)	141 (94.6)	
	> 15	38 (55.1)	31 (44.9)		6 (8.7)	63 (91.3)	
Total years of nursing experience in Saudi Arabia	0–5 years	122 (61.6)	76 (38.4)	< 0.001*	8 (4.0)	190 (96.0)	0.112
	6–10 years	43 (43)	57 (57)		11 (11.0)	89 (89.0)	
	11–15 years	15 (35.7)	27 (64.3)		2 (4.8)	40 (95.2)	
	> 15	19 (79.2)	5 (20.8)		1 (4.2)	23 (95.8)	
Current nursing position	Charge Nurse	13 (52)	12 (48)	0.504	2 (8.0)	23 (92.0)	0.782
	Staff Nurse	182 (54.5)	152 (45.5)		20 (6.0)	314 (94.0)	
	Other	4 (80)	1 (20)		0 (.0)	5 (100.0)	
Total years working in the current position	0–5 years	123 (57.7)	90 (42.3)	0.161	6 (2.8)	207 (97.2)	0.002*
	> 5 years	76 (50.3)	75 (49.7)		16 (10.6)	135 (89.4)	
Monthly income (SR)	< 5000	124 (62)	76 (38)	0.005*	7 (3.5)	193 (96.5)	0.079
	5000–10,000	70 (45.8)	83 (54.2)		15 (9.8)	138 (90.2)	
	11,000–15,000	5 (62.5)	3 (37.5)		0 (.0)	8 (100.0)	
	> 15,000	0	3 (100)		0 (.0)	3 (100.0)	

(*) Shows that p-value is significant

dimension makes the strongest contribution to explaining turnover intention, our results showed no correlation between QNWL and ATS. On the contrary, prior studies reported that the intention to turnover could be explained by the nurse's satisfaction with QNWL [27, 28]. In previous studies based on 1283 hospital nurses in Taiwan and 740 nurses in Iran reported that nurses' QWLs were significantly negatively associated with nurses' turnover intentions [29, 30].

Efficacious QNWL strategies in healthcare settings can enhance employees' self-esteem and organizational efficiency. Furthermore, QNWL can advance the quality of care provided in addition to staffing and preservation of the nursing workforce. This high rate of turnover intention ought to motivate the nursing leaders to develop appropriate and efficient strategies to combat this serious issue and improve the nurses work conditions and their QNWL, which consequently,

Table 3 Correlation between QNWL scale and ATS scale

		Cut off Value of QNWL			p-value
		< 4.2	≥ 4.2	Total	
Cut off Value of ATS	≤ 3.5	11(5.5)	11(6.7)	22(6.0)	0.206
	> 3.5	188(94.5)	154(93.3)	342(94.0)	
	Total	199(54.7)	165(45.3)	364(100.0)	

will enable the nurses to perform better care for their patients.

The strengths of the study that it can be generalizable to the nursing staff working at tertiary hospitals in Riyadh city as the study was conducted at two out of four reputable tertiary hospitals in Riyadh city, Saudi Arabia. Furthermore, the possibility of non-response bias is very little as the response rate is high (91%). While, the limitations that the study is a cross-sectional and data collected using self- administer scales. Therefore, further studies should be carried out with more objective instruments.

Further studies are needed to understand and improve nurses' QNWL and retention. It would be valuable to conduct longitudinal and interventional studies to assess the definite turnover amongst nurses paralleled with described turnover intention in the present study. Additional an in-depth study is required to explore the effect of social and cultural norms on the perception of expatriate nurses towards QNWL and turnover intention.

Conclusions

The QNWL and nurse turnover are challenging issues for healthcare organizations because of the consequences and impact on patient care. Our study provides critical findings low indication satisfaction of nurses with their QNWL and a high turnover intention. The results of this study could be used as a guide for the development of regulations and practical strategies to enhance QNWL and to decrease the turnover.

Abbreviations
ATS: Anticipated Turnover Scale; KFMC: King Fahad Medical City; KFSH: King Faisal Specialized Hospitals; QNWL: Quality of Nursing Work Life; QWL: Quality of Work Life

Acknowledgments
We would like to express their gratitude and appreciation to Research Center, King Fahad Medical City, Riyadh, Saudi Arabia for providing the research grant. Also, we thankfully appreciate Mr. Isamme AlFayyad for his assistance and support in revising and updating the statistical analysis and improving the quality of the manuscript.

Funding
The study funded by the Research Center, King Fahad Medical City, Riyadh, Saudi Arabia. The funding body doesn't have any role in: the design of the study; the collection, analysis, and interpretation of data; and the writing of the manuscript.

Authors' contributions
BK and MA substantial contributed to conception and design and acquisition of data. BK, MA and AA analyzed and interpreted the data. BK, MA and AA drafted the article and revised it critically for important intellectual content. All authors read and approved the final manuscript.

Competing interests
The authors declare that they have no competing interests.

Author details
[1]Ambulatory Care Centre, Executive Administration of Nursing Services, King Fahad Medical City, Riyadh, Saudi Arabia. [2]Research Center, King Fahad Medical City, Riyadh, Saudi Arabia.

References
1. Eren H, Hisar F. Quality of work life perceived by nurses and their organizational commitment level. JHS. 2016;13:1.
2. Huang T-C, Lawler J, Lei C-Y. The effects of quality of work life on commitment and turnover intention. Soc Behav Pers. 2007;35(6):735–50.
3. Buchan J, Aiken L. Solving nursing shortages: a common priority. J Clin Nurs. 2008. https://doi.org/10.1111/j.1365-2702.2008. 02636.x.
4. Yang J, Liu Y, Huang C, Zhu L. Impact of empowerment on professional practice environments and organizational commitment among nurses: a structural equation approach. IJNP. 2013;19:44–55.
5. Coomber B, Barriball KL. Impact of job satisfaction components on intent to leave and turnover for hospital-based nurses: a review of the research literature. Int J Nurs Stud. 2007;44(2):297–314.
6. Aiken LH, Sloane DM, Bruyneel L, Van den Heede K, Griffiths P, Busse R, Sermeus, W. Nurse staffing and education and hospital mortality in nine European countries: A retrospective observational study. Lancet. 2015; doi: https://doi.org/10.1016/s0140-6736(13)62631-8.
7. Duffield CM, Roche MA, Homer C, Buchan J, Dimitrelis S. A comparative review of nurse turnover rates and costs across countries. J Adv Nurs. 2014. https://doi.org/10.1111/jan.12483.
8. Lee Y-W, Dai Y-T, Chang MY, Chang Y-C, Yao KG, Liu M-C. Quality of Work Life, Nurses' Intention to Leave the Profession, and Nurses Leaving the Profession: A One-Year Prospective Survey. J Nurs Scholarsh. 2017. https://doi.org/10.1111/jnu.12301.
9. Brooks BA, Anderson MA. Defining quality of nursing work life. Nurs Econ. 2004;23(6):319–26.
10. Flinkman M, Laine M, Leino-Kilpi H, Hasselhorn M, Salanterä S. Explaining young registered Finnish nurses' intention to leave the profession: a questionnaire survey. Int J Nurs Stud. 2008;45(5):727–39.
11. Al-Nuaim LA. Views of women towards cesarean section. Saudi Med J. 2004; 25(6):707–10.
12. Alamri AS, Rasheed MF, Alfawzan NM. Reluctance of Saudi youth towards the nursing profession and the high rate of unemployment in Saudi Arabia: causes and effects. Riyadh: King Saud University; 2006.
13. Alhusaini HA. Obstacles to the efficiency and performance of Saudi nurses at the Ministry of Health, Riyadh region: analytical field study. Ministry of Health: Riyadh; 2006.
14. Brooks BA. Development of an instrument to measure quality of nurses' worklife. United States, Illinois: Ph.D. Thesis, University of Illinois at Chicago, Health Sciences Center; 2001.
15. Gerber RM, Hinshaw AS, Atwood JR. Anticipated turnover among nursing staff. Ariz Nurse. 1983;36(4):5 8.

16. Armstrong RA. Mandated staffing ratios: effect on nurse work satisfaction, anticipated turnover, and nurse retention in an acute care hospital. Virginia: Ph.D. Thesis, George Mason University; 2004.

17. Brooks BA Storfjell J, Omoike O, Ohlson S, Stemler I, Shaver J, Brown A. Assessing the quality of nursing work life. Nurs Adm Q. 2007;31(2):152–157.18.

18. Bluedorn A. A unified model of turnover from organizations. Hum Relat. 1982. https://doi.org/10.1177/001872678203500204.

19. Almalki MJ, FitzGerald G, Clark M. The relationship between quality of work life and turnover intention of primary health care nurses in Saudi Arabia. BMC Health Serv Res. 2012;12:314.

20. Rudman A, Gustavsson P, Hultell D. A prospective study of nurses' intentions to leave the profession during their first five years of practice in Sweden. Int J Nurs Stud. 2014. https://doi.org/10.1016/j.ijnurstu.2013.09.012.

21. Li J, Galatsch M, Siegrist J, Muller BH, Hasselhorn HM, European NEXT Study Group. Reward frustration at work and intention to leave the nursing profession—Prospective results from the European longitudinal NEXT study. Int J Nurs Stud. 2011. https://doi.org/10.1016/j.ijnurstu.2010.09.011.

22. Sharhraky Vahed A, Mardani Hamuleh M, Asadi Bidmeshki E, Heidari M, Hamedi Shahraky S. Assessment of the items of SCL90 test with quality of work life among Amiralmomenin Hospital Personnel of Zabol City. Sci J Hamdan Univ Med Sci. 2011;18(2):50–5.

23. Dargahi H, Changizi V, Jazayeri GE. Radiology employees' quality of work life. Acta Med Iran. 2012;50(4):250–6.

24. Nayeri ND, Salehi T, Noghabi AA. Quality of work life and productivity among Iranian nurses. Contemp Nurse. 2011a;39(1):106–18.

25. Boonrod W. Quality of working life: perceptions of professional nurses at Phramongkutklao Hospital. J Med Assoc Thail. 2009;92(Suppl 1):7–15.

26. MCarthy G, Tyrrell MP, Lehane E. Intention to 'leave' or 'stay' in nursing. J Nurs Manag. 2007;15(3):248–55.

27. Gregory DM, Way CY, LeFort S, Barrett BJ, Parfrey PS. Predictors of registered nurses' organizational commitment and intent to stay. Health Care Manag Rev. 2007;32(2):119–27.

28. Khani A, Jaafarpour M, Dyrekvandmogadam A. Quality of nursing work life. J Clin Diagn Res. 2008;2(6):1169–74.

29. Lee YW, Dai YT, Park CG, McCreary LL. Predicting quality of work life on nurses' intention to leave. J Nurs Scholarsh. 2013. https://doi.org/10.1111/jnu.12017.

30. Mosadeghrad AM, Ferlie E, Rosenberg D. A study of relationship between job stress, quality of working life and turnover intention among hospital employees. HSMR. 2011. https://doi.org/10.1258/hsmr.2011.011009.

20

Advancing mobile learning in Australian healthcare environments: nursing profession organisation perspectives and leadership challenges

Carey Ann Mather[1]* (iD), Elizabeth Anne Cummings[2] and Fred Gale[3]

Abstract

Background: Access to, and use of, mobile or portable devices for learning at point of care within Australian healthcare environments is poorly governed. An absence of clear direction at systems, organisation and individual levels has created a mobile learning paradox, whereby although nurses understand the benefits of seeking and retrieving discipline or patient-related knowledge and information in real-time, mobile learning is not an explicitly sanctioned nursing activity. The purpose of this study was to understand the factors influencing mobile learning policy development from the perspective of professional nursing organisations.

Methods: Individual semi-structured interviews were undertaken with representatives from professional nursing organisations in December 2016 and January 2017. Recruitment was by email and telephone. Qualitative analysis was conducted to identify the key themes latent in the transcribed data.

Results: Risk management, perceived use of mobile technology, connectivity to information and real-time access were key themes that emerged from the analysis, collectively identifying the complexity of innovating within an established paradigm. Despite understanding the benefits and risks associated with using mobile technology at point of care, nursing representatives were reluctant to exert agency and challenge traditional work patterns to alter the status quo.

Conclusions: The themes highlighted the complexity of accessing and using mobile technology for informal learning and continuing professional development. Mobile learning cannot occur at point of care until the factors identified are addressed. Additionally, a reluctance by nurses within professional organisations to advance protocols to govern digital professionalism needs to be overcome. For mobile learning to be perceived as a legitimate nursing function requires a more wholistic approach to risk management that includes all stakeholders, at all levels. The goal should be to develop revised protocols that establish a better balance between the costs and benefits of access to information technology in real-time by nurses.

Keywords: Agency, Continuing professional development, Digital professionalism, Governance, Mobile learning, Mobile technology, Nursing, Point of care

* Correspondence: Carey.Mather@utas.edu.au
[1]School of Health Sciences, College of Health and Medicine, University of Tasmania, Locked Bag 1322, Launceston, TAS 7250, Australia
Full list of author information is available at the end of the article

Background

The use of mobile technology to access information in real-time is ubiquitous in modern life. Digital knowledge transfer is an outcome of using mobile technology that is currently underutilised in Australian healthcare settings [1]. Harnessing mobile learning to augment traditional andragogies in healthcare environments by stakeholders, especially nurses, has been slow. Previous studies to explore the lack of mobile learning at point of care by nurses have been undertaken [1–4]. Focus group studies with nurse supervisors and online surveys with students have uncovered barriers, challenges, risks and benefits to nurses and undergraduate students of being able to access and use mobile technology for learning at point of care [3–5]. Analysis of the Registered Nurse Standards for Practice [6] and professional Codes of Conduct [7, 8] have revealed an absence of guidance to support this adjunct method of learning.

The aim of this study was to explore the factors influencing the governance of mobile technology at point of care for informal learning and continuing professional development (CPD) from the perspectives of representatives of professional nursing organisations. Barriers, risks, challenges and benefits to using mobile technology by nurses at point of care have been previously been identified in the international literature at individual, organisational and systems levels [9–12]. Inadequate governance and lack of understanding within registered health professions regarding the potential of accessing and using mobile technology for learning has created further disruption to healthcare provision both within Australia and internationally [13–15]. The resultant inability of nurses to use mobile technology for informal learning and CPD at point of care in Australia hinders them meeting the annual learning requirements for registration as a nurse [16, 17]. Additionally, the lack of legitimate access to mobile learning prohibits nurses from guiding and supporting student nurses and modelling digital professionalism, while undertaking work integrated learning within healthcare environments.

Clear direction regarding governance of mobile technology for leisure and learning within healthcare settings remains unaddressed at a systems level in nursing, with flow-on effects impacting at the organisation and individual levels. While nursing informatics is now an essential component of the undergraduate nursing curriculum [18, 19], students and registered nurses are not formally or consistently taught digital professionalism. In the resulting confusion regarding appropriate and safe use of mobile technology at point of care, opportunities arise for advertent and inadvertent professional transgressions to occur [20]. The blurring of public-private boundaries in healthcare environments generates organisational risks and potential adverse media attention if nurses make poor choices regarding access and use of mobile technology. Fear of litigation has negatively impacted the ability of nurses to access mobile technology in the workplace as organisations have dissuaded its use. Paradoxically, however, nursing is consistently reported to be the most trustworthy profession [21], with nurses depended on to provide complex nursing care and administer controlled substances, yet not trusted with carrying a mobile device to access information at point of care [2, 22].

Nurses are the largest group within the registered health professions in Australia [23], making it costly for organisations to educationally prepare their nursing workforce to become proficient in using mobile technology at point of care. However, a digitally capable workforce will be also be able guide the new generation of nurses to become digitally professional and minimise the potential risks associated with using digital media. Upskilling the nursing workforce will also contribute to lessening the current confusion whereby undergraduate students can use mobile technology for learning [11, 24] except during work integrated learning [25]. Promotion of congruency in mobile learning opportunities across the profession is now necessary if nursing is to remain contemporary and continue to be viewed by the public as a trustworthy profession [21, 26].

Research on generational cohorts has previously focused on the retiring 'Baby Boomers' (1946–1964) who were vested with the responsibility of initiating digital technology into occupations [27] and 'Generation Y' (1982–1995) who have grown up with access to digital technology and are currently entering the workforce [28, 29]. However, there is now research indicating 'Generation X' (those born between 1965 and 1982) are hindering the installation of mobile technology into healthcare environments. Christopher and colleagues [30] report Generation X nurses in senior management positions believe they have insufficient formal powers to be innovative within healthcare environments. This lack of influence may manifest as an inability to promote mobile learning as a legitimate nursing function [31]. Research about 'Generation Y' indicates a dislike of hierarchy [29, 32]. This aversion exhibits as Generation Y being reluctant to challenge existing work structures, including those activities that could promote a 'learning organisation' [30, 33] This generational dissonance regarding structural empowerment may contribute to the lack of agency demonstrated by nurses to lead implementation of mobile learning as a legitimate nursing function.

Mobile technology enables individuals to seek and retrieve information in real-time that can aid in decision-making that could potentially improve patient outcomes

[34, 35]. Access to information at point of care also has the potential to improve workflow. Westbrook and colleagues [36] quantified patterns of task time distribution and found nurses completed an average of 72.3 tasks per hour which over time became more fragmented and interrupted, creating potential safety concerns. Deployment of mobile learning has the potential to reduce this fragmentation by enabling continuity of care of patients, as nurses would not need to leave the bedside to check or clarify information. This study targeted representatives from nursing profession organisations to better understand from their perspective the factors influencing the use of mobile technology for informal learning and CPD.

Methods

Design

This research uses interpretive description as discussed by Thorne [37]. It draws on the work of Creswell [38], and Strauss and Corbin [39] by using purposive sampling and employing a reflexive approach within a systematic framework to code, label and categorise the data to enable analysis.

Participants and recruitment

Purposive sampling was used to recruit participants from a range of nursing profession organisations. Inclusion criteria for interview were being a nurse employed or belonging to a nursing profession organisation senior enough to be able to represent the organisation from a policy or guideline perspective and having expertise in nursing practice. A potential list of organisations was generated (CM and EC) that included National ($n = 7$) and Coalition of National Nursing and Midwifery Organisations (CoNNMO) member ($n = 55$) organisations. Invitations were sent to the contact emails provided via the national organisation or CoNNMO website ($n = 52$). If no response was received within two weeks, a follow-up telephone call was made. If there were no telephone contact details available, a further email was sent to the same address. A reminder email was despatched one month after the initial email invitation. An information sheet was provided as an attachment to the email invitation and consent to participate was recorded prior to the beginning of the recorded interview as per ethics protocol for approval H0016097.

Data collection

Interviews with participants were conducted and recorded using Skype for Business™, at a mutually agreeable time using a semi-structured schedule as a guide. The interview schedule question development was informed by previous research [4] and developed by two researchers (CM and EC). Prompts and potential probing questions were included in the schedule to maintain congruency of questioning (Table 1). Interview questions were designed to establish whether the nursing profession organisations had a policy position on mobile technology for informal learning and CPD and then to explore factors impacting the use of mobile technology for learning at point of care.

The interviews were conducted during December 2016 and January 2017, took between 17.29 and 54.29 min (mean 34.05 min) and were transcribed verbatim. Variations in interview length were due to the depth of knowledge of the topic of investigation by individual participants.

Data analysis

A systematic and organised process was developed consisting of trial coding with member checking and development of a codebook that provided a framework of codes. Auditing of codes and reviewing previous interviews to ensure consistency of application of labels across interviews was conducted during the process of coding. Inductive thematic analysis was undertaken by coding 'meaning units' as 'open codes' as described by Elliot and Timulak [40]. 'Meaning units' were tabulated in Microsoft Excel (2016), from which data was labelled

Table 1 Nursing profession representative interview schedule

Number	Question
1	Can you tell me about the overall view of this organisation's position on nurses and midwives using mobile technology for informal learning and CPD in the workplace?
2	If your organisation has a position on mobile technology use for mobile learning, please provide detail about how this position was developed?
3	If your organization has no position on mobile technology use for mobile learning, what do you think this organisation could offer in order to influence the use of mobile technology for informal learning and CPD in the workplace?
4	Can you tell me what your organisation can do to support the development of standards, guidelines or policies about the access and use of mobile technology at point of care?
5	Can you explain to me in your own words how portable or mobile technology could change learning in the workplace?
6	Can you tell me about how your organisation's opinion on access to portable or mobile learning environments impact on patient or client safety?
7	Can you tell me about your organisation's opinion on perceptions of public about nurses and/or midwives using portable or mobile technology in the workplace?
8	Do you have any opinion on perceptions of other health professionals using portable or mobile technology in the workplace?
9	What do you perceive nurses or midwives currently do for continuing professional development to meet the requirements for AHPRA?
10	Do you have any other comments you would like to make regarding nurses using mobile technology for learning?

and reduced from open to axial and finally to selective codes to enable the sub-themes to be revealed. This process of labelling and reducing the phrases by coding enabled further refinement of the data to become four core themes. Constant comparison was undertaken by two of the authors (CM and EC).

Rigour

The interviewer (CM) familiarised herself with the schedule to ensure the interview process flowed and enabled probing questions and prompts to be less rehearsed. The interviewer was aware of the lack of body language cues and maintained a neutral but encouraging dialogue with participants [41]. At the conclusion of each interview, interviewees were asked if they had any further information they would like to add. This opportunity enabled participants to raise any issues or information that had not been discussed during the interview. The accuracy of the transcriptions were confirmed, by reading and listening to the audio recordings of the interviews simultaneously by the interviewer. At the conclusion of each interview, participants were offered the opportunity to check the transcription for errors. This process minimised potential for error and ensured accuracy of the data transcription.

Ethics

Ethics approval was gained from The University of Tasmania Social Sciences Human Research Ethics Committee (H0016097) prior to commencement of the study as required under Australia's National Statement on Ethical Conduct in Human Research [42].

Results

Participant demographics

Six interviews were conducted during the study period (Table 2) Participants were senior registered nurses holding executive positions who through their careers had a broad range of nursing experiences in a variety of healthcare settings. They were paid employees or were

volunteers within Australian nursing specialty organisations that were members of CoNNMO.

Gaining access to appropriate nursing representatives to seek participation proved problematic owing to the complexity of the national organisations targeted or voluntary nature of the membership to nursing specialty organisations. The lead time required to obtain national organisation permission to interview varied. Requests for interviewing a representative from the organisation needed to be taken to appropriate internal meetings to be considered. Feedback from organisations was sought, after meetings were held to discuss the interview request. However, reaching an appropriate representative for interview remained complicated. One organisation declined to participate due to a decision made by the organisation Director. Access to nursing speciality organisation representatives affiliated with CoNNMO was ad hoc, owing to the volunteer nature of many nursing specialty organisations. The voluntary nature of these organisations was apparent by irregular monitoring of email accounts, so non-acknowledgement or response from point of entry was common. However, initial and follow-up contact was undertaken as per ethics protocol. The complexity of gaining access to National representatives and the poor response from voluntary organisations impacted the capacity to recruit interviewees. In addition, the release of the Australian College of Nursing, Health Informatics Society of Australia and Nursing Informatics Australia joint draft position statement on health informatics in February 2017 resulted in cessation of recruitment as the researchers believed it could influence the responses of future participants.

Themes

Four key themes emerged from the data analysis, revealing the complexity of factors that influence governance of mobile learning at point of care in healthcare environments in Australia. These themes were: 1) risk management; 2) perceived use of mobile technology; 3) connectivity to information; and 4) real-time access.

Table 2 Participant demographics

Interview	Nursing organisation	Nurse role	Source of recruitment	Gender
1	National representative (Executive)	Administration	Direct email to organisation	F
2	Specialty nursing Executive position (volunteer organisation)	University academic and clinician	Via email from CoNNMO secretariat[a]	M
3	National representative (Executive)	University academic	Direct email to organisation	F
4	Specialty nursing Executive position (volunteer organisation)	Clinician	Via email from CoNNMO secretariat	F
5	Specialty nursing Executive position (volunteer organisation)	Administration and clinician	Via email from CoNNMO secretariat	M
6	National representative (Executive)	Administration	Direct email	F

CoNNMO[a] Coalition of National Nursing and Midwifery Organisations

Addressing all four themes was found to be imperative for enabling mobile learning at point of care.

Risk management

Participants identified numerous potential risks in employing mobile technology at point of care that required management to minimise adverse or unintended consequences. Participants acknowledged there was a lack of governance at a wider systems level that negatively impacted their capacity to use mobile technology at point of care. They indicated the belief that mobile technology was not allowed within healthcare settings. The belief was expressed that the non-use of mobile technology had developed historically, with one participant stating:

"We also had, I think we've still got some of the misconceptions around the risks with mobile devices and medical devices" (Participant 2).

Another influence on the lack of direction regarding mobile learning within organisations was attributed to generational cohorts. One participant reported:

"But we have to overcome the establishment, the bureaucracy in the health system that actually sees this as a bad thing, that oh no, they're going to be on social media and they're all going to be doing bad things and this instant thought that the internet is just this bad place and no good will come of it. I think some of the older directors of nursing and all that sort of stuff, who are all basically starting to retire now sort of are making way for a younger generation of directors of nursing who we hope is going to have a better or a more positive approach to this" (Participant 5).

Representatives described factors that have influenced organisations to implement policies or local rules within organisations excluding the use of mobile technology. Participants cited organisations formally and informally dissuading nurses from using mobile technology at point of care. This was expressed by one representative who stated:

"But the nurses I find, whether it's just that they're more regulated, are not encouraged to use their phones in the actual clinical environment" (Participant 4).

Interviewees reported there was inconsistency of access and use, which created confusion for nurses within organisations as shown by this comment:

"But unfortunately, it's such a reactive approach rather than proactive approach, in that they're not - it's actually," "Well, the technology's great, most people are using it appropriately, but you can't stop every -

you know, don't stop everybody from using it because some people have been not doing the right thing" (Participant 3).

They acknowledged incongruency with using mobile technology for patient care, clinical decision-making and the lack of capacity for seeking and retrieving information at point of care. Nurses expressed concern over the lack of direction provided to the profession at a National level, which then impacted at an organisation level. Participants provided examples of other health professionals' expectations of nurses being able to access mobile technology even when organisational policy precluded its use. One participant stated:

"But then, as I said, there's that conflict between, we're encouraged to have those things on our phone, but we're not allowed to really use them on the ward. So, there is an issue around that, that you will send a photo to a consultant and actually, that is written into policy that that's a breach of that particular policy; you're not allowed to send patient's photos on personal devices" (Participant 4).

Interviewees revealed that although there was little formal direction at a systems level on whether mobile technology could be used, some nursing staff were beginning to challenge the apparent edict to drive change:

"What they have now, so we're living in a bit of a fantasy world at the moment where people say there's no mobile phones allowed, when in fact everyone has a mobile phone in their pocket" (Participant 2).

A participant indicated another influence on practice was previous breaches of patient confidentiality or privacy, which motivated organisations to limit access to mobile technology:

"I think it will be when - we've had - the reason it's come about unfortunately, is because of the opposite reason, in that people's photos have got out onto Facebook and to general internet public forums and there's been people that have been sued" (Participant 4).

Cyberloafing behaviour was cited as a reason for preventing legitimate access to mobile technology while at work. One representative expressed:

"And I don't know whether it's a different generation or different - that people think that they might be checking Facebook, or they might be misusing their mobile devices rather than using them for education" (Participant 4).

Participants offered potential workarounds to resolve the current impasse regarding legitimate use of mobile technology at point of care, indicating they believed nurses were capable of discerning when mobile learning could be deployed:

"We're good at coming up with solutions to things. And I think that's part of our learning" (Participant 6).

One participant summed up the current situation related to guidance of mobile learning at point of care within Australian healthcare environments by stating:

"So, it is a real messy minefield" (Participant 2).

Interviewees raised the importance of appropriate use of mobile technology for informal learning and CPD. This addresses the concept of digital professionalism, which embodies ethical use and maintenance of professional boundaries when using mobile technology within healthcare environments. One participant suggested learning about safe and appropriate use was a risk management strategy to ameliorate the current circumstances:

"But of course, that's again, I don't think - I think that's the risk but I - my philosophy is let's train people, let's have a policy, let's train people in safe, responsible mobile use" (Participant 2).

Another participant pointed out nurses need to know their professional boundaries regarding seeking and retrieving information, and users must be able to critically reason when it is appropriate to use mobile technology for learning:

"But as I said, nurses need to learn what they need to learn when they need to learn it. This can augment that process but again we're not going to learn how to do open heart surgery just because we've got a new device that's got it there for us. We still have to have appropriate use" (Participant 6).

Within the theme of risk management, it became apparent that nurse representatives belonging to nursing profession organisations acknowledged there was an issue in the workplace. However, due to the volunteer nature or absence of priority to enable informal learning of CPD at point of care within these organisations, there was a lack of agency to drive change, to enable mobile learning to become a legitimate nursing function. A representative indicated:

"I think that we could - and we're doing it at the moment, slowly, as you know, these volunteer

organisations and colleges are slow-moving ships but we are trying to develop a policy, not so much about - it probably won't be specific about mobile learning" (Participant 2).

Interviewees indicated from their comments that despite the lack of congruency about mobile technology use at point of care, they did not view themselves as responsible for solving the current paradox. Representatives discussed the issue as though it was outside the aim and scope of their professional organisation to effect change. There was no acknowledgement of the capacity of their organisations to advocate for a change in the status quo or to show leadership in the National arena relating to accessing mobile learning even though it could potentially benefit their members and patients. One participant stated:

"But we specifically don't have a position statement on it, it's just something that we recognise is a minimum standard that it must be" (Participant 5).

Perceived use of mobile technology

From the comments by representatives of nursing profession organisations it was clear that non-use of mobile learning in nursing healthcare environments is commonplace. Statements by interviewees indicated that healthcare lags behind other industries in harnessing emerging technology and nursing is hindered by groups, within and external to the profession. Representatives provided a range of examples where other stakeholders including the medical profession were using mobile technology. Stakeholders in this context were individuals and organisations that interact with, or impact the opportunities of, participants to access or use mobile technology at point of care. For example, one participant indicated junior medical officers (JMOs) could access mobile learning at point of care:

"Well yeah, it certainly seems to be that it's - I see certainly - I guess, I'm getting a little bit older - see a lot new, younger - you know, the JMOs and even some of the residents coming though and they use their phones constantly and it doesn't seem to be seen as an issue" (Participant 5).

Participants indicated there was a need to address how patients perceive mobile learning by nurses if mobile technology is to be used at point of care. A participant indicated they perceived patients were unaccepting of nurses using mobile technology:

"Because I think that there is perhaps a perception and as I said particularly from older people out there that we're using phones merely to communicate with

our friends as opposed to actually looking up things that are useful for the conversation at hand" (Participant 3).

Another representative commented they believed patients would be accepting if the purpose of using the technology was explained:

"However, from a patient's perspective, also from the perspective on a personal level, if you use it with them and you explain what you're doing they'll often be quite accepting of that" (Participant 4).

Additionally, interviewees indicated there was fear of reputational damage, if nurses were accused of misuse by other stakeholders. This risk influenced whether nurses accessed mobile technology at point of care. One representative indicated:

"I think they've felt - well, there's been complaints from a patient perspective that nurses seem to be on their phones, using their phones. They see it as patient perception, that nurses in particular aren't working, they're using their mobile devices for personal use in the workplace rather than using it for work purposes" (Participant 4).

Participants indicated generational cohorts of patients and co-workers behaved differently and this behaviour needed to be taken into account when using mobile technology for learning:

"But we've got - it's perception from a different generation that doesn't see it the same way necessarily, so there needs to be education around 'this is what's happening with these mobile devices' as well. Whereas, I certainly see the younger generations now - so, gen Y will often use online learning. So, not necessarily mobile technology as such but they will use Internet learning far more readily" (Participant 4).

Furthermore, they suggested that access to mobile technology varied depending on the role of the nurse. One interviewee stated:

"But the nurses, just generalist nurses, certainly aren't able to use their - or are discouraged from having their phones on them when they're with patients" (Participant 4).

Participants believed historical circumstances contributed to the current situation where the nursing profession trails other health professions in using mobile learning. For example, one representative stated:

"And I think that while there might be a little bit of a backlash from people who are yearning for a bygone time, the reality going forward is that this reflects well on nursing, showing that nursing is very professional, that they are engaging in and embracing technology" (Participant 6).

Connectivity to information

Connectivity to information was viewed by interviewees as crucial for enabling informal learning and CPD at point of care. Connectivity to information in this context includes the tangible and intangible consequences of stakeholder interactions using mobile technology for information transfer. Representatives indicated they believed it was detrimental to the work of nurses to block access to information transfer for the purpose of connecting with others, or for seeking and retrieving information via the Internet. Nurses needed to demonstrate they were professional, capable and contemporary in their role as one participant stated:

"If in the aviation industry, if our bookings were done by paper we'd be going what's going on here?...I think most people prefer, to have a nurse turn up with a digital device or something to be accessing information" (Participant 6).

Statements by participants indicated Internet connectivity to undertake their clinical role was hidden. For example, one participant provided an explanation about why they perceived nurses were unable to harness mobile learning at point of care:

"I wonder whether nurses tend to be seen as giving that hands on physical care, so they can't pull their phone out and use it, whereas doctors if they're consulting and so it's all right for them to be looking at their phone and that they're being seen to use it for work purposes" (Participant 4).

The inability of nurses to promote their knowledge and skills hinders their access to this vital resource in the new learning age. Nurses are viewed as caring and compassionate and their high level of clinical skills that can be augmented by knowledge management through connection to the Internet, is less overt. As stated by one participant the need for access to mobile learning tools and resources to improve patient outcomes is invisible.

"Anyway, it's actually detrimental because it's a really useful tool, these mobile devices, for our staff" (Participant 2).

Real-time access

Real-time access refers to whether participants have the ability to connect at the actual time to transfer information using mobile technology. Interviewees were enthusiastic about the potential of mobile learning at point of care from the perspective that information was available when required. One participant stated:

"I mean, I've worked in nursing for a hell of a long time and I think I would have given my left arm for that type of ability to look things up then and there at the time" (Participant 3).

Participants recognised the convenience of being able to access information as required without leaving the patient. One representative reported:

"Because we're busy working. We haven't got time to be always stopping to do things. We're busy. And the modern life is busy. And I actually think that nurses find out what they need to know when they need to know it" (Participant 6).

Similarly, another representative revealed the belief that slow acceptance of mobile learning into healthcare environments hindered the advance of nursing practice:

"And in health, I think technology generally in health is really underutilised and I think that we could become far more efficient with education and in improved patient care by using it more appropriately" (Participant 4).

Comments about the inability to harness mobile learning at point of care indicated that stakeholders were missing vital information and interactions that could improve patient outcomes. One example demonstrates the broad scope of mobile learning for clinicians in practice:

"Whereas we are looking up, we should be looking up blood results and then checking it on an app on your phone and finding out what that could be and looking at with your patient symptoms would be fantastic if nurses were doing that and I think would save a huge amount of patient deterioration and improve care" (Participant 4).

Additionally, participants recognised the benefits for nursing students of being able to learn in real-time:

"So, it is really that point at which they know that it's going to be significant for them [students] and if they were to like make a note for themselves like we used to do when we were on clinical placement to go and look

it up at home. Well sometimes you don't get there, don't do it for one reason or another you forget" (Participant 3).

Interviewees also realised that over time learning in real-time at point of care will become more commonplace:

"Yes, I think so. You've got to move with the times. I realise that, over the next decade or so, we've got an older patient group but my mother's downloaded recipes off the internet. I think that's an excuse. I think we have to move. It's in the banking industry. Every other industry That's just part of society. I don't think it's any different in nursing. I think though that nurses in the public image are a little bit caught in time, in a bit of a time capsule. And we're not allowed to grow up" (Participant 6).

Participants recognised that access to learning in real-time will take leadership and concerted effort by stakeholders:

"But I think there's still a lot of work to be done in being able to do it, I don't think there's a magic bullet that will make it happen but rather a sort of concerted effort over a period of time" (Participant 5).

One representative summed up the future of mobile learning by stating:

"Easily accessible up to date information on the device in your hand at the time you're standing by the patient" (Participant 1).

Discussion

The emergent themes of risk management, perceived use of mobile technology, connectivity to information and real-time access in this research confirm Fixsen and colleagues' [43] framework that mobile learning is stalled at the adoption point in the Stages of Implementation (Fig. 1). The four themes support the contention that nurses within nursing profession organisations are currently unwilling to lead on installing mobile learning at a systems level. This reluctance to advance access and use of mobile technology for learning within national healthcare environments then flows over to organisational and individual levels. The absence of clear direction within the Registered Nurse Standards for Practice [6] and new draft Codes of Professional Standards [44] illustrates the issue and compounds the problem of lack of governance. The leadership vacuum within and outside the nursing profession in favour of reform is perpetuating the mobile learning paradox.

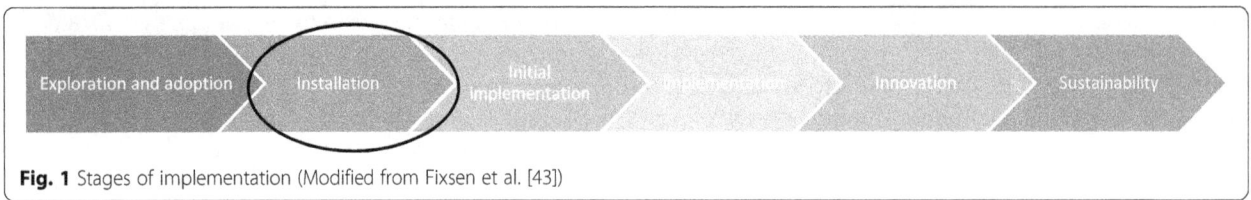

Fig. 1 Stages of implementation (Modified from Fixsen et al. [43])

Action across all four themes is necessary to enhance governance for mobile learning at point of care. As long as the identified limitations persist, nurses will be hindered in their access to mobile learning for informal learning and CPD. Additionally, nurses cannot support, guide or model digital professionalism to nursing students undertaking work integrated learning. The unwillingness of senior nurses to lead on mobile learning is a cause for concern since it is required to overcome the observed stalled implementation [3, 43]. For progress to be made, developing protocols that address the four identified themes will be required.

The release of Australia's National Digital Health Strategy [45] and review of Registered Nurse Accreditation Standards [46] has created opportunities to remedy the current situation by establishing a governance structure within organisations that individuals can implement. Strategy 6 of the Digital Health Strategy acknowledges that Australia requires a health workforce that can confidently use digital health technologies to deliver health and care [45]. Support for change management, training, resources and clear direction are outlined. Additionally, the Australian Nursing and Midwifery Accreditation Council Consultation Papers 1 and 2 provide opportunity to feed forward information about supporting health informatics and mobile learning within the undergraduate nursing curriculum [46, 47].

Nurses are bound by National Standards and Codes which provided detailed cues about expected knowledge, skills, attitudes and behaviour of nurses. The new Registered Nurse Standards for Practice [6] and revised Codes [44] are more generic, giving organisations and individuals more autonomy to determine expectations of nursing practice [16]. However, the lack of explicit information regarding mobile technology in these documents appears to be discouraging its use in healthcare environments because nurses are not yet conversant with the new Standards and Codes and the level of autonomy they provide [48]. The research has demonstrated that senior nurses are unwilling to lead workplace change and have little enthusiasm for being involved in the change process.

Most participants did not view themselves as playing an advocacy role within their nursing profession organisation with regard to mobile learning. Those who did thought that change within professional organisations was slow because it usually relied on volunteer labour,

which waxed and waned depending on individual circumstances. Volunteer 'burnout' led to inconsistency in progressing the aims and objectives of the nursing profession organisation. In addition, the main focus of specialty organisations is advancing specific clinical information and advocating for new platforms to convey that information is not envisaged. Finally, nurses who hold executive positions within nursing profession organisations often do not provide direct care and thus lack contemporary experience of the new ways information can be integrated into nursing practice and transferred at point of care. Thus, until there is a greater appreciation of the issues, the current lack of leadership will continue to hinder progress towards implementation [41].

It is also evident there is a lack of consistency in knowledge, attitudes and behaviour within the nursing profession regarding the use of mobile technology. Resistance to changing workflows [36] owing to inadequate educational preparation and fear of inappropriate use of mobile technology was reported [3, 20]. Representatives provided examples where inappropriate behaviour resulted in the 'banning' of mobile technology at the workplace and anecdotal evidence of previous inappropriate behaviour of health professionals [20, 49, 50] has shaped the current situation. Interviewees justified the inequity of access by claiming adverse media attention was responsible [20, 51, 52]. Participants mentioned cyberloafing and unprofessional behaviour such as using social media while at the workplace contributed to the inability to use mobile technology [53, 54]. All representatives narrated stories of inappropriate behaviour by nurses while admitting they had not witnessed it themselves.

Direct care nurses were unable to access mobile technology, whereas nurses in other roles were allowed to carry a mobile device. This shifting access to mobile technology perpetuates confusion between leisure and learning and will only be ameliorated when mobile learning becomes a legitimate nursing function [55]. Continuance of the lack of governance that supports the mobile learning paradox will impede implementation of mobile learning at point of care. Since further innovation in mobile technology is predicted [56, 57], the current mobile learning gap will continue to widen if the status quo remains unchallenged.

Access to learning resources within healthcare environments is an important imperative. Currently, however, seeking and retrieving relevant information in real-time by nurses is hidden. While nurses are viewed by the public as caring and compassionate individuals, their advanced critical thinking and capacity for managing complex nursing care more covert and less recognised [58]. Therefore, clinical skill enhancement by accessing information in real-time is underappreciated by organisations and nurses. The difficulty in demonstrating the value of access to information transfer in real-time is also arresting progress towards the implementation phase.

As highly skilled clinicians, nurses are constantly analysing and altering their planned schedule of care as new information or events require [36]. Constant interruptions to established workflows require critical thinking and an ability to be flexible. As interruptions to workflow increase, the fragmentation of nursing care creates the need for workarounds. Nurses modify the way they think and behave when practices no longer work as intended, become redundant or opportunities occur to incorporate new work practices that benefit workflow. This adaptation process includes recognising the new intervention's benefits and investing in learning about the new process to enable integration into routine work patterns. Sustaining change occurs when the benefits outweigh non-use [59]. This process is being attenuated with regard to mobile technology and mobile learning, however. From the interviews, nurse leaders appear to absolve themselves of responsibility for advocating within the profession to advance nursing practice. Nurses continue to support a historically hierarchical system that justifies their lack of inclusion in decision-making and are consequently unable to articulate the importance of mobile learning for enabling informal learning and CPD [58]. This apparent inability to communicate the value of access to mobile technology is hindering nurses' capacity to demonstrate how mobile learning improves workflow, promotes continuity of care and potentially improves patient outcomes. It also prevents the modelling of digital professionalism to undergraduate nurses perpetuating the status quo. The current deficiency in the capacity of nurses to influence the direction of mobile learning policy at system and organisation levels further marginalises them within the registered health professions [16, 60].

The casualties of this failure to embrace the mobile learning era include a range of stakeholders. An inability to engage in mobile learning at point of care is a lost opportunity for experienced nurses to lead learning in real-time at the workplace. Being able to legitimately access information at the bedside has the potential to build capacity with other health professionals, students

and patients [61]. Moreover, accessing mobile technology at point of care could strengthen the nurse-patient relationship by increasing mutuality of understanding [1], enable continuity of care and reduce time away from the patient. Nurse supervisors could capitalise on real-time learning moments by supporting students at point of care by using mobile learning when it is safe and appropriate to do so. Currently, nurses support students in practice because they believe 'it is the right thing to do' [48]. However, although they understand the risks, challenges and benefits, they do not advocate for access to mobile learning to support this activity. This unwillingness to lobby for access to learning resources confirms the noted absence of agency by nurses to contemporise their nursing practice by maximising opportunities for informal learning, CPD [62] and teaching students undertaking work integrated learning.

The inclusion of mobile learning early in the nursing curriculum in the classroom will enable modelling of digital professionalism to occur prior to undertaking work integrated learning [24]. Consistency between learning on campus and being able to continue to use mobile technology during work integrated learning will promote safe and appropriate use by the next generation of nurses. The ADHA Digital Health Strategy [45] acknowledges the need for preparation of the nursing health workforce to become digitally literate. As the nursing workforce is the largest of the registered health professions it is imperative that resources are channelled to upskill the current workforce [63]. It is also imperative that nursing profession organisations recognise that knowledge management relies on connectivity to information and that they have a responsibility to advocate for appropriate governance of mobile learning at point of care for the benefit of all stakeholders. Only when there is greater equity of access to mobile technology will nurses be fully able to participate in informal learning, CPD, and training nursing students in digital professionalism and thus to deliver contemporary nursing practice in real-time.

Impact statement

Lack of governance guiding the use of mobile technology at point of care at a systems level negatively impacts the ability of nurses to legitimately incorporate mobile learning into their nursing practice. The current 'mobile learning paradox' needs to be resolved from within the profession of nursing and healthcare organisations. Perpetuation of the mobile learning paradox has implications for the profession internationally, where governance structures regarding access and use of mobile technology in healthcare environments has not been addressed.

Limitations

Limitations of this study include timing of interviews, which due to the short recruitment period took place during December 2016 – January 2017. Recruitment in the lead up to the Christmas period may have reduced opportunity as potential participants may have organised annual leave during the Australian summer, were required to complete work by the end of the year or work during the traditional holiday shut-down period may not have responded, whereas they have done so if recruitment occurred during another time period. Recruitment ceased when the Health Informatics Society of Australia, Nursing Informatics Australia and Australian College of Nursing released the joint draft position statement on nursing informatics in February 2017, as this could have changed perspectives of future interviewees by raising awareness of the topic.

Strengths

Although recruitment numbers were low, participants were senior nurses, who during their careers had experienced clinical, administration, education and research within the nursing profession. This wealth of knowledge was demonstrated through interview. Timing of the interviews was a limitation, and also a strength. This study was undertaken before the draft position statement on nursing informatics was released, providing baseline understanding of the field that can provide direction for further research.

Future directions

The nursing profession is the largest of the registered health profession. As such, this profession is in a strong position to lead mobile learning at point of care. However, this ascendancy will only be accomplished when nurses marshal their mobile learning agency by taking responsibility for leadership within healthcare environments.

There is an opportunity to achieve this aim by embracing the ADHA National Digital Health Strategy [64] and demanding the profession of nursing is included in decision-making at a systems and organisation level. Involving nurses in systems design and creating positive and supportive environments is instrumental to sustainability of the health workforce [65]. Further research into safe and appropriate use of mobile learning by trialling its use needs investigation. The inclusion of digital professionalism early within the undergraduate nursing curriculum is necessary, as is the educational preparation of undergraduate nurses and nurses currently employed within healthcare settings. It is imperative that nurses develop requisite skills to seamlessly undertake patient care and to guide and support students in using mobile technology for learning at point of care.

Further research into mobile learning at point of care is necessary to ensure standards, guidelines and codes of conduct reflect safe and appropriate use. Usability trials to evaluate quality and safety issues may assist with providing evidence to guide risk management for implementation of mobile learning at point of care. This research will also provide rich data to guide undergraduate nursing curriculum development. Gaining the patient perspective regarding nurses using mobile learning will be beneficial to all stakeholders. Findings can be used to guide patient education about the implementation of mobile learning and be used to guide deployment of mobile learning in health care environments.

Conclusions

There is a gap in the governance of mobile technology for learning by nursing profession organisations. At systems and organisation levels, there is a lack of leadership providing direction for the professional conduct of nurses, which is expressed as the inability for nurses to implement mobile technology for learning as a legitimate nursing function. This shortage of support stalls the capacity for individual nurses to implement and model digital professionalism at point of care. Additionally, there is a deficiency of agency within the nursing profession and healthcare organisations that further hinders the installation or deployment of mobile learning at an individual level within healthcare environments.

Through their narratives participants indicated that an absence of governance within nursing organisations is perpetuated by a lack of inclusion in decision-making at a systems level. It is evident from this study that there is insufficient agency by nurses in leadership positions to influence the installation of mobile technology for informal learning and CPD at point of care in healthcare environments. However, inclusion of nurses in healthcare decision-making at a systems level coupled with promoting digital professionalism within organisations and higher education institutions will foster a more inclusive culture that will contribute to improving patient outcomes.

The installation of digital technology for mobile learning to enable informal learning and CPD to be undertaken at point of care challenges traditional work patterns. There is a lack of leadership by nurses within professional organisations to advance governance of digital professionalism that needs to be ameliorated. Empowerment of members within nursing profession organisations will support mobile learning to become a legitimate nursing function.

Abbreviations
ADHA: Australian Digital Health Agency; CoNNMO: Coalition of National Nursing and Midwifery Organisations; CPD: Continuing Professional Development

Acknowledgements

We would like to acknowledge the participants from nursing profession organisations who contributed to this research by freely giving their time to be interviewed.

Funding

No grant funding was obtained for the conduct of this research.

Authors' contributions

The concept and design were developed by CM and EC. CM had overall responsibility and undertook planning, implementation, analysis, interpretation and writing of the manuscript. EC and FG contributed to analysis, interpretation and editing of the manuscript. All authors have read and approved the final version of the manuscript.

Authors' information

Carey Mather is a lecturer in the School of Health Sciences at the University of Tasmania and has investigated the potential and use of innovative technologies in higher education and healthcare settings. Carey has found installing mobile learning as a legitimate nursing function in healthcare environments has created challenges for leaders within the nursing profession. Elizabeth Cummings is an Adjunct Associate Professor at the University of Tasmania. Elizabeth has been involved in a range of state, national and international research projects in ehealth. She is committed to the integration of nursing informatics into nursing education and has a history of conducting research into the use of technology in relation to the management of chronic conditions and ageing well.
Fred Gale is an Associate Professor at the School of Social Sciences, University of Tasmania. He has a longstanding research interest in private governance via standards, certification and labelling which he has investigated in forestry, fisheries, agriculture and nursing contexts. Published books include *Setting the Standard* (UBC Press 2008), *Global Commodity Governance* (Palgrave Macmillan 2011) and *The Political Economy of Sustainability* (Edward Elgar, 2018).

Ethics approval and consent to participate

Ethics approval was gained from The University of Tasmania Social Sciences Human Research Ethics Committee (H0016097) prior to commencement of the study as required under Australia's National Statement on Ethical Conduct in Human Research.
Participants received information and a consent form prior to participation in the study. Interviews were undertaken by telephone and participant consent was recorded before commencement of the recorded interview. Participants agreed prior to beginning of each interview as per the consent form information to have the material used in scientific articles in a de-identified format. The verbal consent was transcribed as part of the interview data as per ethics committee approval protocol.

Competing interests

The authors declare that they have no competing interests.

Author details

[1]School of Health Sciences, College of Health and Medicine, University of Tasmania, Locked Bag 1322, Launceston, TAS 7250, Australia. [2]School of Health Sciences, College of Health and Medicine, University of Tasmania, Private Bag 135, Hobart, TAS 7001, Australia. [3]School of Social Sciences, College of Arts, Law and Education, University of Tasmania, Locked Bag 1340, Launceston, TAS 7250, Australia.

References

1. Mather C, Cummings E. Empowering learners: using a triad model to promote eHealth literacy and transform learning at point of care. Knowl Manag ELearn: Int J. 2015;7(4):629–45.
2. Mather CA, Cummings E. Unveiling the mobile learning paradox. Stud Health Technol Inform. 2015;218:126–31.
3. Mather C, Cummings E. Issues for deployment of Mobile learning by nurses in Australian healthcare settings. Stud Health Technol Inform. 2016;225:277–81.
4. Mather C, Cummings E. Moving past exploration and adoption: considering priorities for implementing Mobile learning by nurses. Stud Health Technol Inform. 2017;241:63.
5. Mather C, Cummings E, Allen P. Nurses' use of mobile devices to access information in health care environments in Australia: a survey of undergraduate students. JMIR mHealth and uHealth. 2013;2(4):e56 e.
6. Nursing and Midwifery Board of Australia. Registered Nurse Standards for Practice 2016. [Available from: https://www.nursingmidwiferyboard.gov.au/news/2016-02-01-revised-standards.aspx]. Accessed 23 Jan 2018.
7. Nursing and Midwifery Board of Australia. Code of Professional Boundaries 2013. [Available from: https://www.nursingmidwiferyboard.gov.au/news/2016-02-01-revised-standards.aspx]. Accessed 23 Jan 2018.
8. Nursing and Midwifery Board of Australia. Code of Ethics Canberra 2013. [Available from: https://www.nursingmidwiferyboard.gov.au/codes-guidelines-statements/professional-standards.aspx]. Accessed 23 Jan 2018.
9. Lluch M. Healthcare professionals' organisational barriers to health information technologies—a literature review. Int J Med Inform. 2011; 80(12):849–62.
10. Mickan S, Tilson JK, Atherton H, Roberts NW, Heneghan C. Evidence of effectiveness of health care professionals using handheld computers: a scoping review of systematic reviews. J Med Internet Res. 2013;15(10):e212.
11. O'Connor S, Andrews T. Mobile technology and its use in clinical nursing education: a literature review. J Nurs Educ. 2015;54(3):137–44.
12. Raman J. Mobile technology in nursing education: where do we go from here? A review of the literature. Nurse Educ Today. 2015;35(5):663–72.
13. Mather C, Cummings E. Modelling digital knowledge transfer: nurse supervisors transforming learning at point of care to advance nursing practice. Informatics. 2017;4(12):1–14.
14. McBride D, LeVasseur SA, Li D. Nursing performance and mobile phone use: are nurses aware of their performance decrements? JMIR Hum Factors. 2015;2(1):e6.
15. McBride DL, LeVasseur SA, Li D. Non-work-related use of personal mobile phones by hospital registered nurses. JMIR mHealth and uHealth. 2015;3(1):e3.
16. Mather C, Gale F, Cummings E. Governing Mobile technology use for continuing professional development in the Australian nursing profession. BMC Nurs. 2017;16(1–11). https://bmcnurs.biomedcentral.com/articles/10.1186/s12912-017-0212-8.
17. Nursing and Midwifery Board of Australia. Guidelines for Continuing Professional Development 2016. [Available from: https://www.nursingmidwiferyboard.gov.au/codes-guidelines-statements/codes-guidelines/guidelines-cpd.aspx]. Accessed 8 Dec 2017.
18. Australian Nursing and Midwifery Accreditation Council. Australian Nursing and Midwifery Accreditation Council Registered Nurse Accreditation Standards: Australian Nursing and Midwifery Accreditation Council; 2012. [Available from: https://www.anmac.org.au/sites/default/files/documents/ANMAC_RN_Accreditation_Standards_2012.pdf. Accessed 8 Dec 2017.
19. Australian Nursing and Midwifery Accreditation Council. Health informatics and health technology - an explanatory note 2014, : ANMAC; 2014. [Available from: https://www.anmac.org.au/sites/default/files/documents/20150130_Health_Informatics_Technology_Explanatory_Note.pdf. Accessed 8 Dec 2017.
20. Green J. Nurses' online behavior: lessons for the nursing profession. Contemp Nurse. 2017;53(3):355–67.
21. Morgan R. Roy Morgan Image of Professions Survey 2016: Nurses still most highly regarded – followed by Doctors, Pharmacists & Engineers, Article 6797, 2016.
22. Ferguson C. It's time for the nursing profession to leverage social media. J Adv Nurs. 2013;69(4):745–7.

23. Health Workforce Australia. Nurses in Focus 2013. Adelaide: South Australia Health Workforce Australia; 2013.

24. Cummings E, Shin EH, Mather C, Hovenga E. Embedding nursing informatics education into an Australian undergraduate nursing degree. Stud Health Technol Inform. 2016;225:329–33.

25. Mather C, Cummings E. Mobile learning: a workforce development strategy for nurse supervisors. Stud Health Technol Inform. 2014;204:98–103.

26. O'Connor S, Hubner U, Shaw T, Blake R, Ball M. Time for TIGER to ROAR! Technology informatics guiding education reform. Nurse Educ Today. 2017;58:78–81.

27. Skiba DJ. Digital wisdom: a necessary faculty competency? Nurs Educ Perspect. 2010;31(4):251–3.

28. Skiba DJ, Barton AJ. Adapting your teaching to accommodate the net generation of learners. Online J Issues Nurs. 2006;11(2):15.

29. Brunetto Y, Farr-Wharton R, Shacklock K. Communication, training, well-being, and commitment across nurse generations. Nurs Outlook. 2012;60(1):7–15.

30. Christopher SA, Fethney J, Chiarella M, Waters D. Factors influencing turnover in GenX nurses: results of an Australian survey. Collegian. 2018; 25(2):217–25.

31. Carroll CL, Bruno K. Social media and free open access medical education: the future of medical and nursing education? Am J Crit Care. 2016;25(1):93–6.

32. Farr-Wharton R, Brunetto Y, Shacklock K. The impact of intuition and supervisor–nurse relationships on empowerment and affective commitment by generation. J Adv Nurs. 2012;68(6):1391–401.

33. Senge PM. The fifth discipline. New York: Doubleday/Currency; 1990.

34. Cader R, Campbell S, Watson D. Judging nursing information on the WWW: a theoretical understanding. J Adv Nurs. 2009;65(9):1916–25.

35. Kim Y. Trust in health information websites: a systematic literature review on the antecedents of trust. Health informatics journal. 2016;22(2):355–69.

36. Westbrook JI, Duffield C, Li L, Creswick NJ. How much time do nurses have for patients? A longitudinal study quantifying hospital nurses' patterns of task time distribution and interactions with health professionals. BMC Health Serv Res. 2011;11(1):319.

37. Thorne S. Interpretive description: qualitative research for applied practice. Routledge; 2016.

38. Creswell JW, Plano Clark VL, Gutmann ML, Hanson WE. Advanced mixed methods research designs. Handbook of mixed methods in social and behavioral research. 2003;209:240.

39. Corbin J, Strauss A. Basics of qualitative research: techniques and procedures for developing grounded theory, 3rd ed. Los Angeles: Sage Publications; 2008.

40. Elliott R, Timulak L. Descriptive and interpretive approaches to qualitative research. A handbook of research methods for clinical and. Health Psychol. 2005;1:147–59.

41. Alshenqeeti H. Interviewing as a data collection method: a critical review. English Linguistics Research. 2014;3(1):39. https://doi.org/10.5430/elr.v3n1p39.

42. Australian Government. National Health and Medical Research Council, Australian Research Council and Australian Vice-Chancellors' Committee. National statement on ethical conduct in human research. Canberra: Australian Government; 2007.

43. Fixsen DL, Naoom SF, Blase KA, Friedman RM. Implementation research: a synthesis of the literature. 2005. Tampa: University of South Florida, Louis de la Parte Florida Mental Health Institute, National Implementation Research Network; 2005. p. 125.

44. Nursing and Midwifery Board of Australia. Professional Standards: NMBA; 2017. [Available from: https://www.nursingmidwiferyboard.gov.au/codes-guidelines-statements/professional-standards.aspx]. Accessed 23 Jan 2018.

45. Australian Government. Australia's National Digital Health Strategy, Safe, seamless and secure: evolving health and care to meet the needs of modern Australia, Australian Digital Health Agency Executive Team Canberra, 2017. [Available from: https://www.digitalhealth.gov.au/about-the-agency/australian-digital-health-agency-board]. Accessed 8 Dec 2017.

46. Australian Nursing and Midwifery Accreditation Council. Review of registered nurse accreditation standards consultation paper 1. Canberra: Australian nursing and midwifery accreditation council; 2017.

47. Australian Nursing and Midwifery Accreditation Council. Review of registered nurse accreditation standards consultation paper 2. Canberra: Australian nursing and midwifery accreditation council; 2018.

48. Mackay B, Anderson J, Harding T. Mobile technology in clinical teaching. Nurse Educ Pract. 2017;22:1–6.

49. White J, Kirwan P, Lai K, Walton J, Ross S. 'Have you seen what is on Facebook?'the use of social networking software by healthcare professions students. BMJ Open. 2013;3(7):e003013.

50. Mansfield SJ, Morrison SG, Stephens HO, Bonning MA, Wang S-H, Withers A, et al. Social media and the medical profession. Med J Aust. 2011;194(12):642–4.

51. Jones C, Hayter M. Social media use by nurses and midwives: a 'recipe for disaster'or a 'force for good'? J Clin Nurs. 2013;22(11–12):1495–6.

52. Wilson R, Ranse J, Cashin A, McNamara P. Nurses and twitter: the good, the bad, and the reluctant. Collegian. 2014;21(2):111–9.

53. Lim VK, Chen DJ. Cyberloafing at the workplace: gain or drain on work? Behav Inf Technol. 2012;31(4):343–53.

54. Moorhead SA, Hazlett DE, Harrison L, Carroll JK, Irwin A, Hoving C. A new dimension of health care: systematic review of the uses, benefits, and limitations of social media for health communication. J Med Internet Res. 2013;15(4).

55. Alt D. Students' wellbeing, fear of missing out, and social media engagement for leisure in higher education learning environments. Current Psychology. 2018;37(1):128–38.

56. Risling T. Educating the nurses of 2025: technology trends of the next decade. Nurse Educ Pract. 2017;22:89–92.

57. Roberts D, Williams A. The potential of mobile technology (# MoTech) to close the theory practice gap. Nurse Educ Today. 2017;53:26–8.

58. Buresh B, Gordon S. From silence to voice: what nurses know and must communicate to the public. United States of America: Cornell University Press; 2006.

59. May C, Sibley A, Hunt K. The nursing work of hospital-based clinical practice guideline implementation: an explanatory systematic review using normalisation process theory. Int J Nurs Stud. 2014;51(2):289–99.

60. Australian Government. Australian Digital Health Agency Executive Team, 2017 [Available from: https://www.digitalhealth.gov.au/about-the-agency/australian-digital-health-agency-executive].

61. Horstmanshof L, Moore K. Understanding the needs of all the stakeholders: issues of training and preparation for health work students and their clinical educators. Asia-Pacific Journal of Cooperative Education. 2016;17(2):93–100.

62. Moorley C, Chinn T. Using social media for continuous professional development. J Adv Nurs. 2015;71(4):713–7.

63. Duke VJ, Anstey A, Carter S, Gosse N, Hutchens KM, Marsh JA. Social media in nurse education: utilization and E-professionalism. Nurse Educ Today. 2017;57:8–13.

64. Australian Government. Australia's National Digital Health Strategy, safe, seamless and secure: evolving health and care to meet the needs of modern Australia. Canberra: ADHA; 2017.

65. Huryk LA. Factors influencing nurses' attitudes towards healthcare information technology. J Nurs Manag. 2010;18(5):606–12.

Neonatal nasogastric tube feeding in a low-resource African setting – using ergonomics methods to explore quality and safety issues in task sharing

Gregory B. Omondi[1][*] [iD], George Serem[1], Nancy Abuya[1,2], David Gathara[1], Neville A. Stanton[3], Dorothy Agedo[4], Mike English[1,5] and Georgina A. V. Murphy[1,5]

Abstract

Background: Sharing tasks with lower cadre workers may help ease the burden of work on the constrained nursing workforce in low- and middle-income countries but the quality and safety issues associated with shifting tasks are rarely critically evaluated. This research explored this gap using a Human Factors and Ergonomics (HFE) method as a novel approach to address this gap and inform task sharing policies in neonatal care settings in Kenya.

Methods: We used Hierarchical Task Analysis (HTA) and the Systematic Human Error Reduction and Prediction Approach (SHERPA) to analyse and identify the nature and significance of potential errors of nasogastric tube (NGT) feeding in a neonatal setting and to gain a preliminary understanding of informal task sharing.

Results: A total of 47 end tasks were identified from the HTA. Sharing, supervision and risk levels of these tasks reported by subject matter experts (SMEs) varied broadly. More than half of the tasks (58.3%) were shared with mothers, of these, 31.7% (13/41) and 68.3% were assigned a medium and low level of risk by the majority (≥4) of SMEs respectively. Few tasks were reported as 'often missed' by the majority of SMEs. SHERPA analysis suggested omission was the commonest type of error, however, due to the low risk nature, omission would potentially result in minor consequences. Training and provision of checklists for NGT feeding were the key approaches for remedying most errors. By extension these strategies could support safer task shifting.

Conclusion: Inclusion of mothers and casual workers in care provided to sick infants is reported by SMEs in the Kenyan neonatal settings. Ergonomics methods proved useful in working with Kenyan SMEs to identify possible errors and the training and supervision needs for safer task-sharing.

Keywords: Ergonomics, Task analysis, Quality and safety, Nasogastric tube feeding

Background

Neonatal mortality has fallen more slowly than child mortality in the past twenty years in many low- and middle-income countries (LMICs) due to challenges with the provision of high quality care given the resource limited nature of such settings [1]. To improve neonatal survival, the provision of high quality care to small and sick is must improve [2]. Assisted feeding, often by nasogastric tube (NGT), is one of a set of interventions that form an essential package of facility based services. When fully implemented, feeding (oral or nasogastric) has the potential to substantially reduce neonatal mortality and morbidity, especially for low-birth-weight neonates [3]. NGT feeding is typically the formal responsibility of nurses. It is a time-consuming task that may need to be performed every two to three hours for small and sick babies [4]. In resource-limited settings, where the nursing workforce is severely constrained, components of the NGT feeding task may be only partly performed or completely missed, negatively impacting survival and early post-natal growth [5–7].

* Correspondence: GOmondi@kemri-wellcome.org
[1]KEMRI-Wellcome Trust Research Programme, Nairobi, Kenya
Full list of author information is available at the end of the article

Task shifting/sharing has been proposed as an approach for addressing health workforce shortages [8–11]. However, despite the recent launch of task-sharing policies in Kenya, there are no specific guidelines that encompass task sharing between nurses and non-professional cadres in newborn units and no recognised 'healthcare assistants' within Kenyan public health facilities [12]. Anecdotal information suggests however, that nurses informally share tasks with untrained casual workers and babies' family members. The safety and quality of care provided under such conditions is a major concern [13–15]. How key neonatal nursing interventions are performed and shared, which components may be missed, and what safety issues need to be considered when performing and sharing tasks, remain undescribed in such settings.

Given the importance of NGT feeding, its time-consuming nature and the potential risk of serious consequences (for example aspiration) if incorrectly performed, it is imperative to consider safety in cases where it is shared. Our aim was, therefore, to explore this task in detail, gain preliminary information on how it is shared in Kenyan public hospitals and examine potential risks. This will provide preliminary data to conduct a larger study with a larger sample. Knowledge gained will inform discussions on whether and how this task could be formally and safely shared. We employed Ergonomics (or human factors and ergonomics, HFE) methods often helpful in unpacking complexities in the dynamics of task implementation processes.

The Human Factors and Ergonomics Society defines Ergonomics as "...the scientific discipline concerned with the understanding of interactions among humans and other elements of a system, and the profession that applies theory, principles, data and methods to design in order to optimize human well-being and overall system performance." [16] HFE methods have been traditionally used to improve quality and eliminate errors in various industries predominantly the aviation, nuclear, manufacturing and oil and gas industries [17]. In healthcare, HFE has the potential to make work practices simpler and therefore have a direct impact on the quality of care provided [18]. A number of studies have looked at how HFE methods can be used to gain insights into the dynamic nature of patient care, improve patient safety, analyse problems to generate solutions, calculate/predict risk levels as well as design solutions to mitigate medication administration errors. However, others argue that HFE methods are currently underutilised in healthcare in exploring issues of quality and safety [15, 19, 20].

In this study, we use Hierarchical Task Analysis (HTA) which is a flexible and structured technique to provide an exhaustive description of tasks in a hierarchical manner [21], and the Systematic Human Error Reduction and Prediction Approach (SHERPA) to describe the errors that might occur in each step of the HTA, the consequences, probability and criticality of such errors, and the remedial steps to be taken to reduce them [21, 22]. Healthcare Failure Mode and Effects Analysis (HFMEA) is a similar method to HTA and SHERPA and has also been used to identify potential failures and their causes before future services are provided and/or to improve current services. While both methods have the ultimate goal of improving patient safety, HFMEA has been shown to have validity challenges [23, 24]. SHERPA's reliability and validity is consistently high, ranging between 0.65–0.9 and 0.74–0.8, respectively, and higher than other human error identification techniques [25–27].

Methods
Subject matter experts
Data collection for this study was conducted and facilitated by three researchers with direct experience in providing care, including NGT feeding, to sick and or premature infants in inpatient neonatal care settings in Kenya. Two of these researchers (GBO, GS) are registered nurses and one (NA) is a medical doctor; all were trained on HTA and SHERPA techniques by a Professor of ergonomics (NS).

Two groups of subject matter experts (SMEs) composed of four nurses (SME1) and eight nurses (SME2), respectively, were constituted for this study. Experts were purposefully selected based on their experience in frontline neonatal nursing practice, teaching and advisory roles on neonatal nursing care policy. SME members across both groups were drawn from five public sector facilities in Nairobi and Kiambu counties in Kenya admitting between 300 and 4500 babies to their neonatal units each year. Such public facilities are characterised by high patient to nurse ratios and provide the great majority of inpatient neonatal care to Kenya's population, especially its poor. (*Murphy* et al, *PLoS One, under review*).

Hierarchical task analysis (HTA)
HTA was initially used by three trained researchers to create a detailed description of the tasks and sub-tasks performed by nurses while carrying out NGT feeding for sick infants. This was done based on their professional experience and information from the Manual of Clinical Procedures, 3rd Edition by the Nursing Council of Kenya [28]. Standard guidelines on performing HTA were followed [19, 22]. Briefly, the purpose of the analysis was defined and boundaries were set; system goals and sub-goals were described for the NGT feeding task; and the goal was then broken down into sub-goals with emerging operations/actions identified at each step [29]. The researchers aimed to limit the number of sub-goals under any super-ordinate goal to between 3 and 10 by grouping them into clusters of operations. The

description of sub-goals ceased after consensus among the researchers was reached that the operations has become sufficiently detailed for the intended purpose of describing NGT feeding. The final operations of a sub-goal that were not broken down any further are referred to as 'end tasks'. Further analysis was based on these end tasks (tasks in boxes with a line under them) and not the super-ordinate tasks (tasks in unshaded boxes, *see* Fig. 1).

SME1 was taken through a day-long workshop on ergonomics methods facilitated by the researchers. They were introduced to the concept of ergonomics in health and taught how to conduct a HTA and validate HTA outputs. SME1 was presented with the draft NGT feeding HTA to review and propose changes. The review was done in pairs, suggested changes were then discussed among all SMEs until consensus was reached on a relevant, clear and meaningful final version [30].

Systematic human error reduction and prediction approach (SHERPA)

SHERPA analysis was done on the HTA end tasks by the three researchers [30]. One researcher (GBO) led the drafting of the first version, this was then reviewed iteratively by the other two researchers (GS and NA) until a consensus was reached for the final draft. For each of the tasks, the error mode/code, description, consequence, recovery, probability, criticality and remedial measures were formulated (*see* Additional file 1: Table S2). For the error modes/codes, SHERPA's predefined human error taxonomy and associated codes classified under the six behaviour categories were used [19]. Probability and criticality levels used were defined as shown in Table 1 [31]. This version of SHERPA was reviewed by an expert neonatal nurse trainer (DA), changes made, and thereafter, adopted as the final version of SHERPA for the NGT feeding HTA.

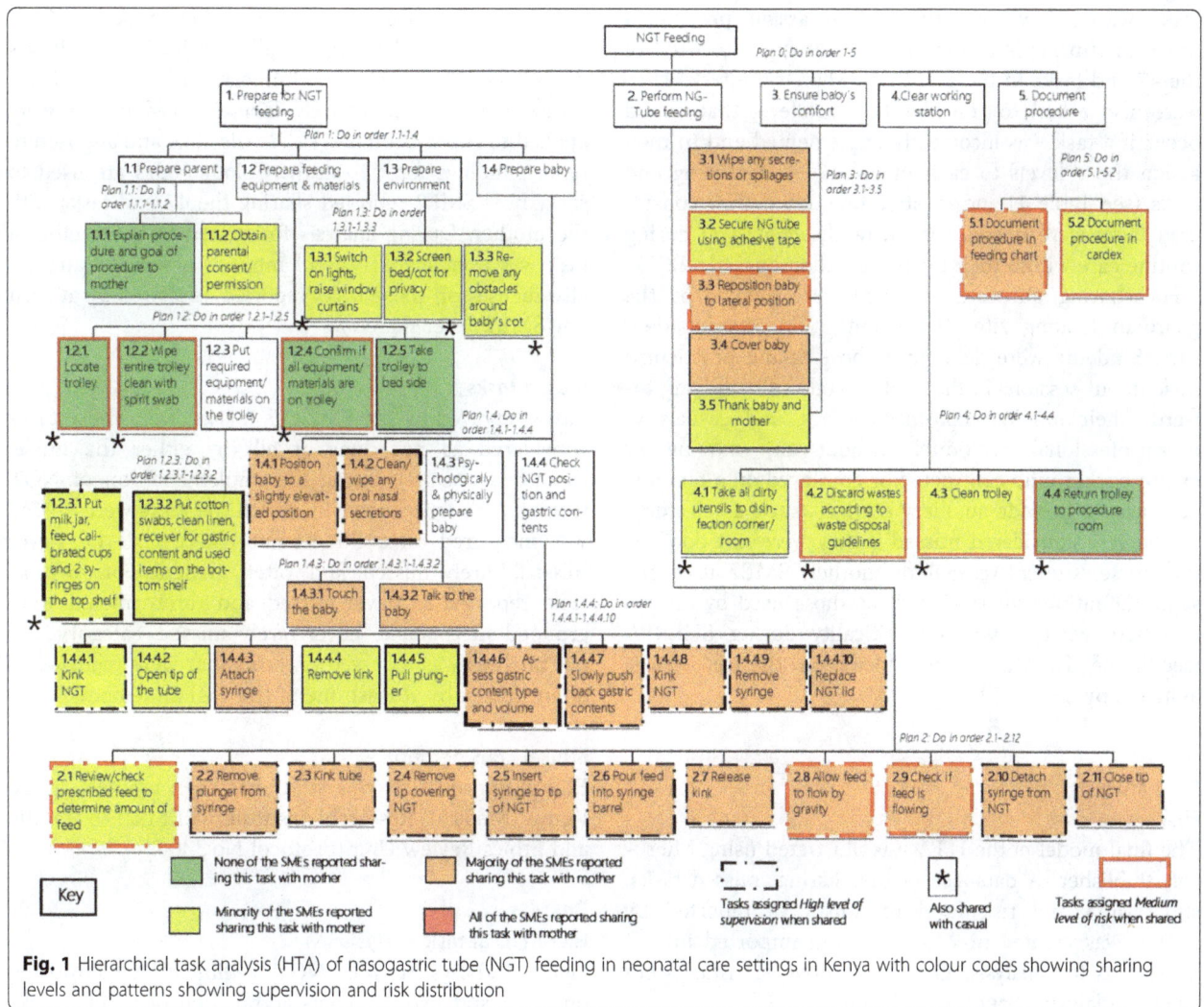

Fig. 1 Hierarchical task analysis (HTA) of nasogastric tube (NGT) feeding in neonatal care settings in Kenya with colour codes showing sharing levels and patterns showing supervision and risk distribution

Table 1 Definition of probability, criticality and supervision levels

Task attribute	Low	Medium	High
Probability	Never known to happen	Known to happen occasionally	Known to happen frequently
Criticality/risk	No risk of injury to patient if task is incorrectly done or missed	Risk of minor injury to patient if task is incorrectly done or missed	Risk of serious injury or death of patient if task is incorrectly done or missed
Supervision[a]	Supervision done by the nurse for only part of the implementation process of the task	Supervision done by the nurse for about half of the implementation process of the task	Supervision done by the nurse for the entire implementation process of the task

[a]During analysis, 'low' and 'medium' levels of supervision were combined into one category of 'low/medium'

Classification of supervision, sharing and risk level of tasks

SME2 was convened for a day-long workshop with the aim to discuss and share their expert opinion on the usual practice of NGT feeding within their settings. This did not aim to reach consensus but instead to illustrate possible variations in opinion and practice, recognising that there were only two representatives from each of the four public hospital settings and that any findings may not be regarded as representative of the wider health system in Kenya. SME2 members were asked to: i) give their opinions on who they share NGT feeding tasks with. They were then asked assign predefined levels of supervision (low, medium or high) to each of the 47 end tasks in the event they shared the task. They were also asked to consider the risk level that would occur if a task was incorrectly implemented and to then assign those levels to each of the 47 NGT feeding end tasks (see Table 1) and to state how often they considered tasks were missed (never, rarely or always) during routine care within their hospitals (Additional file 2).

For sharing purposes, mothers were defined as the guardian looking after the infant during its inpatient care. Students were defined as those taking practicum/attachment sessions in the facility while still studying towards their nursing diplomas/degrees, and casuals as non-professional personnel without any nursing or health background contracted or employed on a temporary basis to provide auxiliary services, such as cleaning. Tasks were considered missed if they were not done by the nurse, student, casual or mother. SME2 used the same definitions for risk levels as those used by the researchers when describing criticality during SHERPA (see Table 1). Our results focus on the risk levels assigned by SME2.

Data analysis
HTA
The final model of the HTA was illustrated using Microsoft Publisher. A database of the sharing, missed tasks, supervision and risk level responses as reported by SME2, was created in MS Excel and imported into R Version 3 for analysis. Only descriptive statistics were used in analysing data for this study.

Sharing, supervision and risk levels
Simple descriptive statistics were used to calculate the proportion of tasks shared with mothers, students and casuals, for example 6 out of the 47 tasks shared would equate to 12.8% of the tasks. Responses from SME2 on sharing, supervision and risk levels were thereafter organised into four response groups according to the number of SME2 members reporting these levels. If, for example, a task was reported to be shared with the mothers by none of the SMEs, then for the purpose of analysis, that task was considered as shared by 'none'. However, if the task was reported as shared with the mother by between one and three; four and seven, and all eight SMEs, then it was considered as shared by a 'minority', majority' and 'all' SME2 members, respectively. These considerations were applied to supervision and risk levels alike and are used to report findings for this study. Colour codes are used to show how SME2 reported sharing the 47 end tasks with the mother. During analysis for shared tasks, whether a task was ever shared was of interest, hence the analysis also focuses on those tasks reported as shared by at least one SME2 ('ever shared').

Missed tasks
Tasks reported by the SME2 as missed were those tasks considered as not done at all (by either the nurse, mother or casual) during the implementation of NGT feeding. The frequency with which the tasks were missed was measured on a three-point Likert scale of 'never missed', 'rarely missed' and 'often missed'. For analysis, tasks reported as 'never missed' and 'rarely missed' were grouped in a single 'never/rarely missed' category and our analysis was focussed on tasks that were reported as often missed by at least one of the SME2 members.

Ethical consideration
Ethical approval for this study has been granted by the Kenya Medical Research Institute (KEMRI) Scientific and Ethics Review Unit (protocol No.3366).

Results
Hierarchical task analysis
Figure 1 shows the final NGT feeding HTA comprising one goal and five sub-goals and a total of 47 end tasks

(i.e. those at the bottom of the hierarchy/tasks that are not described in further sub-tasks). Subsequent results and analysis hereafter focus on these 47 end tasks.

Sharing

Sharing tasks with mothers and students was commonly reported by SME2 members as compared to sharing with casuals (57.3, 39.6 and 7.3% of tasks on average, respectively). All tasks were reported by at least one member of SME2 as ever shared with the students. Nearly all tasks (41/47) were reported as ever shared with the mothers whereas only a small proportion of tasks (23%, *marked with an asterisk in* Fig. 1) was reported as ever shared with the casuals. For six end tasks, none of the SME2 members reported sharing those with the mother.

There was considerable heterogeneity in the tasks reported as shared with mothers, with no task being reported as shared by all eight members of SME2 (Table 2). Slightly more than half (51.1%, $n = 47$) of the tasks were reported as shared with the mothers by a majority of SME2 members.

Missed tasks

Four tasks were reported as often missed by the majority of SME2 while the remaining tasks (91.5%, $n = 47$) were reportedly never/rarely missed. Those tasks reported as often missed were under the sub-goals 'prepare for NGT feeding', and 'ensure infant's comfort' (see Additional file 3: Figure S1*).* There was clear consensus among all SME2 that 16 of the 47 tasks were never/rarely missed, while for the remaining 31 tasks at least one SME2 member reported the task was often missed.

Risk levels

Overall, there was considerable heterogeneity in the reported levels of risk by SME2. Thirteen tasks were assigned medium level of risk by the majority (≥ 4 of 8) SME2 members. These 13, plus an additional five tasks, were assigned medium level of criticality by the

researchers during SHERPA analysis (see Additional file 4: Table S1), demonstrating high concordance in the levels of risk assigned to the tasks by the two groups. None of the 47 tasks were given a high criticality rating by the researchers or SME2 members.

Overlap between task sharing, risk levels and missed tasks

Nine tasks (22%) reported as shared with the mother by at least one of the SME2 were assigned a medium level of risk by a majority (≥ 4 of 8) of SME2 members. Of the nine tasks, three were under 'perform NGT feeding', two under 'ensure baby's comfort', two under 'clear working station' and two under 'document procedure'. Twenty-seven (27/41) of the tasks reported as shared with the mother by at least one SME were also reported to be missed by at least one SME (see Fig. 2a).

Supervision

Considerable heterogeneity was observed in the reported supervision and risk levels of the tasks reported as shared with mothers. Twenty-two tasks were assigned high supervision levels by the majority (≥4 of 8) of SMEs; of these tasks, five were reported as having medium risk (see Fig. 2b). Those tasks reported as highly supervised were predominantly under the sub-goals 'perform NGT feeding' (11/22) and 'prepare for NGT feeding' (9/22).

SHERPA

The most common type of error mode assigned was 'operation omitted', with 44 tasks assigned this error (92%). Forty-four percent (21/47) and 32% (15/47) were assigned medium level of probability and medium level of criticality by the researchers, respectively. Key approaches stated for remedying these medium risk and medium probability errors were linked to training and provision of a checklist for NGT feeding tasks (see Additional file 1: Table S2).

Table 2 Proportions of task sharing with mothers, students and casuals by subject matter expert group 2

Subject matter experts	Current care setting	Proportions of tasks shared with:		
		Mother	Student	Casual
Expert 1a	County referral hospital, approx. 300 annual neonatal admissions, 2 nurses on a typical day shift,15 cots and 52% average occupancy	12.8%	NA[a]	14.9%
Expert 1b		51.1%	NA[a]	8.5%
Expert 2a	Large maternity hospital, approx. 4200 annual neonatal admissions, 3 nurses on a typical day shift, 63 cots and 73% average occupancy	55.3%	63.8%	14.9%
Expert 2b		19.1%	97.9%	0.0%
Expert 3a	County referral hospital, approx. 1800 annual neonatal admission, 2 nurses on a typical shift, 40 cots and slightly above 100% average occupancy	53.2%	61.7%	12.8%
Expert 3b		12.8%	95.7%	6.4%
Expert 4a	National referral hospital, approx. 3200 annual neonatal admissions, 9 nurses on a typical day shift, 56 cots and 117% average occupancy.	61.7%	0.0%	0.0%
Expert 4b		57.4%	31.9%	2.1%

[a]Not applicable (NA): No students come for practicums or are taught at this facility

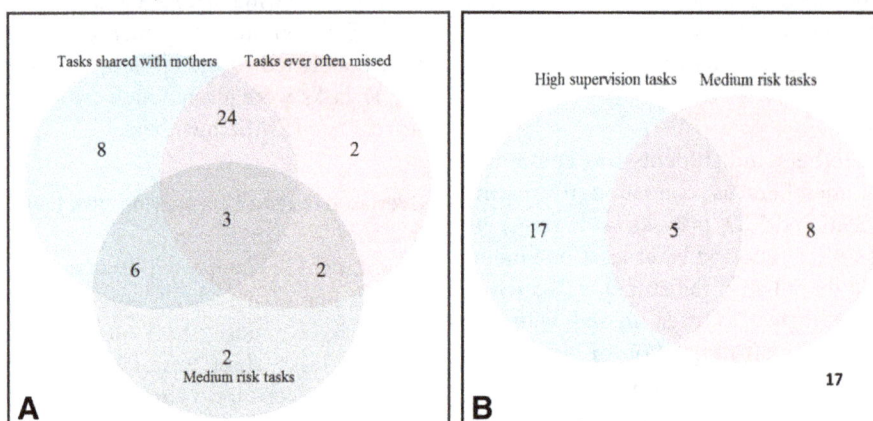

Fig. 2 a Venn diagram showing the overlap between tasks reported as shared and often missed by at least one of the SME, and tasks assigned medium risk level by the majority of SMEs. **b** Venn diagram showing the overlap of tasks reported as highly supervised and those assigned medium risk level by the majority of SMEs. 17 tasks were neither assigned a high supervision nor medium risk level

Discussion

Understanding how humans interact with elements of a system, such as technologies, is important in designing fully functional, effective and safe systems [16, 20]. Patient safety, in the healthcare setting, largely depends on carefully thought out ergonomics of the workplace processes implemented during care provision [32]. HFE, in the healthcare setting, has mostly focussed on the design of medical devices and other aspects of Information Technology for health to increase patient safety and reduce prevalence of medical errors [19, 33]. The focus of HFE in the healthcare is now shifting towards improving human wellbeing through identifying ways to improve work processes and reduce workloads, especially for already resource constrained settings such as infant inpatient settings in LMICs, and more so in Kenya [20]. In this paper we focus on the nursing aspect of care provision in inpatient neonatal care settings in Kenya.

Outcomes of inpatient care for small and sick infants are highly dependent on nursing care, with better outcomes correlated with low patient to nurse ratios [34]. Meeting recommended nurse to patient ratios is still a challenge in most low- and middle-income countries, including Kenya, leading to some tasks being informally shared with unskilled personnel and the infant's mother. The nature of care required to improve patient outcomes in neonatal settings is intricate and time consuming. In this study, we explore the complexity of performing NGT feeding, one of the many key tasks that nurses do while providing care to small and sick infants in inpatient settings [35]. Reported sharing, supervision and risk levels of the 47 tasks in NGT feeding varied widely in this study, despite SMEs coming from fairly similar care settings serving the poor and this could be suggestive of differences in perception and practice.

If not undertaken correctly, NGT feeding can have many serious consequences [36]. However, the greatest risks lie during NGT insertion, a task that precedes NGT feeding. Perforations and incorrect placement of the NGT can occur [37]. The task of NGT insertion was recognised solely as a professional role by the SMEs, undertaken only by qualified and competent personnel and was not the focus of this study. Findings from this study indicated that 'moderate risk' was the highest level of risk assigned to tasks during NGT feeding. None of the tasks was deemed of 'high risk' by either the researchers or the SME, suggesting considerable consensus. The tasks identified as 'medium risk' can be targeted for specific training and/or supervision efforts to reduce risk and increase safety during NGT feeding.

We noted that sharing was mostly reported to be with the mothers. There is growing appreciation of the importance of involving family members and patients in care management, so called patient-family-centred care, as it positively influences neonatal care [38]. In high-income countries, this concept of care has developed over the years, placing parents/family members at the centre of care provision and promoting individualised and tailored health care services. Previous studies have shown that 80–95% of families prefer this kind of care, especially when teaching and discussion on the care of the infant occur at the bedside. [39] This highlights the health benefits of involving mothers or other family members in care of children, including neonates and has led to the development of recommendations on integrating patient-family-centred care by the American Academy of Paediatricians [40–42]. We also noted considerable heterogeneity in how sharing was reported by the experts. There were significant differences in the proportion of tasks reported as shared with either the mother, casual or students, despite the experts coming from fairly similar settings. Similar observations were also noted for reported supervision and risk levels of tasks. These differences could be due to the subjective nature of the perceptions and practice of task sharing by each expert in their respective settings and shows a gap in terms of clear and practical guidelines on how sharing of tasks should be implemented and which specific tasks should be shared, especially in the neonatal care context. One expert, for example, reported not sharing any of the tasks with the students, despite students being present in this setting, while the other expert (from the same setting) shared a considerable amount of tasks with the students (31.9%). We observed that some nurses were uncomfortable with or strongly opinionated against task sharing with students or other unqualified staff. These nurses often held policy or teaching roles that were somewhat removed from the real and practical frontline challenges in delivering nursing care in the context of limited human resources for health, among other challenges [43]. Anecdotal evidence, from other studies we are conducting in similar settings, also suggests that nurses tend to maintain a distinctive identity and therefore wield authority as to whom tasks can be shared with in their settings. This could explain why some experts will share tasks with the mother and not the students or the casuals, hence the heterogeneity in reported sharing proportions with the students, mothers and casuals. This shows a need for practical guidelines for task sharing currently not addressed in Kenya's task sharing policy [12].

The use of HTA and SHERPA revealed the value of the HFE approach in eliciting these differences in perceptions that have direct effects on the quality and safety of NGT feeding. The involvement of mothers and unskilled personnel such as casual workers, in the provision of care for sick infants through task-sharing may help in ensuring that most, if not all the care that the neonate requires is provided. Tasks considered to be low risk can be reassigned to lower cadre workers within the neonatal setting, while high/medium risk tasks can be performed by the nurses; potentially managing the high workload that nurses have, especially in resource constrained settings like Kenya. In addition, nurses may have more time to provide the much needed critical care often associated with high/medium risk tasks. Those tasks reassigned should also be supervised in such a way as to reduce, if not eliminate, risks for undesirable outcomes during their implementation by the lower cadre. Careful consideration is necessary to ensure that the additional supervision responsibility on the nurses' part does not become counterproductive. A delicate balance should be upheld to ensure that safety and quality of care is not compromised. Task sharing has the potential to help mitigate the health worker force shortages in LMICs, however, if undertaken without proper measures

to ensure safety and quality, patient outcomes might be undesirable due to the potential likelihood of provision of low quality of care by whom the task is shared with. Therefore, provisions for standardised and detailed guidelines on training and supervision must be made for safe task-sharing and family-patient-centred care. Ergonomics methods have demonstrated to be useful in unpacking and understanding tasks in a way that can be applied to training and supervision needs, while at the same time highlighting focus areas of potential risks [18, 19]. During the course of the research, a novel way of annotating the HTA to show the task sharing and supervision was developed. This shows the flexibility of the method in being easily adaptable for new analyses.

A very small proportion (8.5%) of the 47 NGT feeding tasks were reported as often missed by the majority of the SMEs in this study. Contrary to the commonly used missed care definition however, and while fully aware of the risk of incorrect implementation of NGT feeding tasks, the SMEs did not consider a task as missed if it was performed by unskilled persons (casuals or mothers). Therefore, despite NGT feeding being an important aspect of care for sick neonates, nurses may often, knowingly, miss parts of the process or delegate to unskilled personnel. This can have significant effects on the recovery time and outcome of the infant [29, 44, 45]. Missed nursing care for sick infants has also been reported in other settings and is often related to support and comfort care [44]. Similarly, in this study we found that screening the bed/cot for privacy, talking to the infant and thanking the infant/mother were some of the tasks related to psychosocial elements of care that were reported as often missed by majority of the SME members.

This study has both strengths and limitations. We used two small groups of SMEs to unpack the complex nature of NGT feeding. Engaging SMEs in discussions on the selected aspects of NGT feeding implementation showed that there was an established implicit understanding of the task. These experts were chosen based on their experience rather than aiming to have a representative sample of care providers in public sector hospitals. The use of SMEs and involvement of small groups of experts in ergonomics methods research is the norm and is valued due to its efficiency in enabling in-depth focus on specific performance issues [21, 22]. The sample size may not be sufficient and lacks power statistically with regard to the task sharing aspect of the study. Our aim for doing this, however, was to gain a preliminary understanding of the norms and practices of task sharing in the SMEs' care settings, and as part of ongoing work to understand the tasks done by nurses to inform future work on task sharing and measuring the work done by nurses [46]. These findings should therefore be interpreted with caution. We plan, in the near future, to share findings from a larger study exploring task sharing in neonatal settings in different hospitals in Kenya using a larger sample size. SME discussions were conducted in groups, which may have led to biased responses of individual experts when reporting on norms within their facilities and convergence of opinions. Furthermore, the provision of two experts from each of the four facilities in SME2, suggests they should not be thought of as independent respondents. Nonetheless, we report high heterogeneity in responses from individual experts in sharing, supervision and risk levels for NGT feeding. Further exploring the origins of the observed heterogeneity would have provided a better explanation to the observations, we, however, did not do this. Almost twice as many tasks were reported as highly supervised as those deemed as of medium risks, whether this increased demand for supervision had implications on the nurses' workload was not further explored. Some tasks, such as 'Insert syringe to tip of NG tube' and 'Pour feed into the syringe' under the sub-goal 'Perform NGT feeding' were reported as often missed by minority of the SMEs yet the subsequent tasks were reported as never missed by all SMEs. This introduces some ambiguity given that the tasks are performed in sequence. One cannot, for example, 'Allow the feed to flow by gravity' if they missed pouring the feed into the syringe in the first place. Some of the noted discrepancies can best be disambiguated through observations. Observational work is often used to complement HTA in ergonomics methods, we plan, in future detailed reports, to share findings from in-depth ethnographic and other methods to explore missed care in Kenya.

To our knowledge, this is the first application of HFE methods to neonatal care research and healthcare in a low-resource setting. A significant number of systems used to report patient safety dwell on analysis of adverse events after they occur, however, there is a shift to focus more on proactive and progressive systems that enable identification of system weaknesses before tragic outcomes and thus avoiding failure modes [47]. Among such methods include HFMEA and HTA/SHERPA. In this study however, we chose to use HTA and SHERPA given our expertise and experience with the methods and their flexibility in their implementation across different teams. HFE methods have previously been shown to be valuable in highlighting patient safety issues during care provision [15, 19, 20]. In our setting, local researchers and SMEs found the methods engaging and easy to grasp [27, 48]. The SMEs welcomed the use of HFE to better understand and articulate the complexity of tasks that hitherto had been a form of implicit knowledge in Kenya making it difficult to share tasks or have standards that comprehensively guide task sharing. This positive experience is contrary to previous reports that healthcare professionals usually have an initial scepticism for these methods [49].

Conclusion

Sharing tasks with lower cadre workers or even with a patient's family in low-resourced healthcare settings may help ease the pressure of high workloads and nursing shortages. However, little is known about how task-sharing might impact safety and quality of care, particularly for neonatal patients where informal task-sharing seems common and not standardised. The novel use of HTA and SHERPA in this study to analyse NGT feeding in a low income neonatal setting revealed the value of these methods to describe the complexity and elicit quality and safety concerns in preforming routine nursing tasks. Our findings could lead to targeted, evidence-based local policy on reorganisation of tasks and detailed training and standard guidance for NGT feeding in neonatal care in LMIC as part of efforts to improve quality of care and reduce neonatal mortality. More widely HTA could help to formalise approaches to task sharing as well as identifying the training needs for non-professional carers, whereas SHERPA could help to assess the risks associated with sharing tasks. Together, these methods offer a way to help improve mortality rates in low-resource intensive settings.

Additional files

Additional file 1: Table S2. Systematic human error reduction and prediction approach analysis table of the 47-nasogastric tube feeding tasks. (PDF 304 kb)

Additional file 2: HFE questionnaire. (DOCX 245 kb)

Additional file 3: Figure S1. Color coded NGT feeding HTA for missed task steps showing distribution of consensus among the SMEs for the tasks reported as often missed. (PNG 274 kb)

Additional file 4: Table S1. Systematic human error reduction and prediction approach (SHERPA) table of selected tasks assigned medium probability and criticality levels showing risks and supervision levels as reported by subject matter experts. (PDF 177 kb)

Acknowledgments
We would like to thank the following people/groups for their contribution towards this study: Odessa Omanyo (Kenyatta National Hospital); Bredget Wesonga and Orina Nyakina (Pumwanin Maternity Hospital); Winnie Nduta and Anne Kawira (Mama Lucy Kibaki Referral Hospital); Beatrice N. Njoroge and Winfred Gichovi (Kiambu Teaching and Referral Hospital). We are grateful for the ongoing support and intellectual contributions to this project from Nairobi City County government, the Ministry of Health Kenya, and the Kenya Paediatric Association.

Funding
This work was supported by a Health Systems Research Initiative joint grant provided by the Department for International Development, UK (DFID), Economic and Social Research Council (ESRC), Medical Research Council (MRC), and Wellcome Trust, grant number MR/M015386/1. ME is supported by a Wellcome Trust Senior Fellowship (#097170). The funders had no role in study design, data collection and analysis, decision to publish, or preparation of the manuscript.

Authors' contributions

GM, ME and NS substantially contributed to the conception and designed the study. GBO, GS, DG and NA made substantial contributions to the acquisition of data by leading data collection activities with the subject matter experts. GBO, GS, NA, DA and GM contributed substantially to the analysis and interpretation of data. GBO drafted the manuscript with support from GM, ME and DG. All authors (GBO, GS, NA, DA, NS, DA, ME, GM) substantially contributed to the interpretation of the results and the implications of the findings. GM, ME, DG and DA were involved in critical review of the manuscript for important intellectual content. All authors critically reviewed drafts of the manuscript and gave final approval before submission.

Ethics approval and consent to participate

Ethical approval for this study was granted by the Kenya Medical Research Institute (KEMRI) Scientific and Ethics Review Unit (protocol No.3366). Written informed consent was not sought during this study, instead, completion of the questionnaire and voluntarily returning it was interpreted as provision of consent. However, the questionnaire handed over to the participants included a cover information, typical to the information provided in a consent form information sheet, explaining that their participation was completely voluntary and that there would be no negative repercussions from participating, declining to participate or giving a particular response and how their data would be confidentially stored and used. The participants were encouraged to remove and keep this information sheet.

Competing interests

The authors declare that they have no competing interests.

Author details

¹KEMRI-Wellcome Trust Research Programme, Nairobi, Kenya. ²Nairobi City County Government, Nairobi, Kenya. ³Faculty of Engineering and the Environment, University of Southampton, Southampton, UK. ⁴Kenyatta National Hospital, Nairobi, Kenya. ⁵Nuffield Department of Medicine, University of Oxford, Oxford, UK.

References

1. Liu L, Oza S, Hogan D, et al. Global , regional , and national causes of child mortality in 2000 – 13 , with projections to inform post-2015 priorities : an updated systematic analysis. Lancet. 2015;385(9966):430–40. https://doi.org/10.1016/S0140-6736(14)61698-6.
2. Bhutta ZA, Das JK, Bahl R, et al. Can available interventions end preventable deaths in mothers, newborn babies, and stillbirths, and at what cost? Lancet. 2014;384(9940):347–70. https://doi.org/10.1016/S0140-6736(14)60792-3.
3. World Health Organization. Guidelines on optimal feeding of low birth-weight infants in low-and middle-income countries. Geneva: WHO; 2011. p. 16–45.
4. Murphy, Georgina A V, Gathara, David, Mwachiro, Jacintah et al. Effective coverage of essential inpatient care for small and sick newborns in a high mortality urban setting - A cross-sectional study in Nairobi City County, Kenya.
5. Papastavrou E, Andreou P, Tsangari H, Merkouris A. Linking patient satisfaction with nursing care: the case of care rationing - a correlational study. BMC Nurs. 2014;13(1):26. https://doi.org/10.1186/1472-6955-13-26.
6. Tubbs-Cooley HL, Pickler RH, Meinzen-Derr JK. Missed oral feeding opportunities and preterm infants' time to achieve full oral feedings and neonatal intensive care unit discharge. Am J Perinatol. 2015;32(1):1–8. https://doi.org/10.1055/s-0034-1372426.
7. Jones TL, Hamilton P, Murry N. Unfinished nursing care, missed care, and implicitly rationed care: state of the science review. Int J Nurs Stud. 2015; 52(6):1121–37. https://doi.org/10.1016/j.ijnurstu.2015.02.012.
8. Tubbs-Cooley HL, Pickler RH, Mark BA, Carle AC. A research protocol for testing relationships between nurse workload, missed nursing care and

neonatal outcomes: the neonatal nursing care quality study. J Adv Nurs. 2015;71(3):632–41. https://doi.org/10.1111/jan.12507.
9. Fulton BD, Scheffler RM, Sparkes SP, Auh EY, Vujicic M, Soucat A. Health workforce skill mix and task shifting in low income countries: a review of recent evidence. Hum Resour Health. 2011;9(1):1. https://doi.org/10.1186/1478-4491-9-1.
10. Callaghan M, Ford N, Schneider H. A systematic review of task- shifting for HIV treatment and care in Africa. Hum Resour Health. 2010;8(1):8. https://doi.org/10.1186/1478-4491-8-8.
11. Campbell C, Scott K. Retreat from Alma Ata? The WHO's report on task shifting to community health workers for AIDS care in poor countries. Glob Public Health. 2011;6(2):125–38. https://doi.org/10.1080/17441690903334232.
12. Republic of Kenya. Ministry of Health. In: Task sharing policy 2017–2010: expanding access to quality health services through task sharing; 2017.
13. Gurses AP, Ozok AA, Pronovost PJ. Time to accelerate integration of human factors and ergonomics in patient safety: table 1. BMJ Qual Saf. 2012;21(4): 347–51. https://doi.org/10.1136/bmjqs-2011-000421.
14. Greig PR, Higham H, Vaux E. Lack of standardisation between specialties for human factors content in postgraduate training: an analysis of specialty curricula in the UK: table 1. BMJ Qual Saf. 2015;24(9):558–60. https://doi.org/10.1136/bmjqs-2014-003684.
15. Hignett S, Jones EL, Miller D, et al. Human factors and ergonomics and quality improvement science: integrating approaches for safety in healthcare. BMJ Qual Saf. 2015;24(4):250–4. https://doi.org/10.1136/bmjqs-2014-003623.
16. Human Factors and Ergonomics Society.
17. Wolf LD, Potter P, Sledge JA., Boxerman SB, Grayson D, Evanoff B. Describing nurses' work: combining quantitative and qualitative analysis. Hum Factors 2006;48(1):5-14. doi:https://doi.org/10.1518/001872006776412289.
18. Leatt P, Baker GR, Halverson PK, Aird C. Downsizing, reengineering, and restructuring: long-term implications for healthcare organizations. Front Health Serv Manag. 1997;13(4):3–37.
19. Lane R, Stanton NA, Harrison D. Applying hierarchical task analysis to medication administration errors. Appl Ergon. 2006;37(5):669–79. https://doi.org/10.1016/j.apergo.2005.08.001.
20. Carayon P, Xie A, Kianfar S. Human factors and ergonomics as a patient safety practice. BMJ Qual Saf. 2014;23(3):196–205. https://doi.org/10.1136/bmjqs-2013-001812.
21. Stanton NA, Salmon PM, Rafferty LA, Walker GH, Baber C, Jenkins DP. Human factors methods: a practical guide for engineering and design. 2nd ed; 2005. https://www.scopus.com/record/display.uri?eid=2-s2.0-84900228923&origin=inward&txGid=30bb73a639d23d64d82cf5dcd18ba117.
22. Stanton NA. Hierarchical task analysis: developments, applications, and extensions. Appl Ergon. 2006;37(1 SPEC. ISS):55–79. https://doi.org/10.1016/j.apergo.2005.06.003.
23. Shebl NA, Franklin BD, Barber N. Failure mode and effects analysis outputs: are they valid? BMC Health Serv Res. 2012;12:150. https://doi.org/10.1186/1472-6963-12-150.
24. Wetterneck TB, Skibinski K, Schroeder M, Roberts TL, Carayon P. CHALLENGES WITH THE PERFORMANCE OF FAILURE MODE AND EFFECTS ANALYSIS IN HEALTHCARE ORGANIZATIONS: an IV medication administration HFMEA. PROCEEDINGS of the HUMAN FACTORS AND ERGONOMICS SOCIETY 48th ANNUAL MEETING. 2004:1708.
25. Baber C, Stanton NA. Human error identification techniques applied to public technology: predictions compared with observed use. Appl Ergon. 1996;27(2):119–31. https://doi.org/10.1016/0003-6870(95)00067-4.
26. Kirwan B. Human error identification in human reliability assessment. Part 2: detailed comparison of techniques. Appl Ergon. 1992;23(6):371–81. https://doi.org/10.1016/0003-6870(92)90292-4.
27. Stanton NA, Stevenage SV. Learning to predict human error: issues of acceptability, reliability and validity. Ergonomics. 1998;41(11):1737–56. https://doi.org/10.1080/001401398186162.
28. Manual of Clinical Procedures. Nursing Council of Kenya. Nairobi; 2009. 3rd ed; 2009.
29. Annett J, Duncan KD. Task analysis and training design. Occup Psychol. 1967;41(July):211–21.
30. Shepherd A. Hierarchical task analysis. In: Hierarchical Task Analysis. ; 2000: 296. doi:https://doi.org/10.1016/j.apergo.2005.06.003
31. Embrey DE. SHERPA. A systematic human error reduction and prediction approach. Proc Int Top Meet Adv Hum factors Nucl power Syst. 1986;I:184–93. https://doi.org/10.1201/9780203489925.ch37.

32. Dul J, Bruder R, Buckle P, et al. A strategy for human factors/ergonomics: developing the discipline and profession. Ergonomics. 2012;55(4):377–95. https://doi.org/10.1080/00140139.2012.661087.

33. Leape LL, Bates DW, Cullen DJ, et al. Systems analysis of adverse drug events. ADE Prevention Study Group Jama. 1995;274(1):35–43. https://doi.org/10.1001/jama.275.1.33.

34. Aiken LH, Sloane DM, Bruyneel L, et al. Nurse staffing and education and hospital mortality in nine European countries: a retrospective observational study. Lancet. 2017;383(9931):1824–30. https://doi.org/10.1016/S0140-6736(13)62631-8.

35. Moxon SG, Lawn JE, Dickson KE, et al. Inpatient care of small and sick newborns: a multi-country analysis of health system bottlenecks and potential solutions. BMC Pregnancy Childbirth. 2015;15(S2):S7. https://doi.org/10.1186/1471-2393-15-S2-S7.

36. Stayner JL, Bhatnagar A, McGinn AN, Fang JC. Feeding tube placement: errors and complications. Nutr Clin Pract. 2012;27(6):738–48. https://doi.org/10.1177/0884533612462239.

37. Metheny NA, Meert KL, Clouse RE. Complications related to feeding tube placement. Curr Opin Gastroenterol. 2007;23(2):178–82. https://doi.org/10.1097/MOG.0b013e3280287a0f.

38. Fegran L, Fagermoen MS, Helseth S. Development of parent-nurse relationships in neonatal intensive care units - from closeness to detachment. J Adv Nurs. 2008;64(4):363–71. https://doi.org/10.1111/j.1365-2648.2008.04777.x.

39. Staniszewska S, Brett J, Redshaw M, et al. The POPPY study: developing a model of family-Centred Care for Neonatal Units. Worldviews Evidence-Based Nurs. 2012;9(4):243–55. https://doi.org/10.1111/j.1741-6787.2012.00253.x.

40. De Man J, Mayega RW, Sarkar N, Waweru E, Leyse M, Van Olmen J, Criel B. Patient-centered care and people-centered health Systems in sub-Saharan Africa: why so little of something so badly needed? Int J Pers Cent Med. 2016;6(3):162–73.

41. Medicine I of. Committee on Quality of Health Care in America.Crossing the quality chasm: A New Health System for the 21st Century.; 2001.

42. Family-Centered Care Committee on Hospital Care and Institute for Patient Care. Patient- and Family-Centered Care and the Pediatrician's Role. Pediatrics. 2012;129:394–404. https://doi.org/10.1542/peds.2011-3084.

43. Tsofa B, Goodman C, Gilson L, Molyneux S. Devolution and its effects on health workforce and commodities management - early implementation experiences in Kilifi County, Kenya Lucy Gilson. Int J Equity Health. 2017. https://doi.org/10.1186/s12939-017-0663-2.

44. Tubbs-Cooley HL, PRH& M-DJK. Missed oral feeding opportunities and preterm infants' time to achieve full oral feedings and NICU discharge. Am J Perinatol. 2014;32(1):1–8.

45. Tubbs-Cooley HL, Pickler RH, Younger JB, Mark BA. A descriptive study of nurse-reported missed care in neonatal intensive care units. J Adv Nurs. 2015;71(4):813–24. https://doi.org/10.1111/jan.12578.

46. Gathara D, Serem G, Murphy GAV, et al. Quantifying nursing care delivered in Kenyan newborn units: protocol for a cross-sectional direct observational study. BMJ Open. 2018. https://doi.org/10.1136/bmjopen-2018-022020.

47. DeRosier J, Stalhandske E, Bagian JP, Nudell T. Using health care failure mode and effect analysis™: the VA National Center for patient Safety's prospective risk analysis system. Jt Comm J Qual Improv. 2002. https://doi.org/10.1016/S1070-3241(02)28025-6.

48. Stanton NA, Young MS. Giving ergonomics away? The application of ergonomics methods by novices. Appl Ergon. 2003;34(5):479–90. https://doi.org/10.1016/S0003-6870(03)00067-X.

49. Waterson P, Catchpole K. Human factors in healthcare: welcome progress, but still scratching the surface. BMJ Qual Saf. 2016;25(7):480–4. https://doi.org/10.1136/bmjqs-2015-005074.

Permissions

The contributors of this book come from diverse backgrounds, making this book a truly international effort. This book will bring forth new frontiers with its revolutionizing research information and detailed analysis of the nascent developments around the world.

We would like to thank all the contributing authors for lending their expertise to make the book truly unique. They have played a crucial role in the development of this book. Without their invaluable contributions this book wouldn't have been possible. They have made vital efforts to compile up to date information on the varied aspects of this subject to make this book a valuable addition to the collection of many professionals and students.

This book was conceptualized with the vision of imparting up-to-date information and advanced data in this field. To ensure the same, a matchless editorial board was set up. Every individual on the board went through rigorous rounds of assessment to prove their worth. After which they invested a large part of their time researching and compiling the most relevant data for our readers.

The editorial board has been involved in producing this book since its inception. They have spent rigorous hours researching and exploring the diverse topics which have resulted in the successful publishing of this book. They have passed on their knowledge of decades through this book. To expedite this challenging task, the publisher supported the team at every step. A small team of assistant editors was also appointed to further simplify the editing procedure and attain best results for the readers.

Apart from the editorial board, the designing team has also invested a significant amount of their time in understanding the subject and creating the most relevant covers. They scrutinized every image to scout for the most suitable representation of the subject and create an appropriate cover for the book.

The publishing team has been an ardent support to the editorial, designing and production team. Their endless efforts to recruit the best for this project, has resulted in the accomplishment of this book. They are a veteran in the field of academics and their pool of knowledge is as vast as their experience in printing. Their expertise and guidance has proved useful at every step. Their uncompromising quality standards have made this book an exceptional effort. Their encouragement from time to time has been an inspiration for everyone.

The publisher and the editorial board hope that this book will prove to be a valuable piece of knowledge for researchers, students, practitioners and scholars across the globe.

List of Contributors

Glenn Larsson
Department of Ambulance and Prehospital Care, Region Halland, Health Centre Nyhem, 302 49 Halmstad, Sweden

Glenn Larsson, Cecilia Rogmark and Anna Nilsdotter
Department of Orthopaedics, Lund University, Lund, Sweden

Cecilia Rogmark
Skane University Hospital, Malmö, Sweden

Ulf Strömberg and Anna Nilsdotter
Department of R&D, Sahlgrenska University Hospital, Göteborg, Sweden

Irit Titlestad, Anne Haugstvedt, Jannicke Igland and Marit Graue
Faculty of Health and Social Sciences, Western Norway University of Applied Sciences, Postbox 7030, N-5020 Bergen, Norway

Irit Titlestad
Kleppestø Nursing Home, Askøy Municipality, Bergen, Norway

Jannicke Igland
Department of Global Public Health and Primary Care, University of Bergen, Bergen, Norway

Susan Jones
School of Human and Health Sciences, University of Huddersfield, Queensgate, Huddersfield HD1 3DH, UK

Somasundari Gopalakrishnan, Charles A. Ameh, Brian Faragher and Nynke van den Broek
Centre for Maternal and Newborn Health, Liverpool School of Tropical Medicine, Pembroke Place, Liverpool L3 5QA, UK

Betty Sam
Centre for Maternal and Newborn Health, Liverpool School of Tropical Medicine, Wilkinson Road, Freetown, Sierra Leone

Roderick R. Labicane
Welbodi Partnership, Ola During Children's Hospital, Freetown, Sierra Leone

Hossinatu Kanu, Makally Mansary and Rugiatu Kanu
Ministry of Health and Sanitation, Youi Building, Freetown, Sierra Leone

Fatmata Dabo
School of Midwifery, Makeni, Sierra Leone

Amanuel Kidane Andegiorgish and Eyob Azeria Kidane
Department of Epidemiology and Biostatistics, Asmara College of Health Sciences, School of Public Health, Asmara, Eritrea

Merhawi Teklezgi Gebrezgi
Department of Epidemiology, Robert Stempel College of Public Health and Social Work, Florida International University, 11200 SW 8th St, Miami, FL 33199, USA

Zukiswa Brenda Ntlokonkulu, Ntombana Mc'deline Rala and Daniel Ter Goon
Department of Nursing Science, Faculty of Health Sciences, University of Fort Hare, East London, South Africa

Demlie Belete Endeshaw
Maternal and Child Survival Program (MCSP), Community Based Newborn Care (CBNC) Coordinator, Save the children, Woldia, Ethiopia

Lema Derseh Gezie
Department of Epidemiology and Biostatistics, Institute of Public health, University of Gondar, Gondar, Ethiopia

Hedija Yenus Yeshita
Department of Reproductive Health, Institute of Public health, University of Gondar, Gondar, Ethiopia

Christiane Schaepe and Michael Ewers
Charité – Universitätsmedizin Berlin, corporate member of Freie Universität Berlin, Humboldt-Universität zu Berlin, and Berlin Institute of Health, Institute of Health and Nursing Science, Berlin, Germany

Ali Soroush, Bahare Andayeshgar and Afsoon Vahdat
Clinical Research Development Center of Imam Reza Hospital, Kermanshah University of Medical Sciences, Kermanshah, Iran

Alireza Abdi
Students Research Committee, School of Nursing and Midwifery, Kermanshah University of Medical Sciences, Kermanshah, Iran

Alireza Khatony
Social Development and Health Promotion Research Center, Kermanshah University of Medical Sciences, Kermanshah, Iran
Nursing Department, School of Nursing and Midwifery, Doolat Abaad, Kermanshah, Iran

Nadine Saladin
Institute of Applied Nursing Science IPW-FHS, FHS St.Gallen, University of Applied Sciences, Rosenbergstrasse 59, 9001 St. Gallen, Switzerland

Wilfried Schnepp
Faculty of Health, Department of Nursing Science, Chair of Family Oriented and Community Based Care, Witten/Herdecke University, Stockumer Strasse 12, .58453 Witten, Germany

André Fringer
Institute of Nursing, School of Health Professions, ZHAW Zurich University of Applied Sciences, Technikumstr. 81, CH-8400 Winterthur, Switzerland

Rekha Timalsina and Sarala K.C.
Patan Academy of Health Sciences, School of Nursing and Midwifery, Lalitpur Nursing Campus, Lalitpur, Nepal

Nilam Rai
Dristi Nepal, Kathmandu, Nepal

Anita Chhantyal
Tribhuvan University Teaching Hospital, Maharajgunj, Kathmandu, Nepal

Heather Moquin, Cydnee Seneviratne and Lorraine Venturato
Faculty of Nursing, University of Calgary, 2500 University Dr NW, Calgary, AB T2N 1N4, Canada

Olivier Anne Blanson Henkemans and Anna Dijkshoorn
TNO, Child Health, Schipholweg 77-89, 2316 ZL, Leiden, The Netherlands

Marjolein Keij
Pharos, Arthur van Schendelstraat 620, 3511, MJ, Utrecht, The Netherlands

Marc Grootjen
Eaglescience B.V., Naritaweg 12K, 1043, BZ, Amsterdam, The Netherlands

Mascha Kamphuis
JGZ Zuid-Holland West, Croesinckplein, 24-26 2722, EA, Zoetermeer, The Netherlands

Bernard Atinyagrika Adugbire
Nurses' Training College, Zuarungu, Ghana

Lydia Aziato
Department of Adult Health, School of Nursing, College of Health Sciences, University of Ghana, Legon, Accra, Ghana

Genevieve Currie and Aliyah Dosani
School of Nursing and Midwifery, Mount Royal University, 4825 Mount Royal Gate SW, Calgary, Alberta T3E 6K6, Canada

Aliyah Dosani, Shahirose S. Premji and Sandra M. Reilly
O'Brien Institute of Public Health, University of Calgary, Calgary, Alberta, Canada

Shahirose S. Premji and Sandra M. Reilly
Faculty of Nursing, University of Calgary, 2500 University Drive NW, Calgary, Alberta T2N 1N4, Canada

Abhay K. Lodha
Department of Paediatrics, Section of Neonatology, Alberta Health Services, Foothills Medical Centre, 1403 29th Street NW, Calgary, Alberta T2N 2T9, Canada
Alberta Children's Hospital Research Institute, Calgary, Alberta, Canada

Marilyn Young
Prenatal & Postpartum Services, Public Health
Calgary Zone, Alberta Health Services, 1430, 10101
Southport Road SW, Calgary, Alberta T2W 3N2,
Canada

Ditte Maria Sivertsen
Optimed, Clinical Research Centre (Section 056),
Copenhagen University Hospital Hvidovre,
Kettegård Allé 30, DK-2650 Hvidovre, Denmark

Louise Lawson-Smith
Novo Nordisk A/S, Vandtårnsvej 114, 2860 Søborg,
Denmark

Tove Lindhardt
Department of Internal Medicine, Copenhagen
University Hospital Herlev, Herlev Ringvej 75, 2730
Herlev, Denmark

**Michelle Lobchuk, Lisa Hoplock, Christina
West, Cheryl Dika, Terri Ashcroft, Kathleen and
Jocelyne Lemoine**
Rady Faculty of Health Sciences, College of Nursing,
University of Manitoba, Room 315 – 89 Curry Place,
Winnipeg, MB R3T 2N2, Canada

Gayle Halas
Max Rady Faculty of Health Sciences, College
of Medicine, University of Manitoba, P228-770,
Bannatyne Avenue, Winnipeg, MB R3E 0W3,
Canada

Wilma Schroeder
Red River College, Nursing, 2055 Notre Dame
Avenue, Winnipeg, MB R3H 0J9, Canada

Chambers Clouston
Department of Surgery, Section of General Surgery,
University of Manitoba, 770 Bannatyne Avenue,
Winnipeg, MB R3E 0W3, Canada

**Katarina Kornaros, Eva Nissen and Björn
Salomonsson**
Department of Women's and Children's Health,
Karolinska Institutet, Stockholm, Sweden

Sofia Zwedberg
Sophiahemmet Högskola, Stockholm, Sweden

Joana Agyeman-Yeboah
International Maritime hospital, Tema, Ghana

Kwadwo Ameyaw Korsah
School of Nursing, University of Ghana, Legon,
Ghana

Bayan Kaddourah
Ambulatory Care Centre, Executive Administration
of Nursing Services, King Fahad Medical City,
Riyadh, Saudi Arabia

Amani K. Abu-Shaheen and Mohamad Al-Tannir
Research Center, King Fahad Medical City, Riyadh,
Saudi Arabia

Carey Ann Mather
School of Health Sciences, College of Health and
Medicine, University of Tasmania, Locked Bag
1322, Launceston, TAS 7250, Australia

Elizabeth Anne Cummings
School of Health Sciences, College of Health and
Medicine, University of Tasmania, Private Bag 135,
Hobart, TAS 7001, Australia

Fred Gale
School of Social Sciences, College of Arts, Law and
Education, University of Tasmania, Locked Bag
1340, Launceston, TAS 7250, Australia

**Gregory B. Omondi, George Serem, Nancy Abuya,
David Gathara, Mike English and Georgina A. V.
Murphy**
KEMRI-Wellcome Trust Research Programme,
Nairobi, Kenya

Nancy Abuya
Nairobi City County Government, Nairobi, Kenya

Neville A. Stanton
Faculty of Engineering and the Environment,
University of Southampton, Southampton, UK

Dorothy Agedo
Kenyatta National Hospital, Nairobi, Kenya

Mike English and Georgina A. V. Murphy
Nuffield Department of Medicine, University of
Oxford, Oxford, UK

Index

A

Acute Hospitalisation, 134
Advanced Home Care, 51-54, 56-59
Ambulance Nurse, 1-3, 5-6, 8
Axial Coding, 54, 71

B

Birth Attendant, 43-44, 47, 49
Birth Preparedness, 42-44, 46, 49-50
Breast Cancer, 27-33
Breast Lump, 29-30

C

Cancer Screening, 27-28, 31-33
Clinical Breast Examination (CBE), 27
Clinical Empathy, 143-152
Community Health Care, 126
Complication Readiness, 42-44, 46, 49-50

D

Danger Sign, 43, 46
Diabetes, 10-17, 64, 153
Digital Professionalism, 178, 183, 186-188
Discharge Planning, 117-118, 125, 131, 140-142

E

Eclampsia, 19
Electrocardiogram, 2, 8
Episteme, 160-161
Ergonomics, 191-193, 196-197, 199-200
Esmoe, 36, 40

F

Family Caregivers, 48, 51-60, 139, 141-142, 153
Family-centred Care Approach, 101-102

H

Haemorrhage, 19, 35-36, 40
Hastened Death, 68-70, 80
Health-care Utilization, 134
Healthcare Assistants (HCA), 39
Heart Health Whispering, 143, 145, 150-152
Herbal Medicines, 65-66
Hermeneutics, 37, 154, 156, 163

Hip Fracture, 1-5, 7-9
Home Mechanical Ventilation, 51, 59-60
Hypoglycaemia, 11-15

I

Interpretative Phenomenological
Analysis, 34-35, 40

L

Long-term Care, 17, 68, 70-72, 74-76, 79, 91, 96, 99-100

M

Mammogram, 27
Mastectomy, 29
Medium-fidelity Simulation, 34-36, 40
Mhealth Intervention, 101
Motherhood, 42-43, 50, 163

N

Nasogastric Tube Feeding, 191, 198
Neonatal Mortality, 48, 191, 198
Nurse Education, 18, 25, 35, 40, 153, 190
Nurse Turnover, 171, 176
Nursing, 1-19, 22, 24-26, 29, 32, 34-36, 39-41, 51-68,
70-75, 77-94, 100, 110, 116-119, 123-128, 132, 138-145,
147, 149, 151-153, 157, 159-160, 163-192, 194, 196-200
Nursing Home, 10-17, 81, 139
Nursing Personnel, 10-17

O

Obstetric Emergency, 34-36, 38, 40-41, 43-44, 46-48
Oral Contraceptives, 27

P

Palliative Care, 68, 70, 73, 79, 81, 91
Parent Empowerment, 101, 106-107
Patient Safety, 10-17, 34-35, 40, 51-52, 54, 57-60, 125,
170, 192, 196, 198-200
Patient Safety Culture, 10-11, 13-17
Patient Satisfaction, 1-5, 7-9, 116, 125
Perinatal Care, 133, 154
Personal Hygiene, 117, 123, 138
Point of Care, 178-189
Postnatal Child Health Care, 154
Postpartum Depression, 154, 162-163

Prehospital Fast Track Care, 1-3
Preterm Infant, 128, 131-133
Psychotherapist Competence, 154
Psychotherapy, 116, 154-157, 159, 162-163
Public Health Nurse, 118, 132

S
Self-medication, 61-67
Student Satisfaction, 18-21, 26

T
Task Analysis, 191-194, 199
Techne, 160-161

Tertiary Care, 67, 171, 173
Tracheostomy, 52, 57

U
Unsafe Abortion, 19

V
Vsed, 68-79

W
Wound Care, 117-118, 120-121, 123
Wound Infection, 117-118, 121-123

www.ingramcontent.com/pod-product-compliance
Lightning Source LLC
Chambersburg PA
CBHW082026190326
41458CB00010B/3289